ICSU Short Reports Volume 4

ADVANCES IN GENE TECHNOLOGY: MOLECULAR BIOLOGY OF THE ENDOCRINE SYSTEM

Proceedings of the Eighteenth

Miami Winter Symposium

Miami, Florida, U.S.A.

February 3-7, 1986

Edited by David Puett, Fazal Ahmad,

Sandra Black, Diana M. Lopez, Michael H. Melner,

Walter A. Scott and William J. Whelan

The right of the University of Cambridge to print and sell all manner of books was granted by Henry VIII in 1534. The University has printed and published continuously since 1584.

CAMBRIDGE UNIVERSITY PRESS
Cambridge
London New York New Rochelle
Melbourne Sydney

Published by the Press Syndicate of the University of Cambridge, The Pitt Building, Trumpington Street, Cambridge CB2 1RP, UK; 32 East 57th Street, New York, NY 10022, USA; 10 Stamford Road, Oakleigh, Melbourne 3166, Australia

First published 1986

Printed in the United States of America

Library of Congress catalogue card number: 85-31332

ISBN 0 521 32658 3

This is ICSU Short Reports, Volume 4. All have been published for the ICSU Press by Cambridge University Press Other volumes in the series are:

ICSU Short Reports, Volume 1
Advances in Gene Technology: Human Genetic Disorders, 1984
ISBN 0 521 26749 8

ICSU Short Reports, Volume 2
Advances in Gene Technology: Molecular Biology of the Immune System, 1985
ISBN 0 521 30486 5

ICSU Short Reports, Volume 3
Third European Bioenergetics Conference, 1985
ISBN 0 521 30813 5

ICSU Short Reports, Volume 5
Fourth European Bioenergetics Conference
To appear in August 1986

ICSU Short Reports, Volume 6
Fourth Congress, Federation of Asian and Oceanian Biochemists
To appear in December 1986

Contents

SYMPOSIUM PRESENTATIONS

PEPTIDE AND POLYPEPTIDE HORMONES

GROWTH FACTORS AND ONCOGENES

PEPTIDE AND PROTEIN RECEPTORS

GLYCOPROTEIN HORMONES

STEROID RECEPTORS AND GENE REGULATION

LYMPHOKINES, INTERLEUKINS, INTERFERONS AND RECEPTORS

PREFACE

This is the record of the 18th Miami Winter Symposium, the joint venture of the Department of Biochemistry of the University of Miami School of Medicine and the Papanicolaou Cancer Research Center. The Symposium was held at the Hyatt Regency Hotel/University of Miami/James L. Knight International Center, during February 3-7, 1986.

This annual event is dedicated to exposing advances in gene technology, highlighting each year a fast-growing area of the new biology and honoring the leaders in the field by the Lynen Medal Lecture, given this year by Stanley Cohen (Vanderbilt University) and the Distinguished Service Award, presented to Herbert W. Boyer (University of California, San Francisco) and Stanley N. Cohen (Stanford University). We gratefully acknowledge the financial support for these awards, provided respectively by GIBCO/BRL Research Products Division of Division of Life Technologies and the Biomedical Division of Elsevier Science Publishers.

The proceedings are published in the ICSU Short Reports format and are arranged in the same six sections as were presented in the Symposium. In each section the 4-page Reports from invited speakers are followed by the relevant 2-page Reports that correspond to the record number of poster presentations, 129 in all, that the Symposium attracted.

Each presentation is intended to be a complete and original communication that may be cited in the literature as forming part of ICSU Short Reports, Volume 4, 1986.

The ICSU Short Reports represent a new method of reporting Symposia proceedings. This volume was part of the registration package for Symposium attendees, in a paperback version, and simultaneously placed on open sale in a hardback version by Cambridge University Press on behalf of the ICSU Press. We are grateful to Schleicher and Schuell Inc. for meeting the cost of publishing the paperback edition, as noted on page xxv.

This reporting format began in 1984 with the 16th Miami Winter Symposium. It was intended to address the problem associated with the widespread use of posters to present short communications at scientific meetings. These posters are extremely informative. They are put together with a great deal of pains, but the poster is displayed for only a few hours, and, in a large meeting, is often not seen by many of the Symposium participants. All that remains for posterity is the abstract that was prepared many months before the meeting, which was already out-of-date at the time of the meeting, and which was contained in a book of abstracts which does not find its way into libraries and therefore the information cannot be retrieved.

The new format used here is an attempt to allow the presenter to commit the poster to paper. The two-page spread can be used to convey a great deal of information by way of introduction, methodology, results, conclusions, bibliography, diagrams, figures and tables. Produced to a very tight deadline, only 2 months before the meeting, the Short Report acts as an up-to-date, permanent record of the poster. The simultaneous availability of the volume of Short Reports to libraries and persons who could not attend the meeting places the report in the body of retrievable literature.

Along with these advantages is the inclusion of four-page reports from the invited speakers, produced to the same deadline and available at the time of the Symposium, not, as is customary, many months later. What is presented here is a succinct but complete and documented statement. Via the bibliography, the reader is directed to explore the subject in more depth by being referred to the original seminal papers on which the speaker's contribution is based.

We have been much encouraged by the reception accorded to the Short Reports, of which this is the fourth volume. The series to date is listed elsewhere in the frontispiece. We regard this as the beginning of a new form of rapid communication which is certain to attract its imitators.

The ICSU Press, as a very new publishing house, which began publishing in 1984, merits mention, and more details are to be found on page xxiii. It is the publishing house of ICSU, the International Council of Scientific Unions, an international non-governmental, scientific organization made up of 20 international scientific unions together with more than 80 national members, scientific and national associates. More familiar than ICSU itself are the individual members such as the International Union of Biochemistry, a union member, or the Royal Society of London, a national member. ICSU is the "United Nations" umbrella organization that allows these different unions and national members to come together to confront problems of common interest, and take advantage of opportunities for collaboration that are only possible on an international, interdisciplinary scale.

ICSU's headquarters are located at 51 Bd. de Montmorency, 75016 Paris, France.

THE ICSU PRESS

The ICSU Press, the publishing house of the International Council of Scientific Unions, was founded in 1983 to serve the publishing needs of ICSU and the ICSU family. Many of these family members are already heavily engaged in publishing, but the need was felt for a central service within ICSU to carry out the following functions:

Undertaking publication projects for any ICSU family member, initiating interdisciplinary projects on behalf of a group of ICSU members; advising on publication activities both for technical and contractual matters and providing written recommendations and guidelines for these purposes; acting as an expert negotiator on behalf of ICSU members; producing service publications for them and studying new communications technologies.

Since it began publishing in 1984, the ICSU Press has published seven symposia. It has launched two journals, BioEssays and the Journal of Tropical Ecology. It has initiated a new rapid-communication format embodied already in four volumes of "Short Reports". Educational texts, monographs and semi-popular expositions of the work of the ICSU family are in preparation.

ICSU Press activities are made known in its Newsletter, distributed twice yearly to the ICSU family and cooperating bodies. Further information about the ICSU Press may be had from the office of the Chairman at P.O. Box 016129, Miami, Florida 33101, U.S.A.

ICSU PRESS

THE ICSU PRESS

The ICSU Press [illegible] of the International Council of Scientific Unions, [illegible] ICSU family. [illegible] are already heavily engaged in publishing, but the need was felt for a central service within ICSU to carry out the following functions:

Undertake publication projects [illegible] members [illegible] recommendations and guidelines [illegible] providing services [illegible] technical and [illegible]

Since it began publishing in 198[illegible] the ICSU Press has published [illegible] launched [illegible] Processes and the [illegible] communication format [illegible] volumes [illegible] reports [illegible] texts, monographs and semi-popular [illegible] the work of the ICSU family of organisations.

ICSU Press [illegible] made known [illegible] distributed [illegible] ICSU family and [illegible] Further information about the ICSU Press may be had from [illegible] at the [illegible] Miami, Florida [illegible] U.S.A.

ACKNOWLEDGEMENT

The organizers of the Miami Winter Sympoisa are pleased to acknowledge the generosity of Schleicher & Schuell, Inc., in underwriting the cost of printing the edition of this volume that was given to the Symposium participants. The fact that a simultaneous print run was made of the Symposium edition and the library edition lowered the unit cost of each version of the Symposium.

Peptide and Polypeptide Hormones

MOLECULAR BIOLOGY AND POST-TRANSLATIONAL PROCESSING OF ENDOCRINE HORMONES.

P.C. Andrews, Ourania Andrisani, Tim Hayes, Marie Tavianini and Jack E. Dixon
Department of Biochemistry, Purdue University, West Lafayette, Indiana 47907

The genes of the endocrine pancreas are responsible for the synthesis of several peptide hormones which have pronounced effects on the overall homeostasis of the animal. One of these genes encodes the small peptide somatostatin, which regulates insulin and glucagon secretion. This hormone also has important regulatory effects on numerous other gastrointestinal hormones. We have examined both the gene expression and post-translation processing of the preprohormone.

The gene encoding rat somatostatin has been isolated from a λ phage gene library. Phage harboring the gene were identified by plaque hydribization using a nick-translated fragment derived from the cDNA for rat somatostatin. The transcriptional unit includes exons of 238 and 367 base pairs (bp) separated by one intron of 621 bp. The intron is located between the codons for Gln (-57) and Glu (-56) of prosomatostatin. Analysis of the nucleotide sequence 5' to the start of transcription reveals a number of sequences which may be involved in the expression of somatostatin. A variant of the "TATA" box, TTTAAA, lies 26 bp upstream from the start of transcription, and a sequence homologous to the "CAAT" box (GGCTAAT) is 92 bp upstream from the transcription start. A long alternating purine-pyrimidine stretch $(GT)_{25}$, which is similar to Z DNA-forming sequences in other genes, lies 628 bp 5' to the transcription start and is flanked by small repeats. Hybridization analysis shows that this region is highly repeated in the genome and that homologous sequences are located approximately 2 kilobase pairs downstream from the poly(A) addition site. Southern hybridization of the λ clone with probes derived from brain or liver poly(A+) RNA demonstrates that another transcribed sequence lies about 7 kilobase pairs downstream from the poly(A) addition site of the rat somatostatin gene.

In order to define the sequences which are involved in the expression of the rat somatostatin gene, a fragment corresponding to 750 bp 5' to the start of transcription was fused with the bacterial chloramphenicol acetyl transferase (CAT) gene, resulting in plasmid pUCB'sst. Promoter deletions were constructed using conveniently located restriction sites or by Bal 31 nuclease digestion. The activity of the somatostatin promoter and its deletions were tested in two cell lines; Hela cells which do not express any endogenous somatostatin, and CA-77 cells (derived from a rat medullary thyroid carcinoma) which produces endogenous somatostatin. Plasmid DNA was introduced into the Hela and CA-77 cell lines by calcium phosphate precipitation and electroporation, respectively. Briefly, the following results were obtained:

1. The 750 bp fragment harboring the somatostatin promoter (+1 to -750) is transcriptionally inactive in Hela cells, but is active in CA-77 cells.

2. The plasmid containing the promoter sequences between +1 and -250 is active in CA cells but not in Hela cells.

3. Removal of the sequences between -200 and -750 renders the somatostatin promoter active in Hela cells.

4. All the deletions show promoter activity in CA-77 cells, except the deletion which contains sequences between +1 and -43.

In conclusion, the deletion analyses of the somatostatin promoter demonstrate that it shows tissue specific expression. In addition, removal of the sequences harboring a "negative element" results in activation of the somatostatin promoter in Hela cells.

We have also examined the post-translation modifications which the larger precursor protein, preprosomatostatin, undergoes to ultimately produce the biologically active peptide. We have utilized the anglerfish pancreas as a model system to develop procedures for rapidly identifying post-translational processing events. The anglerfish pancreas is particularly attractive because two cDNAs encoding different somatostatin precursors have been cloned and sequenced. One of the precursors (preprosomatostatin I) contains at its carboxyl-terminus a 14-residue peptide identical to the mammalian somatostatins (SST-14). This peptide has been isolated from the anglerfish and other species, and its amino acid sequence is invariant. The second anglerfish mRNA (preprosomatostatin II) codes for a preprosomatostatin which has at its carboxyl-terminus a peptide which differs from SST-14 at 2 sites, Tyr-7 and Gly-10.

We have utilized gas-phase sequencing and fast atom bombardment mass spectrometry (FAB•MS) as well as additional analytical methods to identify proteolytic processing sites as well as other post-translational modifications. Peptides of interest were purified using classical chromatographic methods and reversed-phase HPLC. The purified peptides are identified by immunoreactivity and/or structural characteristics. Tryptic digests analyzed by FAB•MS have proven useful in verifying peptide structures and identifying peptides whose masses deviate from the mass based upon deduced protein sequence. Deviations may be due to the presence of modified amino acid side chains, or to DNA sequencing errors.

Naturally occurring cleavage products resulting from proteolytic processing were obtained for both prosomatostatins. Analysis of these peptides allow us to suggest processing pathways for the two prosomatostatins. Cleavage of the signal peptide from preprosomatostatin-I occurs between Cys-25 and Ser-26 (numbering relative to preprosomatostatin). Both somatostatin-14 and the dodecapeptide preceding it are then rapidly cleaved from prosomatostatin-I. A slower cleavage occurs at Arg-53. Similarly, somatostatin-28 is rapidly cleaved from prosomatostatin-II but not processed to somatostatin-14. An additional slower cleavage at residues Lys-61, Arg-62 also occurs. The terminal basic residues presumed to be produced as a result of endoproteolytic processing were not present for any of the peptides isolated. Their removal is presumed to occur as a result of exopeptidase activity specific for basic residues.

TRANSCRIPTIONAL AND POST-TRANSCRIPTIONAL REGULATION OF NEUROENDOCRINE GENE EXPRESSION. Stuart E. Leff, Christian Nelson, E. Bryan Crenshaw, III, Harry Elsholtz, Harry Mangalam, Andrew Russo, *Ronald M. Evans, and Michael G. Rosenfeld. Howard Hughes Medical Institute, Eukaryotic Regulatory Biology Program, School of Medicine, University of California, San Diego, La Jolla, CA 92093, and *The Salk Institute, La Jolla, CA 92037.

The central research theme in these laboratories is to identify regulatory mechanisms critical for the developmental and physiological expression of neuroendocrine genes in the unique, restricted fashion characteristic of each gene in the neuroendocrine system.

I. CALCITONIN GENE EXPRESSION. We provided the initial demonstration that certain genes of the neuroendocrine system contain discrete hormone-encoding or neuropeptide-encoding domains or exons, whose expression is dependent on alternative RNA processing events (1-5). Extensive evidence documents the physiological operation of these events in expression of the gene encoding calcitonin, a 32 amino acid calcium-regulatory hormone. The consequence of these alternative RNA processing events is the production of an mRNA in neuronal tissue, distinct from the predominant species in thyroid C-cells, which encodes a novel neuropeptide referred to as calcitonin gene-related peptide (CGRP).

The predominant thyroidal mRNA product of calcitonin gene expression encodes a 17.5 kDa precursor of calcitonin, while that in neural tissue generates a 16 kDa protein with 76 N-terminal acids in common with the calcitonin precursor and a unique 42 amino acid C-terminal region with processing signals predicting the excision of a novel 37 amino acid neuropeptide (CGRP). The distribution of CGRP mRNA and peptide in brain and other tissues, in concert with studies of biological actions of the synthetic peptide, suggests functions for CGRP in nociception, ingestive behavior, and modulation of cardiovascular homeostasis (5); these predictions are supported by initial physiological studies (e.g., 6,7). An approach combining immunocytochemistry and RNA structural analysis was used to identify CGRP in the brain (5).

The two mature transcripts of the calcitonin gene share the identical 5′ CAP site but utilize discrete 3′ polyadenylation sites adjacent to calcitonin or CGRP exons, respectively. Selection of alternative polyadenylation sites appears to be a critical event responsible for the alternative RNA processing events (8). However, it has not been conclusively determined if alternative polyadenylation site selection occurs independently of alternative splicing pathways. Termination of RNA transcription has been mapped to a point >1 kb downstream from the 3′ (CGRP) poly(A) site, irrespective of whether calcitonin or CGRP mRNA is the predominant product of calcitonin gene expression. Transfection of the cloned rat calcitonin gene into heterologous cell lines results in a cell-specific pattern of RNA processing. Calcitonin mRNA is the sole mature transcript in lymphocyte cell lines, while CGRP mRNA is the predominant mature transcript in certain carcinoma cell lines (9). These data are consistent with a model in which a trans-acting factor(s) regulates the alternative RNA processing events in brain. The introduction of mutant calcitonin transcription units into cell lines should aid in determining the cis-active elements that mediate cell-specific patterns of alternative RNA processing.

II. HORMONAL REGULATION OF PROLACTIN AND GH EXPRESSION. Analysis of the tissue-specific pattern of prolactin and growth hormone gene expression and their homeostatic regulation provides a model for definition of the molecular mechanisms by which neuropeptides and other regulatory molecules dictate and modulate the pattern of neuroendocrine gene expression. We have demonstrated that thyrotropin releasing hormone (TRH), epidermal growth factor (EGF), and agents which produce elevated intracellular cAMP levels exert rapid transcriptional effects (within 60 seconds) on prolactin gene transcription using a clonal rat pituitary cell line (GH) as the model system (10-13). Growth hormone releasing factor (GRF), glucocorticoids, and thyroid hormones regulate the transcription of the growth hormone gene (14,15). The 5′ flanking portion of the prolactin gene contains the structural determinants which permit the transfer of hormonal and cAMP regulation of prolactin gene transcription to heterologous transcription units, as documented using chimaeric genes for DNA-mediated gene transfer (16). Detailed analysis reveals that a region (<60bp) of 5′-flanking prolactin genomic information transfers EGF, TRH, phorbol ester, and cAMP regulation to fusion genes in GH cells (17). Similarly, the glucocorticoid and thyroid hormone regulating sequences have been localized to 200 bp of 5′-flanking growth hormone information (18).

III. MOLECULAR BASIS OF HERITABLE PATTERNS OF NEUROENDOCRINE GENE EXPRESSION. The recent development of methods for introducing foreign genes into the germ line of mice and Drosophila provides an in vivo approach for studying the mechanisms underlying developmental and inducible gene regulation. It is important to utilize this type of technology, in concert with DNA-mediated gene transfer into heterologous cultured cell lines, to determine the rules underlying neuron-specific expression of specific genes. This approach was utilized in a series of collaborative experiments to address questions concerning the genetic basis of development and differentiation which restricts the expression of neuroendocrine genes to defined sets of neurons and endocrine cells. Transgenic offspring, resultant from introduction into fertilized eggs of a fusion gene containing 5′ flanking mouse metallothionein-I gene sequences and the coding portion of the rat growth hormone, were shown to express the encoded gene product and to develop as large mice with massively elevated plasma growth hormone levels (19). This genetic trait is transmitted to the offspring, which exhibit an apparently stable heritable pattern of tissue-specific gene expression. In the brain of a number of pedigrees carrying the MGH gene, the growth hormone product of the fusion gene is expressed in restricted groups of neurons in highly localized regions that include magnocellular neurosecretory neurons of the hypothalamus, pyramidal cells in layer V of the neocortex and CA_3 of the hippocampus, neurons in the suprachiasmatic nucleus, the central nucleus of the amygdala, the pars compacta of the substantia nigra and adjacent neurons in the ventral tegmental area, and the dorsal motor nucleus of the vagus (20). Neither growth hormone nor metallothionein genes are normally expressed in these cells. It is, therefore, tempting to propose a model that requires sequences within both the 5′ flanking and the 3′ structural regions of the fusion gene for the observed cellular specificity. According to this hypothesis, sequences present in the growth hormone chromosomal fragment are capable of promoting expression outside of the anterior pituitary, which appears to be the only localization for endogenous growth hormone gene expression. However, this expression occurs only when 5′ flanking growth hormone sequences are replaced by the metallothionein promoter. This interpretation is supported by the observations that transgenic animals containing either the intact GH gene, or a metallothionein-GRF fusion gene that has been cloned and structurally characterized in our laboratories by K.E. Mayo(21,22), exhibit no neuronal GRF expression. Chromosomal position of the fusion genes as a means to control growth hormone expression in brain is excluded because of the identical pattern of expression of the fusion gene in an identical neuronal distribution in unrelated strains of transgenic animals. These observations provide the conceptual basis for a series of experiments designed to elucidate the "developmental code" for neuronal gene expression.

In the case of the rat prolactin and growth hormone genes, we have recently identified regions of <200 bp which confer the tissue-specific pattern of expression characteristic of the genes. This sequence results in markedly enhanced expression of fusion genes in cells of pituitary origin, but not other cell types including fibroblasts, lymphocytes, hepatocytes, mammary epithelium, islet cells, or thyroid "C" cells. The identification of the precise sequences responsible for the heritable pattern of growth hormone and prolactin gene expression permit the direct inquiry into their actions on fusion genes during normal pituitary and brain development of transgenic animals.

REFERENCES

1. Rosenfeld, M.G., S.G. Amara, B.A. Roos, E.S. Ong, and R.M. Evans (1981) Nature 290, 63.
2. Amara, S.G., et.al. (1982) J. Biol. Chem. 257, 2129.
3. Rosenfeld, M.G., et. al. (1982) Proc. Natl. Acad. Sci. USA 79, 1717.
4. Amara, S.G., V. Jonas, M.G. Rosenfeld, E.S. Ong, and R.M. Evans (1982) Nature 298, 240.
5. Rosenfeld, M.G., et. al. (1983) Nature 298, 240.
6. Fisher, L.A., et. al. (1983) Nature 305, 354.

7. Brain, S.D., T.J. Williams, J.R. Tippins, H.R. Morris and I. MacIntyre (1985) Nature 313, 54.
8. Amara, S.G., R.M. Evans, and M.G. Rosenfeld (1984) Mol. and Cell. Biol. 4, 2151.
9. Leff, S.E., S.G. Amara, R.M. Evans, and M.G. Rosenfeld, in preparation.
10. Potter, E., A.K. Nicolaisen, E.S. Ong, R.M. Evans (1981) Proc. Natl. Acad. Sci. USA 78, 6662.
11. Murdoch, G.H., E. Potter, A.K. Nicolaisen, R.M. Evans, and M.G. Rosenfeld (1982) Nature 300, 192.
12. Murdoch, G.H., M.G. Rosenfeld, and R.M. Evans (1982) Science 218, 1315.
13. Murdoch, G.H., R. Franco, R.M. Evans, and M.G. Rosenfeld (1983)J. Biol. Chem. 258, 15329.
14. Evans, R.M., N.C. Birnberg, and M.G. Rosenfeld (1982) Proc. Natl. Acad. Sci. USA 79, 7659.
15. Barinaga, M., L.M. Bilezikjian, W.W. Vale, M.G. Rosenfeld, and R.M. Evans (1985) Nature 314, 279.
16. Supowit, S., E. Potter, R.M. Evans, and M.G. Rosenfeld (1984) Proc. Natl. Acad. Sci. USA 81, 2975.
17. Elsholtz, H., Potter, E., H. Mangalam, R. Evans, and M.G. Rosenfeld, manuscript in preparation.
18. Miller, D., E.S. Ong, M.G. Rosenfeld, I.M. Verma, and R.M. Evans (1984) Science 225, 994.
19. Palmiter, R.D., et. al. (1982) Nature 300, 611.
20. Swanson, L.W., et. al. (1985) Nature 317, 363.
21. Mayo, K.E., et. al. (1985) Proc. Natl. Acad. Sci. USA 82, 63.
22. Mayo, K.E., G.M. Cerelli, M.G. Rosenfeld, and R.M. Evans (1985) Nature 314, 464.

TISSUE-SPECIFIC HORMONAL REGULATION OF PROOPIOMELANOCORTIN GENE EXPRESSION

Michael H. Melner,[1,2,3] Steven L. Young,[2,3] Frank S. Czerwiec,[2,3] Deborah Lyn,[2,3] Arthur E. Jackson,[2,3] David Puett[2,3] and Robert D. Koos[3,4]

[2]Department of Biochemistry, [3]The Reproductive Sciences and Endocrinology Laboratories, [4]Departments of Obstetrics and Gynecology and of Anatomy and Cell Biology, University of Miami, School of Medicine, Miami, FL 33101

[1]To whom inquiries should be addressed.

Proopiomelanocortin (POMC) is the single polypeptide precursor which undergoes post-translational processing to yield a number of bioactive peptides including adrenocorticotropic hormone (ACTH), β-endorphin, and α,β, and γ melanocyte stimulating hormone (MSH) (1,2). The gene encoding POMC is present as a single-copy gene in some species including human, rat and bovine (3). Initial evidence indicated that the POMC gene is expressed in multiple tissues including the anterior and neurointermediate lobes of the pituitary and the hypothalamus, and that hormonal control of its expression is tissue-specific. In the anterior lobe of the pituitary, glucocorticoids negatively regulate POMC expression while corticotropin-releasing factor (CRF) positively regulates its expression (7). In the neurointermediate lobe of the pituitary, these hormones are ineffectual while dopamine negatively regulates POMC expression (8). Recent evidence has demonstrated expression of the POMC gene in reproductive tract cells of both males and females including testicular Leydig cells (4-6) and ovarian granulosa cells (11). We describe herein the unique regulation of POMC gene expression in reproductive tract cells and the potential mechanisms involved. This system is unique in that the same gene is under different hormonal regulation in the different cell types where it is expressed.

Regulation of POMC gene expression in ovarian granulosa cells. Granulosa cells of developing ovarian follicles respond to complex hormonal regulation by differentiation and the production of steroids and peptides (9). These cells offer advantages for in vitro studies as they can be placed in primary culture under serum-free conditions and yet maintain many of their differentiated functions, including hormonal responsiveness (9). To obtain sufficient cells for these studies, immature 25-day female rats were primed with 20 IU pregnant mare's serum gonadotropin (PMSG), and the granulosa cells were isolated as described previously (10), and placed in serum-free culture in Medium 199. Using similar cultures, we have previously shown that follicle stimulating hormone (FSH) dramatically stimulates granulosa cell POMC mRNA levels (11). In the present experiments we were interested in extending these earlier observations to include potential regulation by other hormones known to regulate granulosa cell function and differentiation. Androgens of theca cell origin are normally present within the ovary and are known to regulate granulosa cell steroidogenesis (9). In addition, the ovulatory surge of luteinizing hormone

(LH) plays a pivotal role in inducing the differentiation of granulosa cells to luteal cells (9). Granulosa cells were cultured at a density of 1.5 x 10^6 viable cells/35 mm dish for 48 hours under basal conditions, and with either 10^{-7}M androstenedione, 100 ng/ml LH, or LH plus androstenedione. Following incubation, the cells were washed in cold PBS, scraped, and centrifuged in microfuge tubes. Cytoplasmic dot hybridization was performed using the method of White and Bancroft (12). Hybridizations were effected using a nick translated (1 X 10^8 cpm/μg) cDNA probe for the rat pituitary POMC sequence (8). As shown in Figure 1, treatment with LH alone elicited small increases in POMC mRNA. Androstenedione alone stimulated POMC mRNA to a greater extent than LH while a combination of LH plus androstenedione had a dramatic effect on POMC mRNA levels. Scanning laser densitometric analyses of the dot-blot autoradiographs are shown in Figure 2. These data demonstrate an approximate 5-fold increase in POMC mRNA levels with LH treatment, a 10-fold increase with androstenedione, and a 47-fold increase with the combination treatment. This suggests a possible synergistic effect with the combination of gonadotropin and androgen treatment.

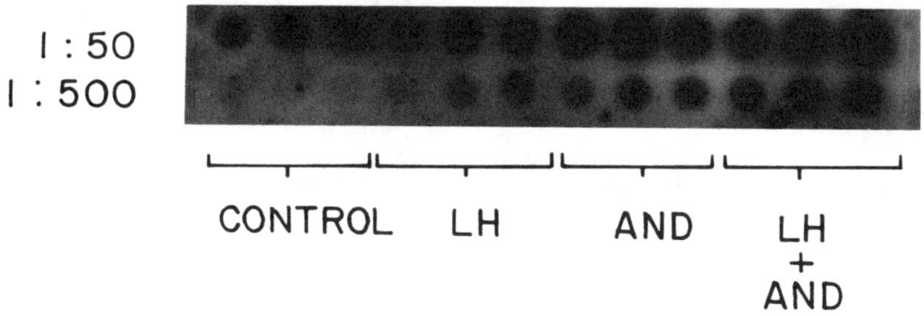

Figure 1. Cytoplasmic dot-blot hybridization analysis of cultured rat granulosa cells 48 hours following addition of PBS (central), LH (100 ng/ml), androstenedione (10^{-7}M) or LH + androstenedione. The numbers refer to dilutions of the cytoplasmic extract. Each dot represents a dilution from cells in an individual culture dish.

Since androstenedione is a substrate for aromatase, which is present in granulosa cells, and can be converted into an estrogen, it was of interest to test the effects of a non-aromatizable androgen on POMC mRNA expression. Granulosa cells prepared as before were incubated for 48 hours with 10^{-7}M dihydrotestosterone (DHT), a potent androgen which is not a substrate for aromatization. DHT, either alone or in combination with LH, had a marked stimulatory effect on POMC mRNA expression. Together, these data suggest that granulosa cell POMC gene expression can be regulated by androgens.

This finding may have clinical significance in women with polycystic ovary (PCO) syndrome. Women with PCO often have elevated levels of androgens of ovarian origin and elevations in serum LH (13). Interestingly, these patients display elevated plasma levels of β-endorphin, α-MSH, and β-lipotropin (14,15). It is conceivable that ovarian androgens could increase POMC gene expression in humans and that this may play a role in the etiology of this syndrome.

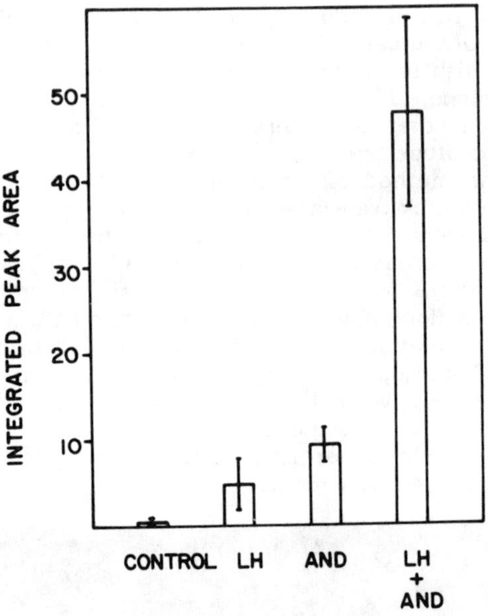

Figure 2. Integrated peak areas from scanning laser densitometric analysis of the dot-blot autoradiographs in Figure 1. The bars represent the mean ± standard error from triplicate samples.

Assay of DNA sequences which confer hormonal regulation on the POMC gene. We have developed a nonradioactive, HPLC-based assay for the marker gene chloramphenicol acetyl transferase (CAT) in transfection studies (16). This technique is based upon the assay of Gorman et al. (17) with the alterations of using unlabeled chloramphenicol as a substrate followed by HPLC separation of the acetylated derivatives. The quantitation is then accomplished by monitoring UV absorbance using an in-line spectrophotometer. In our hands this assay is at least as sensitive as the original TLC-based method with the added advantages of using unlabeled chloramphenicol and the rapidity of HPLC separations and immediate quantitation. This technique forms the basis of our search for tissue-specific, hormone-specific enhancer-like elements in the human POMC gene. Particular attention is being focused on a region of the gene (-460 to -490) which shares homology with the glucocorticoid-regulatory sites of the mouse mammary tumor virus long terminal repeat (MMTV-LTR) and the rat growth hormone gene (18). These studies address two specific questions: (i) Does the same sequence-specific DNA element function as a hormone regulatory element for all the steroid hormones in a tissue-specific manner? This is intriguing since glucocorticoids are inhibitory to corticotroph POMC expression while androgens appear stimulatory to granulosa cell expression. (ii) Do identical or different sequence-specific DNA elements function as hormone regulatory elements for the hormones with different intracellular mechanisms of action? For example, do FSH and androgens both act via similar or different sequences in enhancing granulosa cell POMC expression? The POMC gene thus offers an excellent system for studying tissue-specific hormonal regulation of gene expression. Further investigations of the mechanisms of hormonal regulation of this gene in the ovary and testis will yield new insights into the general properties of cell-specific gene regulation.

ACKNOWLEDGEMENTS

Supported in part by NSF DCB-8417602, ACS IN 51Y, NIH AM33973, HD17999 and HD07129.

REFERENCES

1. Roberts, J.L., Phillips, M., Rosa, P.A. and Herbert, E. (1978) Biochemistry 17, 3609-3618.
2. Keutmann, H.T., Lampman, G.W., Mains, R.E. and Eipper, B.A. (1981) Biochemistry 20, 4148-4155.
3. Uhler, M., Herbert, E., D'Eustachio, P. and Ruddle, F.D. (1983) J. Biol. Chem. 258, 9444-9453.
4. Melner, M.H. and Puett, D. (1984) Arch. Biochem. Biophys. 232, 197-201.
5. Pintar, J.E., Schachter, B.S., Herman, A.B., Durgerian, S. and Krieger, D.T. (1984) Science 225, 632-634.
6. Chen, C.-L.C., Mather, J.P., Morris, P.L. and Bardin, C.W. (1984) Proc. Natl. Acad. Sci. USA 81, 5672-5675.
7. Birnberg, N.C., Lissitzky, J.-C., Hinman, M. and Herbert, E. (1983) Proc. Natl. Acad. Sci. USA 80, 6982-6986.
8. Chen, C.L.C., Dionne, F.T. and Roberts, J.L. (1983) Proc. Natl. Acad. Sci. USA 80, 2211-2215.
9. Hsueh, A.J.W., Adashi, E.Y., Jones, P.B.C. and Welsh, T.H. (1984) Endocrine Reviews 5, 76-127.
10. Clark, M.R. (1982) Endocrinology 110, 146-152.
11. Melner, M.H., Luo, Y., Koos, R.D., Clark, M.R., Roberts, J.L. and Puett, D. (1984) 7th International Congress of Endocrinology, Excerpta Medica, International Congress Series 654, 1383.
12. White, B.A. and Bancroft, F.C. (1982) J. Biol. Chem. 257, 8569-8572.
13. Barnes, R.B. and Lobo, R.A. (1985) J. Clin. Endocrinol. Metab. 61, 779-782.
14. Givens, J.R., Wiedemann, E., Anderson, R.N. and Kitabchi, A.E. (1980) J. Clin. Endocrinol. Metab. 50: 975-976.
15. Wortsman, J., Wehrenberg, W.B., Gavin, J.R. and Allen, J.P. (1984) Obstet. Gynecol. 63: 630-633.
16. Young, S.L., Jackson, A.E., Puett, D. and Melner, M.H. (1985) DNA, in press.
17. Gorman, C.M., Moffat, L.F. and Howard, B.H. (1982) Mol. Cell. Biol. 2, 1044-1051.
18. Cochet, M., Chang, A.C.Y. and Cohen, S.M. (1982) Nature 297, 335-339.

TRANSCRIPTIONAL REGULATION OF PROOPIOMELANOCORTIN GENE EXPRESSION IN PITUITARY AND BRAIN

James L. Roberts
Center for Reproductive Sciences and
Department of Biochemistry
Columbia University College of Physicians & Surgeons

Proopiomelanocortin (POMC) is the precursor to a number of important biologically active peptides, hormones and neuropeptides. Three of its primary sites of expression are in the corticotrophs and melanotrophs of the pituitary as well as a discrete population of neurons in the periarcuate region of the rat hypothalamus. Interestingly, the peptides derived from post-translational processing of the POMC precursor differ between these three sites of expression, each tissue producing a discrete set of different biologically active peptides. Possibly, because of the difference in biological activities of the peptides produced in these tissues, we observe that the regulation of POMC secretion from these tissues is quite different. For example, glucocorticoids negatively regulate POMC peptide secretion from the anterior pituitary corticotroph, while they have no effect on the intermediate pituitary melanotroph (1-3). Conversely, dopamine inhibits POMC peptide secretion from the melanotroph, with no effect on the corticotroph (4,5). Estrogen has been shown to alter POMC peptide content in hypothalamic neurons with no effects on either of the pituitary POMC cells (6,7).

Thus, these three POMC cell types have evolved a complex machinery for regulating the secretion of their peptide products. As we will show below, they have also evolved a similar complex machinery for regulating expression of the POMC gene. This is not due to the presence of a group of POMC genes, each expressed in a different cell type, since research from several labs has shown that there is only one POMC gene in the rat haploid genome. In some instances the differential regulation relies on th presence or absence of specific receptors in the POMC expressing cells. For example, the intermediate lobe melanotrophs do not express the glucocorticoid receptor, and thus their lack of response is probably due to the fact that they cannot recognize the glucocorticoid receptor (8).

In order to understand how this complex secretory machinery correlates with alterations in expression of the POMC gene we have set about to analyze the effects of various secretagogues on POMC gene transcription, both in the intact animal and in primary pituitary cultures. Adult female Sprague-Dawley rats were used for these studies. After various treatments the animals are sacrificed, brain and pituitaries rapidly dissected, and the tissue fractionated into nuclei and a postnuclear supernatant as previously described (9). The postnuclear supernatant is used for isolation of total cytoplasmic RNA and the amount of POMC mRNAs quantitated by dot blot hybridization (7). The nuclei are used for an in vitro nuclear runon assay, which measures the number of RNA polymerase II molecules which were engaged on the POMC gene at the time of sacrificing the animal.

Secretagogues which interact directly with receptors on the plasma membranes of the cell to stimulate or inhibit secretion of the POMC peptide had rapid and parallel effects on POMC gene transcription. For example, corticotropin releasing hormone (CRH) caused an increase in POMC gene expression, which was detectable within 5 min and maximal after 60 min of CRH treatment. The response was subsequently attenuated, but was still elevated 1.6 fold after 18 hrs of CRH treatment. CRH also had stimulatory effects on the POMC gene expression in the melanotrophs, however, it required an approximately 10 fold higher dosage to elicit the same maximal effect. This observation is in agreement with that previously reported by others for secretory effects in the intermediate lobe cells (10).

Glucocorticoids, which are known to inhibit POMC mRNA levels, have been shown to elicit this effect through a rapid direct inhibition of POMC gene expression. In anterior lobe corticotrophs of intact animals (9) and in primary cultures glucocorticoids elicited an immediate 4-7 fold decrease in POMC gene transcription. The fact that these effects were observed in vitro suggests that the in vivo effects were due to a direct effect of glucocorticoids on the POMC gene. Glucocorticoids we also observed to inhibit CRH stimulated POMC gene expression. When cultures of anterior pituitary cells were treated first with glucocorticoids and then CRH, we found a time dependency of the length of glucocorticoid treatment on the subsequent ability of CRH to stimulate POMC gene expression. These results suggest that the inability of CRH to stimulate POMC gene expression after prior exposure to glucocorticoids is somehow temporally related to the inability of CRH to stimulate secretion of the POMC peptide (1,3), possibly by uncoupling the CRH receptors from the intracellular second messenger machinery. Interestingly, upon culture of intermediate lobe pituitary melanotrophs, the glucocorticoid receptor becomes expressed and these cells become negatively regulated by glucocorticoids. This observation would imply that the only thing the melanotrophs need to respond like corticotrophs in their POMC gene expression is the glucocorticoid receptor.

In the melanotroph, the primary modulators of POMC peptide secretion are catacholamines in which dopamine is inhibitory and norepinephrine is stimulatory. As with peptide hormone secretagogues, we found that stimulation of POMC secretion by norepinephrine was paralleled by a similar stimulation in gene transcription, whereas inhibition of secretion by dopamine agonists, such as 8-bromo-ergocryptine, were inhibitory to transcription. These studies would suggest, again, that regulated secretion of POMC peptides and the associated intracellular events are temporally related in parallel effects on transcription.

POMC gene expression is also regulated in the hypothalamus. Previous studies by others have shown alterations in POMC peptide content in response to castration and sex steroid replacement (6). In these studies analyzing the levels of hypothalamic POMC gene expression we found that, indeed, estrogen treatment of a castrated animal results in a decrease in POMC mRNA (11). Using the in vitro runon nuclear transcription assay we have, as well, identified that POMC gene expression is negatively regulated by estrogen in these tissues.

Thus, we have shown that a variety of secretagogues can regulate POMC gene transcription in a parallel fashion. Our interest was to identify what region of the POMC gene was responsible for this parallel regulation. First, we isolated and completely characterized by sequence analysis, the entire 5' end of the POMC gene. Sequence analysis of this gene showed it to be typical for an RNA polymerase II secretory protein gene. There are two regions which have close homology to glucocorticoid regulatory elements (GRE), as well as one homologous to the recently identified cyclic AMP regulatory element. In collaboration with David Moore of Massachusetts General Hospital, we characterized the glucocorticoid receptor binding sites by filter hybridization assays and identified one of the putative GRE elements in the 5' end of the POMC gene as being a discrete glucocorticoid receptor binding element. A series of deletion mutants in this region of the gene are being analyzed to determine if this region is indeed responsible for conferring glucocorticoid regulation of this particular gene.

We have shown the POMC gene to be regulated by a variety of different types of secretagogues, peptides, catacholamines, and steroids, in parallel with the effects on secretion. These observations would suggest that some event which is associated with secretion is transmitted to the 5' region of the POMC gene in order that transcription is coordinately regulated. From a physiological point of view this makes good sense; as additional peptide is secreted the cell should stimulate the machinery for producing more peptide to maintain stores and the converse being true if secretion were inhibited. Since secretion of POMC peptides in these cells is associated with increased intracellular levels of calcium, increased intracellular levels of cAMP, and stimulation of phosphatidylinositol turnover, any one or all of these three systems could be responsible for generating the secondary (tertiary, etc.) cytoplasmic messenger, which results in modulation of transcription. For example, the stimulation of cAMP production by coupling of the CRH receptor to adenylcyclase can set in motion a chain of events. cAMP binds the cAMP-dependent protein kinase, which dissociates into the now the active catalytic and regulatory subunits. The catalytic subunit subsequently phosphorylates a variety of cytoplasmic and possibly nuclear substrates. It has been hypothesized by other researchers that such cytoplasmic phosphoproteins may then make their way to the nucleus and interact with the specific genes in question, such as the POMC gene in this case, to directly activate or inhibit gene transcription, much like the steroid receptors. Because of its complex physiology, the POMC gene will serve as an excellent model for understanding the molecular mechanisms by which multiple types of hormones and neurotransmitters orchestrate the correct level of expression of genes.

REFERENCES

(1) Bilezikjian, L.M. and Vale, W. (1983) Endocrinology 113, 657-662.

(2) Proulx-Ferland, L., Labrie, F., Dumont, D. and Cote, J. (1982) Science 217, 62-63.

(3) Gilles, G. and Lowry, P.J. (1978) Endocrinology 103, 521-529.

(4) Farah, J.M., Jr., Malcolm, D.S. and Mueller, G.P. (1982) Endocrinology 110, 657-659.

(5) Hollt, V. and Bergmann, M. (1982) Neuropharmacology 21, 147-154.

(6) Wardlaw, S.L., Thoron, L. and Frantz, A.G. (1982) Brain Res. 245, 327.

(7) Chen, C.L.C., Dionne, F.T. and Roberts, J.L. (1982) Proc. Natl. Acad. Sci. USA 80, 2211.

(8) Antakly, T. and Eisen, H.J. (1984) Endocrinology 115, 1984-1989.

(9) Eberwine, J.H. and Roberts, J.L. (1984) J. Biol. Chem. 259, 2166-2170.

(10) Vale, W., Vaughn, J., Smith, M., Yamamoto, G., Rivier, J. and Rivier, C. (1983) Endocrinology 113, 1121-1131.

(11) Wilcox, J.N. and Roberts, J.L. (1985) Endocrinology, in press.

LOCALIZATION AND CHARACTERIZATION OF THE HUMAN PLACENTAL LACTOGEN GENE ENHANCER

Bruce L. Rogers, Mark G. Sobnosky, and Grady F. Saunders
Biochemistry and Molecular Biology, University of Texas System Cancer Center, M.D. Anderson Hospital and Tumor Institute, Houston, Texas 77030.

INTRODUCTION: Human placental lactogen (hPL) and human growth hormone (hGH) are polypeptide hormones closely related in structure (85% homology in amino acid sequence) but differ in both function and expression (1). hGH is involved in the regulation of growth and metabolism during development and hPL stimulates mammary gland development and lactogenesis. hPL is expressed in increasing amounts during pregnancy, accounting for at least 5% of the total poly(A^+)RNA in the placenta during the third trimester of pregnancy (2), whereas hGH is expressed in the anterior lobe of the pituitary. The structure of the hPL/hGH gene cluster is well defined (Fig. 1) with two hGH genes interspersed with three hPL genes, all in the same transcriptional orientation (3). Several of the genes have been cloned (4) and sequenced including the most transcriptionally active members of the multigene family, hPL_3 (5) and hGH_1 (6). The second hGH gene, hGH_2, has been shown to be able to encode a variant peptide in transfection experiments (7) but its role _in vivo_ is poorly defined. The cDNA derived from hPL_4 has been cloned and sequenced (8) and is expressed _in vivo_, whereas the hPL_1 gene, although able to direct transcription initiation _in vitro_ (9), is not expressed in transfected cells.

RESULTS: _Cloning of the Structural Genes and their Flanking Regions: Transfection of JEG-3 Cells._ _EcoRI_ fragments containing the 2.9 kb hPL_3 and hPL_4 as well as the 2.6 kb hGH_1 structural genes were cloned into the vector pSV2gpt (10) or the enhancer-deleted pSER vector (11; see Fig.1). The two possible orientations were designated (+) or (-) relative to the direction of transcription of the gpt gene. The DNA constructs illustrated in Fig.1 were introduced into the placental cell line JEG-3 (12) by the $CaPO_4$ coprecipitation method (13,14). Stably transformed cell lines were obtained from pools of transformants and poly(A^+)RNA was isolated. Northern blot analysis of glyoxalated samples demonstrated that the hPL_3, hPL_4, and hGH_1 exogenous genes were transcribed. The introduced hPL and hGH genes did not exhibit tissue specific expression since hGH_1 was expressed at a level similar to that of hPL_3 and hPL_4 (15).

Detection of an Enhancer Within the hPL_3 3' Flanking Region. The DNA fragments shown in Fig.1 as well as the hPL_3, hPL_4, and hGH_1 structural genes were cloned into pSER and tested for their ability to substitute for the SV40 enhancer. Relative transformation frequencies for the stable transformants were determined for each of the constructs (TableI). Such an assay system has been shown to be a valid test for enhancer activity (11,16,17). One particular construct, pSERfrag1(+), containing a 3.9 kb 3' flanking region of the hPL_3 gene exhibited an almost 10-fold higher transformation frequency compared to the pSER vector (TableI). In this construct the enhancer containing fragment 1 is cloned in the 3' region relative to the direction of the gpt direction of transcription. Another construct, pSER2frag1(+), which has fragment 1 cloned into an EcoRI site 5' to the SV40 promoter exhibited an even higher relative transformation frequency (TableI). It is concluded that fragment 1, a 3' flanking region of hPL_3, contains an active enhancer sequence which can work in a position independent manner. Furthermore, the enhancer can function in an orientation independent manner as indicated by the elevated relative transformation frequencies of pSERfrag1(-) and pSER2frag1(-) (TableI).

Plasmids	Relative Frequency
pSV2gpt	1.0
pSER	<0.03
$pSERhPL_3$(+)	0.02
$pSERhPL_4$(+)	0.02
$pSERhGH_1$(+)	0.02
$pSER2hPL_3$(-)	0.02
$pSER2hGH_1$(-)	0.02
pSERfrag1(+)	0.30
pSERfrag1(-)	0.29
pSER2frag1(+)	1.3
pSER2frag1(-)	2.3
pSERfrag2	0.02
pSERfrag3	0.10
pSERfrag4	0.01
pSERfrag5	0.01
pSERfrag6	0.02
pSERfrag7	0.01
pSERfrag8	0.02
pSERfrag9	0.01

Table I. Relative transformation frequencies of pSV2gpt and derivative plasmids in JEG-3 cells. The transformation frequencies were normalized to the frequency obtained with pSV2gpt ($1.1x10^{-4}$ for JEG-3 cells). All transfections were done in duplicate and in the case of pSV2gpt, pSER, pSERfrag1(+), pSERfrag1(-), pSER2frag1(+) and pSER2frag1(-), the frequencies listed were deduced from at least three different experiments using two different plasmid preparations.

Fig. 1. Restriction map of recombinant clones containing hPL and hGH flanking regions cloned into pSER. The map and gene nomenclature is derived from maps previously published (3,4). The vertical bars each represent an EcoRI site. The structural gene regions are indicated by the open blocks and the numerals indicate the designated fragment (e.g. frag1 throught 9). Frag1 has its orientation indicated by the ClaI endonuclease site. The EcoRI fragments, designated (+) or (-) depending on their orientation relative to the gpt gene, were cloned into the EcoRI site of pSER (11,15).

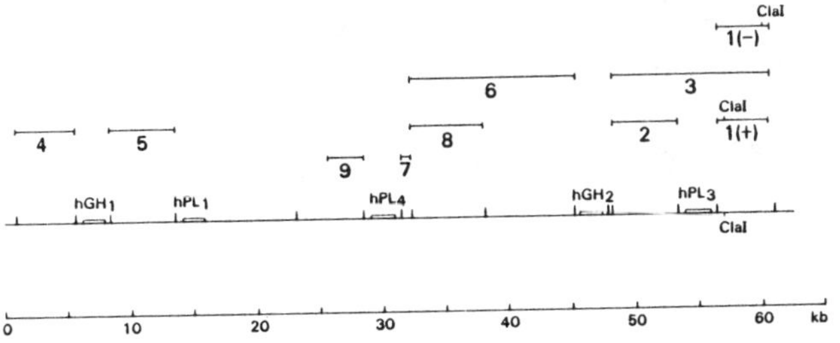

Localization of the Enhancer Within the hPL_3 Flanking Region. Fragment 1 was cloned into the EcoRI site of pSV1CAT and transient chloramphenicol acetyltransferase (CAT) assays (18) demonstrated that fragment 1 contains an enhancer that can act directly to increase transcriptional activity from a heterologous promoter (Fig.2,3). The enhancer containing fragment 1 was digested with a series of restriction endonucleases and a number of smaller subfragments were cloned into the BamHI site of pSV1CAT (Fig.2). CAT assays demonstrated that the enhancer is located within an AccI-SacI generated fragment of approximately 1.0 kb (Fig.2,3; pSV1CATAS). The AccI-SacI fragment is presently being sequenced and when complete should provide interesting data concerning its relatedness to other enhancer sequences of both viral and cellular origin.

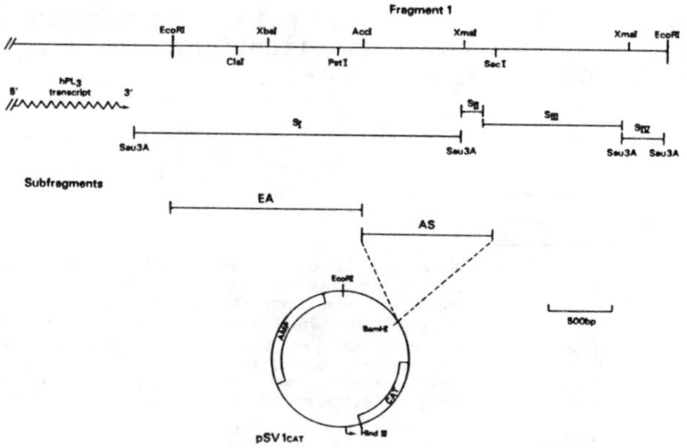

Fig. 2. Subfragments of the enhancer containing hPL_3 3' flanking region cloned into pSV1CAT. Four Sau3A generated fragments, designated S_I through S_{IV}, were cloned into the BamHI site of pSV1CAT (18). None of these fragments proved positive in transient CAT assays. Two fragments, EA and AS, were generated by AccI-SacI digestion of purified fragment 1 and were cloned into the BamHI site of pSV1CAT following fill-in and blunt-end ligation reactions.

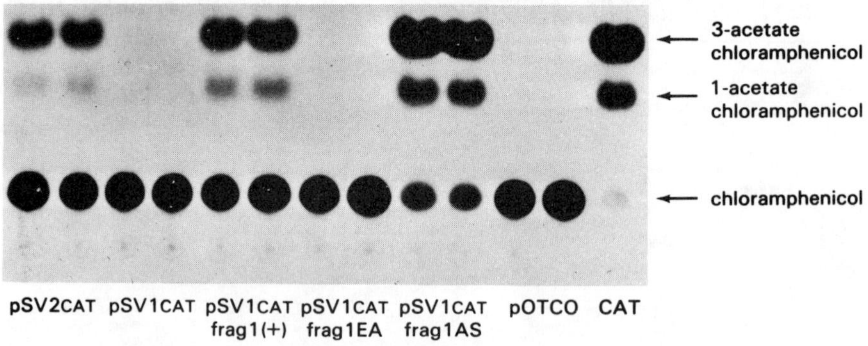

Fig. 3. CAT activity in JEG-3 cells: localization of the hPL_3 enhancer to an AccI-SacI restriction fragment (frag1AS). Cell lysates were assayed for CAT activity (18). Purified CAT enzyme served as a control and the radiolabeled products detected by autoradiography are arrowed.

The hPL_3 Enhancer is Not Strictly Tissue Specific. The hPL_3 enhancer is not strictly tissue specific since it functions in human-cell lines of placental (JEG-3) and pituitary (18-54,SF;19) origin. Nonetheless, the enhancer has a cell-type preference since it functions more efficiently, relative to the SV40 enhancer activity, in JEG-3 cells than in 18-54,SF cells. Other non-placental cell lines are presently being used as recipients in transfection assays to assess whether the enhancer exhibited cell-preference in its activity in other cell lines.

SUMMARY: EcoRI generated fragments containing the hPL and hGH structural genes and their flanking regions have been assayed for enhancer activity. Relative transformation frequencies of pSV2gpt or pSER recombinants containing these DNA have indicated that the hPL_3 3' flanking region contains an active enhancer. This enhancer can function in an orientation and distance independent manner but is not strictly tissue specific. The enhancer has been localized to a 1.0 kb DNA fragment that is 2.0 kb 3' to the end of the hPL_3 structural gene. It is proposed that this enhancer may play a role in the high expression of hPL_3 *in vivo*.

REFERENCES:

(1) Miller, W.L. and Eberhardt, N.L. (1983) Endocrine Rev. 4, 97-130. **(2)** Barrera-Saldana, H., Robberson, D.L. and Saunders, G.F. (1982) J. Biol. Chem. 257, 12399-12404. **(3)** Barsh, G.S., Seeburg, P.H. and Gelinas, E. (1983) Nucl. Acids Res. 11, 3939-3958. **(4)** Kidd, V.J. and Saunders, G.F. (1982) J. Biol. Chem. 257, 10673-10680. **(5)** Selby, M.J., Barta, A., Baxter, J.D., Bell, G.I. and Eberhardt, N.L. (1984) J. Biol. Chem. 259, 13131-13138. **(6)** DeNoto, F.M., Moore, D.D., Goodman, H.M. (1981) Nucl. Acids Res. 9, 3719-3730. **(7)** Pavlakis, G.N., Hizuka, N., Gorden, P., Seeburg, P. and Hamer, D.H. (1981) Proc. Natl. Acad. Sci. USA 78, 7398-7402. **(8)** Barrera-Saldana, H.A., Seeburg, P.H. and Saunders, G.F. (1983) J. Biol. Chem. 258, 3787-3793. **(9)** Selvanayagam, C.S., Tsai, S.Y., Tsai, M.-J., Selvanayagam, P. and Saunders, G.F. (1984) J. Biol. Chem. 259, 14642-14646. **(10)** Mulligan, R.C. and Berg, P. (1981) Proc. Natl. Acad. Sci. USA 78, 2072-2076. **(11)** Gillies, S.D., Morrison, S.L., Oi, V.T. and Tonegawa, S. (1983) Cell 33, 717-728. **(12)** Kohler, P.O. and Bridson, W.E. (1971) J. Clin. Endocrinol. 32, 683-687. **(13)** Graham, F.L. and Van Der Eb, A.J. (1973) Virology 52, 456-467. **(14)** Wigler, M., Pellicer, A., Silverstein, S., Axel, R., Urlaub, G. and Chasin, L. (1979) Proc. Natl. Acad. Sci. USA 76, 1373-1376. **(15)** Rogers, B.L., Sobnosky, M.G., and Saunders, G.F. (submitted). **(16)** Lusky, M., Berg, L., Weiher, H. and Botchan, M. (1983) Molec. Cell. Biol. 3, 1108-1122. **(17)** Gillies, S.D., Folson, V. and Tonegawa, S. (1984) Nature 310, 594-597. **(18)** Gorman, C.M., Moffat, L.F. and Howard, B.H. (1982) Molec. Cell. Biol. 2, 1044-1051. **(19)** Wyche, J.H. and Noteboom, W.D. (1979) Endocrinology 104, 1765-1773.

REGULATION OF PROLACTIN GENE EXPRESSION BY STEROIDS AND CYCLIC AMP

Richard A. Maurer

Physiology and Biophysics, University of Iowa, Iowa City 52242

The production of prolactin by specialized cells of the anterior pituitary is controlled by the interaction of several different hormones. A rather large number of hormones have been shown to alter prolactin production including dopamine, estradiol, glucocorticoids, thyroid hormone, thyrotropin releasing hormone, vasoactive intestinal peptide, epidermal growth factor, somatostatin and others. While all of these hormones can affect prolactin, it seems likely that estradiol and dopamine are the major physiological regulators of prolactin synthesis and secretion.

Estradiol acts to increase prolactin production through stimulation of prolactin gene transcription (1) leading to increased prolactin mRNA levels and increased prolactin synthesis. Estradiol induces a several-fold increase in prolactin transcription which is sufficient to account for the observed changes in mRNA levels and prolactin synthesis. Increased prolactin gene transcription was detected as early as 20 minutes after treatment with the steroid, suggesting that the estradiol receptor may directly regulate the transcription of this gene. Studies utilizing inhibitors of protein synthesis (2) have also provided evidence for a direct effect of the estradiol receptor. These studies suggest that estrogenic regulation of prolactin gene transcription may be the principle mechanism which permits the steroid to alter the biosynthesis of prolactin. Furthermore, the finding that transcription is regulated suggests that the estradiol receptor might interact with the prolactin gene or with elements involved in the transcription of the gene.

Analysis of the interaction of the estradiol receptor with the rat prolactin gene has identified a DNA fragment from the 5' flanking region of the gene which is selectively recognized by the receptor (3). A competition binding assay was used to examine the interaction of the estradiol receptor with specific restriction endonuclease fragments of the prolactin gene. The assay determines the ability of soluble DNA fragments to compete with insoluble DNA-cellulose for receptor binding. Although fragments representing most of the 10 kilobase prolactin gene showed no selective binding, a fragment located between 1.2 and 2.0 kilobases upstream from the transcription initiation site was able to selectively bind the receptor. Although this site is further upstream than has been found for similar receptor binding sites of several other steroid responsive genes, it seems likely that the selective binding may be a part of the mechanism which allows the receptor to stimulate the transcription of the prolactin gene. Current studies seek to further localize the receptor binding sites.

In contrast to estradiol which stimulates prolactin production, dopamine inhibits the synthesis and secretion of prolactin. Furthermore, as dopamine receptors are located on the plasma membrane, the mechanisms involved in the dopaminergic regulation of prolactin are likely substantially different than the mechanism involved in estrogen action. Indeed, it would seem necessary that the dopaminergic regulation of prolactin production should involve an intracellular mediator. At least two lines of evidence suggest that dopamine effects on prolactin synthesis and prolactin mRNA levels are mediated by cAMP. The first line of evidence concerns the fact that dopamine can apparently alter cAMP production by the pituitary. Dopamine and dopamine agonists alter adenylate cyclase activity of pituitary membranes (4) and alter pituitary cAMP levels (5). Interestingly, dopaminergic stimuli decrease cAMP levels. The other line of evidence concerns the fact that cAMP derivatives can stimulate prolactin synthesis and prolactin mRNA levels in cells which have been pretreated with dopaminergic agents (5). Taken together these studies suggest that cAMP is a positive regulator of prolactin gene expression and that dopamine inhibits prolactin production through decreasing the levels of this positive regulator.

The ability of cAMP to alter prolactin mRNA levels appears to be due to changes at the transcriptional levels. Studies in this laboratory (6) and by Murdoch et al. (7) have demonstrated that cAMP stimulates prolactin gene transcription. In both of these studies cAMP was found to induce a several-fold increase in prolactin gene transcription and the magnitude of this effect is sufficient to account for the ability of cAMP to increase prolactin mRNA levels. The kinetics of cAMP effects on transcription are very rapid suggesting that only minimal intervening steps occur between increases in cAMP levels and stimulation of transcription. It seems quite possible that increased transcription could be due to activation of cAMP-dependent protein kinase leading to changes in phosphorylation of specific proteins involved in transcription although other mechanisms cannot be excluded. Murdoch et al. (7) have observed a good correlation between prolactin transcription and the phosphorylation of a specific chromosomal protein which they term "basic regulated protein". However, the functional significance of the phosphorylation of this protein has not yet been determined and further studies are required to elucidate the mechanisms involved in cAMP regulation of gene transcription.

Currently, considerable effort is being focused on analysis of the DNA sequences which mediate the multihormonal regulation of prolactin transcription. These studies utilize fusion genes containing putative regulatory sequences linked to appropriate marker genes. The utility of this approach to analysis of prolactin gene sequences has been demonstrated by recent studies identifying sequences required for epidermal growth factor responsiveness by Supowit et al. (8) and for thyroid releasing hormone responsiveness by Camper et al. (9). Preliminary studies in this laboratory suggest the usefulness of this approach for identifying DNA sequences required for the response to estradiol and analyzing the interaction of these different hormonal regulators.

REFERENCES

(1) Maurer, R.A. (1982) J. Biol. Chem. 257, 2133-2136.
(2) Shull, J.D. and Gorski, J. (1984) Endocrinology 114, 1550-1557.
(3) Maurer, R.A. (1985) DNA 4, 1-9.
(4) De Camilli, P., Macconi, D. and Spada, A. (1979) Nature 278, 252-254.
(5) Maurer, R.A. (1982) Endocrinology 110, 1957-1963.
(6) Maurer, R.A. (1981) Nature 294, 94-97.
(7) Murdoch, G.H., Rosenfeld, M.G. and Evans, R.M. (1982) Science 218, 1315-1317.
(8) Supowit, S.C., Potter, E., Evans, R.M. and Rosenfeld, M.G. (1984) Proc. Natl. Acad. Sci. U.S.A. 81, 2975-2979.
(9) Camper, S.A., Yao, Y.A.S. and Rottman, F.M. (1985) J. Biol. Chem. 260, 12246-12251.

SPECIFIC DNA BINDING PROTEINS AND REGULATION OF TRANSFECTED PITUITARY GENES

CARTER BANCROFT[1], BRUCE A. WHITE[2], THOMAS C. LUFKIN[1,3], AND NANCY Y. IP[3]

[1]Department of Physiology and Biophysics, Mount Sinai Medical School, NY, NY 10029. [2]Anatomy Department, University of Connecticut, Farmington, CT 06032. [3]Molecular Biology Department, Sloan-Kettering Institute, NY, NY 10021

The prolactin and growth hormone genes are subject to tissue-specific regulation, since they are expressed almost exclusively in the pituitary gland. In addition, expression of these genes in pituitary cells or cell lines is regulated by a wide variety of hormones and other factors (1). Each type of regulation is almost surely mediated by interactions between specific regulatory proteins and their cognate regulatory DNA sequences. We describe here our use of a protein blotting technique to search for candidate regulatory proteins for the rat prolactin gene, and of gene transfer experiments to identify genomic DNA sequences responsible for regulation of the rat prolactin and growth hormone genes.

Pituitary cell chromatin proteins which bind specifically to the 5'-flanking region of the rat prolactin gene (2). The protein blotting procedure employed (3) involves SDS-polyacrylamide gel fractionation of proteins, transfer to nitrocellulose, and incubation with various ^{32}P-labeled hybrid plasmids. Two pituitary cell chromatin proteins, NP44 and NP48, were detected by their ability to bind a prolactin genomic clone. These proteins exhibited a pronounced DNA sequence specificity, since they bound strongly to a plasmid containing an upstream flanking sequence of the prolactin gene, but only very weakly to plasmid DNA or to plasmids containing upstream flanking regions of two other rat genes. They also exhibited a partial tissue-specific distribution, since they were detected at high levels in pituitary cells or cell lines and in osteosarcoma cells, but at lower or undetectable levels in glial, liver or kidney cells. Further analysis with prolactin genomic subclones showed that NP44 and NP48 bind to at least two sites, located between -0.4 and -2.0 kilobase-pairs (kbp) (region I) and between -2.0 and -4.8 kbp (region II) relative to the transcription initiation site. End-labeled restriction fragments of one of these subclones were exposed to and recovered from NP44 and NP48, and size fractionated to determine which had bound. This experimental approach yielded a further localization of region I to between -1.27 and -0.62 kbp.

Regulation of expression of a transfected prolactin-CAT chimeric gene. We have investigated whether the 5'-flanking sequence of the rat prolactin (PRL) gene contains information for pituitary cell-specific expression of this gene. The bacterial chloramphenicol acetyltransferase (CAT) gene was removed from pRSV-CAT (4), and cloned downstream of 1.95 kbp of PRL upstream flanking sequence plus about 37 bp of transcribed PRL sequence, to yield plasmid pPRL-CAT. The CAT enzymatic assay (4) was employed to measure the activity of pPRL-CAT in various cell lines during transient expression (5). pPRL-CAT expression was strong in either GH_3 rat pituitary cells or their PRL-negative GC cell variants, but was low or undetectable in rat glial, human or monkey kidney, or mouse fibroblast cell lines. In contrast, neither pRSV-CAT, pSV_2-CAT, nor a mouse metallothionein-CAT plasmid (pmMT-CAT) were expressed especially strongly in GH_3 cells. Similar results were obtained in polyclonal cultures of either GH_3 cells or rat glial cells stably transfected with pPRL-CAT. These results imply that pPRL-CAT contains DNA sequences required for pituitary cell-specific expression of the rat prolactin gene. Furthermore, experiments employing RNAse protection of an SP6-promoted RNA probe (6) showed that transcription of pPRL-CAT in stably transfected GH_3 cells is initiated at the correct site.

To begin to map the prolactin gene promotor region, 5' deletions of the prolactin gene DNA sequence in pPRL-CAT were constructed, and analyzed during transient expression in GH_3 cells. Deletions from -1950 to about -600 bp (relative to the prolactin gene transcription initiation site) yielded a gradual 70% decrease in CAT activity. Further deletions revealed the existence of succesive strong positive, negative, and positive regulatory regions. These results imply that the more proximal binding site for NP44 and NP48 (Region I) may be involved in the tissue-specific expression of the prolactin gene, but that the prolactin gene promotor contains a rather complex regulatory structure which lies downstream of the binding sites for these chromatin proteins.

Regulation of expression of a transfected growth hormone-CAT chimeric gene. We first investigated whether the 5'-flanking sequence of the rat growth hormone (GH) gene contains information for pituitary cell-specific expression of this gene. Plasmid pGH-CAT was constructed by cloning about 580 bp of growth hormone gene flanking sequence plus 13 bp of transcribed sequence upstream of the CAT gene. In polyclonal cultures of stably transfected cells, pGH-CAT activity in GH_3 rat pituitary cells was at least 100-fold higher than in rat glial, human kidney, mouse fibroblast, or rat hepatoma cells. In contrast, pmMT-CAT expression in GH_3 cells was lower than in either mouse fibroblast or rat glial cells. These results imply that pGH-CAT contains DNA sequences required for pituitary cell-specific expression of the rat growth hormone gene. As before, experiments employing RNAse protection of an SP6-promoted RNA probe (6) showed that transcription of pGH-CAT in stably transfected GH_3 cells is initiated at the correct site.

To begin to map the growth hormone gene promotor region, 5' deletions of the growth hormone gene DNA sequence in pGH-CAT were constructed, and analyzed during transient expression in GH_3 cells. Deletion from -550 to -236 (relative to the growth hormone gene transcription initiation site) yielded no decrease in CAT activity, implying that these sequences are not required for pituitary cell expression of the growth hormone gene. Further deletions to about -100 abolished pGH-CAT expression. Hence, there are DNA sequences between -236 and -100 which are apparently required for growth hormone gene expression in pitutary cells.

Glucocorticoid hormones have been shown previously to yield a rapid increase in the transcription by GH_3 rat pituitary cells of the growth hormone gene (7,8). To investigate whether growth hormone gene 5' flanking sequences mediate this glucocorticoid response, we examined regulation of the expression of pGH-CAT, both in stably transfected GH_3 cells and during transient expression by these cells. The synthetic glucocorticoid dexamethasone stimulated pGH-CAT activity in some but not all individual clones of GH_3 cells stably transfected with pGH-CAT. Results with a polyclonal stably transfected culture showed that either dexamethasone or 3,5,3'-triiodo-L-thyronine (T_3) independently regulate expression from both the exogenous and endogenous growth hormone gene promotor. To begin to map glucocorticoid regulatory sites upstream of the growth hormone gene, dexamethasone regulation of transient expression of pGH-CAT and its 5' deletions was examined. Dexamethasone stimulated pGH-CAT expression about eight-fold. Deletion of sequences between -580 and -236 yielded no significant decrease in the stimulation by dexamethasone, implying that these sequences are not required for a glucocorticoid response. Further deletion from -236 to -180 reduced the dexamethasone stimulation about three-fold, while deletion below -180 abolished the dexamethasone response. These results imply that the rat growth hormone gene 5'-flanking region contains at least two regions, one above and one below -180, which function as glucocorticoid regulatory elements.

Conclusions. Analysis by protein blotting of specific DNA-binding proteins, together with transfection experiments of the type described above, should ultimately yield information about: 1. the identity and function of chromatin proteins which mediate cell-type specific expression and hormonal regulation of the rat prolactin and growth hormone genes, and 2. the cognate DNA sequences to which they bind.

References

1. Bancroft, F.C. 1981. GH cells: functional clonal lines of rat pituitary tumor cells, p. 47-59. In G. Sato (ed.), Functionally Differentiated Cell Lines. Alan R. Liss, Inc. New York., New York.
2. White, B.A., Lufkin, T.C., Preston, G.M., and C. Bancroft. 1985. Detection of two chromatin proteins which bind specifically to the 5' flanking region of the rat prolactin gene. Mol. Cell. Biol. 5: 2967-2974.
3. Bowen, B. Steinberg, J., Laemmli, U.K., and Weintraub, H. 1980. The detection of DNA-binding proteins by protein blotting. Nucl. Acids Res. 8: 1-20.
4. Gorman, C.M., Merlino, G.T., Willingham, M.C., Pastan, I., and Howard, B.H. 1982. The Rous sarcoma virus long terminal repeat is a strong promoter when introduced into a variety of eukaryotic cells by DNA-mediated transfection. Proc. Natl. Acad. Sci. USA 79: 6777-6781.
5. Lopata, M.A., Cleveland, D.W., and Sollner-Webb, B. 1984. High level transient expression of a chloramphenicol acetyltransferase gene by DEAE-dextran mediated DNA transfection coupled with a dimethyl sulfoxide or glycerol shock treatment. Nucl. Acids Res. 12: 5707-5717.
6. Zinn, K., DiMaio, D., and Maniatis, T. 1983. Identification of two distinct regulatory regions adjacent to the human b-interferon gene. Cell 34: 865-879.
7. Dobner, P.R., Kawasaki, E.S., Yu, L.-Y., and Bancroft, F.C. 1981. Thyroid or glucocorticoid hormone induces pre-growth-hormone mRNA and its probable nuclear precursor in rat pituitary cells. Proc. Natl. Acad. Sci. USA 78: 2230-2234.
8. Spindler, S.R., Mellon, S.H., and Baxter, J.D. 1982. Growth hormone gene transcription is regulated by thyroid and glucocorticoid hormones in cultured rat pituitary tumor cells. J. Biol. Chem. 257: 11672-11632.

cAMP SUBSTITUTES FOR INSULIN IN EXPRESSION OF THE 25K CASEIN GENE IN MAMMARY EXPLANTS FROM VIRGIN RAT

Piotr Chomczynski
Laboratory of Biochemistry and Metabolism, NIADDK, NIH, Bethesda, MD 20892

Expression of the 25K casein gene in rat mammary gland depends on insulin, prolactin and glucocorticoid. The role of insulin in this multihormonal system has been related to activation of the transcription of the 25K casein gene (1). The mechanism by which insulin influences this nuclear event remains obscure. Substitution of insulin by cAMP in the estrogen-dependent induction of the ovalbumin gene transcription suggests that insulin and cAMP may exert their effects, at least in part, through a common pathway (2). In support of this hypothesis it is reported here that a similar effect of cAMP can be observed in the case of the 25K casein gene.

METHODS. Mammary explants from Sprague-Dawley rats were cultured in Medium 199 for 4 days. Total RNA was isolated from explants by the guanidinium-cesium chloride method and was analysed for the 25K casein mRNA content by hybridization with nick-translated [32P] 25K casein cDNA using the DBM disk method, and by Northern blot analysis. Procedural details are provided in ref. 1.

RESULTS AND DISCUSSION. Mammary explants from virgin rat cultured in the presence of hydrocortisone and prolactin accumulate a small amount of 25K casein mRNA (Fig. 1). Addition of cAMP increases markedly

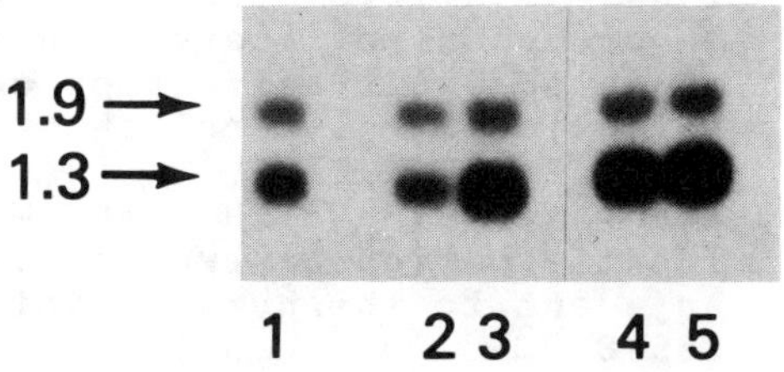

Fig. 1. Northern blot analysis of accumulated 25K casein mRNA (1.3 kb) and β-actin mRNA (1.9 kb) in mammary explants from virgin rats. Explants were cultured with: hydrocortisone (F) and prolactin (P) (lane 2); F, P plus 0.5 mM 8 bromo cAMP (lane 3); F, P plus insulin (I) (lane 4); F, P and I plus 0.5 mM 8 bromo cAMP (lane 5). Lane 1, fresh tissue. Numbers on the left represent kb values.

the level of this mRNA to that observed in the 3-hormone system containing insulin. Stimulation of the 25K casein mRNA accumulation was also observed when cholera toxin (0.5 ug/ml) was added to the FP system (not shown). Both cAMP and insulin stimulate selectively 25K casein mRNA accumulation, but not β-actin mRNA accumulation. Fig. 2 shows that the effect of cAMP is seen only in the FP system. In the FI and PI systems cAMP does not influence the amount of 25K casein mRNA. In addition, cAMP is not effective in the FPI system. Results indicate that cAMP can act as a substitute for insulin, but cannot substitute for hydrocortisone or prolactin in stimulating 25K casein mRNA accumulation in virgin mammary explants. The fact that the

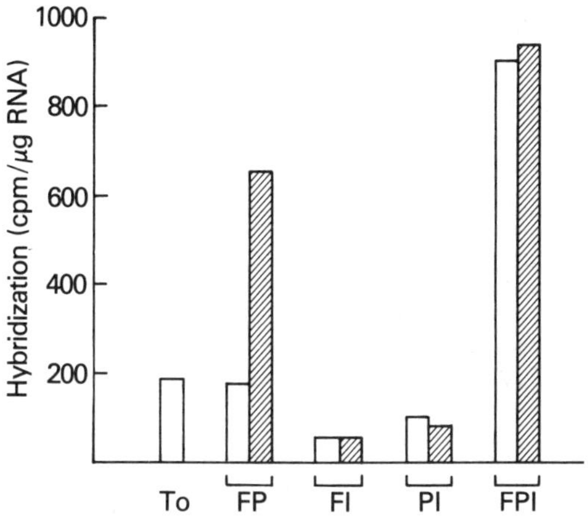

Fig. 2. Substitution of insulin by cAMP in stimulation of 25K casein mRNA accumulation in mammary explants from virgin rats. Culture conditions as described in legend to Fig. 1. Hatched bars, culture systems supplemented with 0.5 mM 8 bromo cAMP. To, fresh tissue.

effects of cAMP and insulin are not additive suggests that both agents may use a common pathway to stimulate 25K casein mRNA accumulation. Since insulin affects transcriptional activity of the 25K casein gene but not stability of the transcript (1), the stimulatory effect of cAMP reported here is most probably related to the transcriptional events, as has been found in other systems (3).

Substitution of insulin by cAMP was also tested in mammary explants from pregnant rats. In this case, no stimulation of 25K casein mRNA was observed upon the addition of cAMP to the FP system. cAMP was unable to stimulate 25K casein accumulation at concentrations up to 1 mM, or when used together with a phosphodiesterase inhibitor (IBMX) (not shown). Thus, substitution of insulin by cAMP in rat mammary gland, with respect to 25K casein gene activation, depends on the physiological state of the gland.

These results suggest that cAMP is not a transmitter of the insulin signal in activating transcription of the 25K casein gene, but rather acts by mechanism which converges with that of insulin, as has been proposed for the expression of the ovalbumin gene.

REFERENCES

(1) Chomczynski, P., Qasba, P. and Topper, Y.J. (1984) Science, 226, 1326-1328.
(2) Evans, M.I. and McKnight, G.S. (1984) Endocrinology 115, 368-377).
(3) Gancedo, J.M., Mazon, M.J. and Erso, P. (1985) Trends Biochem. Sci. 210-212.

STUDY OF THE CONTROL OF PRO-THYROID HORMONE (THYROGLOBULIN) GENE EXPRESSION.

D. Christophe, C. Hansen, F. Libert, A. Bacolla, C. Gerard & G. Vassart*, IRIBHN and *Service de Chimie, Campus Erasme, route de Lennik 808, B-1070 Bruxelles, Belgium.

INTRODUCTION

The thyroid hormones, thyroxine and 3,5,3'-triiodothyronine, are formed through iodination and oxidative coupling of specific tyrosine residues on a large glycoprotein precursor, thyroglobulin (Tg). The synthesis of Tg in the thyroid is under positive control of the pituitary hormone thyrotropin (TSH), the action of which inside the cell is mediated by cyclic AMP (cAMP).

It has recently been demonstrated that the control of Tg production is mainly transcriptional (1) and strong evidence has been gained supporting the view that cAMP is the effective modulator of Tg gene transcription (2). Both human (3,4) and bovine (G. de Martynoff, in preparation) Tg gene promoter regions have been cloned. The availability of these clones allowed us to undertake the study of the mechanisms involved in the regulation of Tg gene expression.

RESULTS

Characterization of promoter regions. In addition to the canonical TATA-Box and a CAAT-Box homology, an unusually long (209 bp) poly(purine)-poly(pyrimidine) sequence has been found in the human Tg gene promoter region. This sequence has been shown to be cleaved by the single-strand specific nuclease S1 when contained in a supercoiled plasmid (4). A similar region, although much shorter (38 bp), was found upstream from the bovine Tg gene (G. de Martynoff, in preparation). This sequence also displayed a high sensitivity to S1 nuclease action under torsional stress. However, apart from the homopurine-homopyrimidine asymmetry, no clear homology with the human counterpart could be detected. Interestingly the most conserved segment between the two promoter regions (1 mismatch/30 bases) includes the CAAT-Box homology. The conservation of these elements could suggest that they represent essential targets for the transcriptional machinery.

Role of DNA methylation. We investigated the possibility that DNA methylation at the 5'end of the gene could be correlated with gene activity. Blots of Hpa II-digested DNA from various human tissues were probed with a labelled 8 kb Eco RI genomic fragment encompassing the 5'end of the human Tg gene (see figure). From the three expected fragments (0.95, 2.9 and 4.9 kb), none was detected in liver, salivary gland and sperm DNA, two (0.95 and 2.9 kb) appeared in thyroid DNA and surprisingly, all three were present in placental DNA. Thus, there is both a specific demethylation event in adult somatic tissue which can be related to the tissue-specific expression of the gene and a general demethylation process in the extraembryonal tissue without any bearing on transcriptional activity (such a phenomenon has been described for other genes too, see ref.(5).

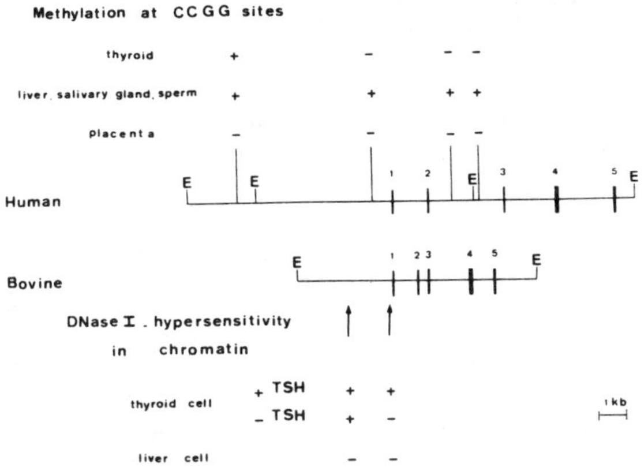

Fig. Maps of human and bovine Tg gene 5' regions. The data on DNA methylation and DNase I-hypersensitivity of chromatin are summarized. E = Eco RI; exons are represented by black boxes and numbered.

Study of chromatin structure. The existence of DNase I-hypersensitive regions in the chromatin at the 5'end of the gene was investigated. Mild DNase I digestion of bovine thyroid cell nuclei revealed the presence of two such hypersensitive tracts. One of these is located about 1.5 kb upstream from the Cap site and the other is just close to it (see figure). None of them was detected in bovine liver cell chromatin. The study of the relationship between the presence of these hypersensitive sites and the expression of the gene was undertaken using primary cultured bovine thyroid cells. TSH deprivation resulted in the disappearance of the hypersensitive site located close to the transcriptional start and the decrease of the Tg mRNA content of the cell. Subsequent stimulation of the cell restored both DNase I-hypersensitivity at this site and detectable Tg mRNA content.

PROSPECTS

The study of the transcriptional control of the Tg gene by means of transfection experiments is underway. As the way by which cAMP regulates transcription in eukaryotes is still unknown, the func tional study of recombinant Tg gene promoters may rank as a good model system to investigate this general phenomenon.

REFERENCES

(1) VAN HEUVERSWYN, B., STREYDIO, C., BROCAS, H., REFETOFF, S., DUMONT, J. & VASSART, G. (1984) Proc. Natl. Acad. Sci., USA 81, 5941-5945.

(2) VAN HEUVERSWYN, B., LERICHE, A., VAN SANDE, J., DUMONT, J.E. & VASSART, G. (1985) FEBS Lett. 188, 192-196.

(3) TARGOVNIK, H.M., POHL, V., CHRISTOPHE, D., CABRER, B., BROCAS, H. & VASSART, G. (1984) Eur. J. Biochem. 141, 271-277.

(4) CHRISTOPHE, D., CABRER, B., BACOLLA, A., TARGOVNIK, H., POHL, V. & VASSART, G. (1985) Nucl. Acid Res. 13, 5127-5144.

(5) SANFORD, J.P., CHAPMAN, V.M. & ROSSANT, J. (1983) Trends in Genetics, 1, 89-93.

DIFFERENTIAL EFFECT OF VARIOUS SECRETOGOGUES ON ß-ENDORPHIN RELEASE AND PRO-OPIOMELANOCORTIN BIOSYNTHESIS IN RAT ANTERIOR PITUITARY CELLS AND AtT-20 CELLS

Jitendra R. Dave, Lee E. Eiden and Robert L. Eskay
Laboratory of Clinical Studies, NIAAA, DICBR and Laboratory of Cell Biology, NIMH, Bethesda, Maryland 20892.

Corticotrophs of the anterior pituitary (AP) gland synthesize the pro-opiomelanocortin (POMC) precursor from which are derived adrenocorticotropin and ß-lipotropin [N-terminally extended ß-endorphin (BE)]. The POMC gene in corticotrophs is known to be regulated by corticotropin-releasing hormone (CRF) and glucocorticoids (1-3). *In vitro* studies have demonstrated the release of POMC-derived peptides from primary-cultured pituitary cells and from a mouse-derived anterior pituitary tumor-cell line (AtT-20 cells). A variety of pharmacological agents which elevate cyclic AMP or intracellular calcium, or which stimulate protein kinase C, as well as the physiological regulator, CRF, enhance hormone release (4). We recently demonstrated that both forskolin and CRF stimulate hormone secretion and POMC biosynthesis, whereas, a phorbol ester (TPA) stimulated only hormone release in AP and AtT-20 cells (5). These data suggested that stimulation of POMC-derived peptide secretion and POMC biosynthesis depends on activation of the adenylate cyclase/cyclic AMP/protein kinase A system. The objective of the present study was to determine if a ß-adrenoceptor agonist, isoproterenol (ISO)(primarily working through activation of the adenylate cyclase/cAMP system), a calcium ionophore, A23187 or barium (Ba^{2+}) would stimulate both hormone release and POMC synthesis in rat AP and AtT-20 cells, as is the case for CRF.

CELL CULTURES: Anterior pituitary (AP) cells were cultured in DMEM media as described earlier (6) and used on day 5 after the dispersion. AtT-20 cells were cultured in DMEM media with 0.1% glucose and used on day 6-8 following plating.

ß-ENDORPHIN (BE) ASSAY: One hour after the addition of various secretogogues, the media was removed from the wells containing AP or AtT-20 cells and immunoreactive BE levels were determined in media aliquots by RIA. The BE-antiserum recognizes ß-lipotropin and BE on an equimolar basis (7).

POMC mRNA QUANTITATION: Twenty-four hr after the addition of various agents, POMC messenger RNA levels were quantitated in cells using Northern-blot and slot-blot techniques as described earlier (8).

RESULTS AND DISCUSSION: ISO, A23187 and Ba produced a dose-related increase in BE release in both AP and AtT-20 cells. In cultured AP cells, ISO at 10^{-6}M, A23187 at 10^{-6}M and Ba^{2+} at 2.5 x 10^{-3}M maximally enhanced BE release by approximately 2.5-fold, 2-fold and 2-fold, respectively (Figure 1). In AtT-20 cells, ISO at 10^{-6}M, A23187 at 10^{-6}M and Ba^{2+} at 2.5 x 10^{-3}M maximally enhanced BE release by approximately 3-fold, 1-fold and 6-fold, respectively (Figure 2). ISO produced a dose-related increase in POMC mRNA levels in both AP and AtT-20 cells; however, A23187 and Ba^{2+} failed to increase POMC mRNA levels in either of the cell types. In AP and AtT-20 cells, ISO at 10^{-6} M concentration increased relative POMC mRNA levels by approximately 2-fold. The maximal stimulatory concentrations of A23187 (10^{-6}M) and Ba^{2+} (2.5 x 10^{-3}M) for BE release did not change POMC mRNA levels in either of the cell types (Figures 1 & 2). These data suggest that stimulation of POMC-derived peptide secretion and POMC biosynthesis depends on activation of the cAMP/ adenylate cyclase system. By contrast, addition of barium in adrenomedullary chromaffin cells stimulates both the release and biosynthesis of enkephalin and its messenger RNA (10). Activation of the protein kinase C or other second messenger systems appears to be linked only to secretion and not to biosynthesis, as described in another system (11). The coupling of secretion and biosynthesis follow-

FIGURE 1

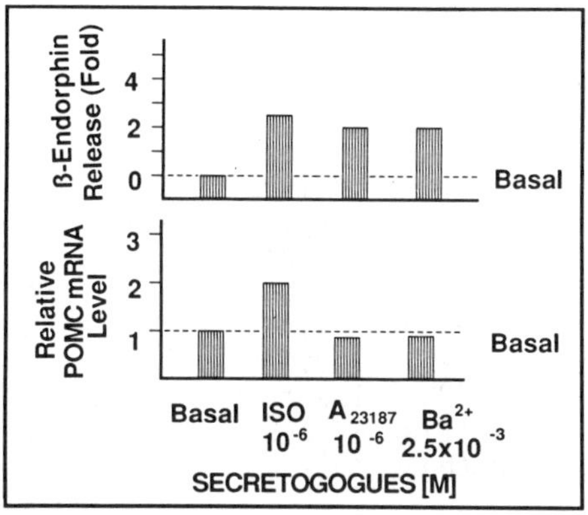

FIGURE 2

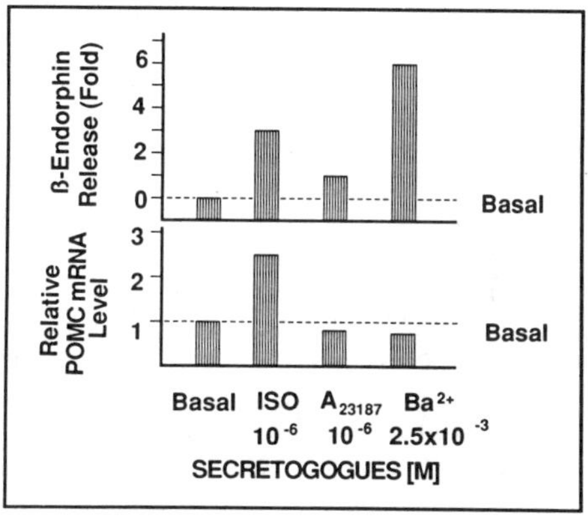

Addition of isoproterenol (ISO), A23187 or barium chloride (Ba^{2+}) to cultured anterior pituitary cells (Figure 1) or to cultured mouse-derived anterior pituitary tumor (AtT-20) cells (Figure 2) produced differential effects on release and biosynthesis of pro-opiomelanocortin- derived peptides. Detailed assay conditions are described in Ref. 5,7 and 8.

---

ing secretogogue activation appears to be a general principle of the regulation of neuropeptide-producing endocrine cells. In corticotrophs of anterior-pituitary origin, this coupling appears to be mediated via the cAMP/adenylate cyclase system.

REFERENCES:

1) Herbert, E., Birnberg, N., Lissitsky, J-C., Civelli, O. and Uhler, M. (1982). In Pituitary Hormones and Related Peptides. Motta, M., Zanisi, M. and Piva, F. Eds. 31-42. Acaemic Press, New York, N.Y.
2) Birnberg, N.C., Lissitsky, J-C, Hinman, M. and Herbert, E. (1983) Proc. Natl. Acad. Sci. U.S.A. 80, 6982-6986.
3) Eberwine, J.H. and Roberts, J.L. (1984) J. Biol. Chem. 259, 2166-2170.
4) Axelrod, J. and Reisine, T.D. (1984) Science. 224, 452-459.
5) Dave, J.R., Eiden, L.E. and Eskay, R.L. (1986) Ann. N.Y. Acad. Sci. (in press).
6) Vale, W., Grant, G., Amoss, M., Blackwell, R. and Guillemin, R. (1972) Endocrinology.91, 562-572.
7) Dave, J.R., Rubinstein, N. and Eskay, R.L. (1985) Endocrinology. 117, 1389-1396.
8) Dave, J.R., Eiden, L.E., Karanian, J.W. & Eskay, R.L. (1986) Endocrinology. 118 (in press)
9) Eiden, L.E., Giraud, P., Affolter, H-U., Herbert, E. and Hotchkiss, A.J. (1984) Proc. Natl. Acad. Sci. U.S.A. 81, 3949-3953.
10) Waschek, J.A. and Eiden, L.E. (1985) 15th Colloquim, French Society of Neuroendocrinology, Gif-sur-Yvette, France, September, 1985 (Abstract).
11) Barinaga, M., Bilezikjian, L.M., Vale, W.W., Rosenfeld, M.G. and Evans, R.M. (1985) Nature. 314, 279-281.

REGULATION OF INSULIN-STIMULATED SUGAR TRANSPORT BY MODULATION OF BASAL SUGAR TRANSPORT

R.J. Germinario, M. Oliveira, and S. Manuel
Lady Davis Institute for Medical Research, 3755 Cote St.Catherine Rd., Montreal, Quebec, Canada H3T 1E2

INTRODUCTION: Recently it has been reported that glucose starvation enhancement of hexose transport in cultured human fibroblasts (1) and 3T3 adipocytes (2) resulted in an inability of insulin to stimulate hexose transport in these cells. This loss of insulin sensitivity was thought to be related to a depletion of intracellular insulin translocatable hexose carriers (1). Thus, we questioned whether other factors that might affect basal hexose transport will similarly affect insulin sensitivity. In this report, we present evidence that short term exposure (i.e. 6h) to cycloheximide (CHX) elevated hexose transport in glucose-fed human fibroblasts resulting in a subsequent loss of insulin-stimulated hexose transport in these cells.

MATERIALS AND METHODS: Details of cell culture and the transport of 2-deoxy-D-glucose (2-DG) and 3-O-methyl-D-glucose (3-OMG), performed under rate-limiting conditions, can be found in (1,3,4)

RESULTS: The data in Table I show that increasing concentrations of CHX directly affect basal 2-DG transport. Upon addition of insulin to these CHX treated cells, the insulin:control transport ratio was indirectly proportional to the basal transport increase. The data is representative of an average of 4 experiments. The inhibition of protein synthesis for 5 μg and 50 μg CHX/ml was 64% and 91%, respectively.

Table I. The effect of CHX exposure for 6 h on basal and insulin-stimulated hexose transport

CHX μg/ml	2-DG transport* Basal	+100 mU insulin/ml**	Ratio (+I/-I)
0	5.45	9.24	1.68
5	8.06	9.54	1.20
50	11.59	12.55	1.06

*nmoles/mg P/2 min, 1 mM 2-DG; **insulin added for the last 2 h of CHX treatment.

To further demonstrate the nature of the CHX effect on these cells as a transport change, the nonmetabolizable glucose analogue 3-OMG was employed. Basal 3-OMG uptake increased in the presence of CHX (0.723 vs 2.598 nmoles 3-OMG/mg P/30 sec, respectively), while the insulin stimulation ratio decreased precipitously, i.e. 3.72 vs 1.09 in the control vs CHX groups, respectively. Additionally, the hexokinase activity of cell-free homogenates ± CHX were not different. We next determined the changes in hexose transport kinetics as affected by CHX treatment. The data in Table II indicate that CHX elevated the V_{max} and not the K_m of hexose transport. The data has been corrected for the diffusional uptake of sugar (3) and the seven 2-DG concentrations employed were from 0.05 mM to 3.0 mM.

Table II. The effect of CHX on the K_m and V_{max} for 2-DG transport

Treatment (6h)	K_m (mM)	V_{max} (nmoles/mg P/min)
Control	3.33	8.0
+50 µg CHX/ml	5.00	24.4

DISCUSSION: The data presented herein lend support to the importance of the regulation of the hexose carrier in the overall sequence of events leading to insulin stimulation of sugar transport. While glucose-starved cells regulate carrier activity by modulating carrier synthesis and turnover (1,5), the results shown in this report were obtained with glucose-fed cells in the presence of CHX. We feel that the CHX is affecting the rate of carrier degradation as suggested by others (5). This is supported in part by our observation that cells exposed to CHX at high concentrations (50 µg.ml) inhibited protein degradation significantly (data not shown). We have not ignored the insulin receptor and preliminary data (not shown) indicate that CHX after 6h can lead to a decrease in insulin binding. This is in agreement with the inverse correlations observed by others showing factors that increase transport decrease insulin binding (1,2). While the importance of the insulin receptor in an insulin response is acknowledged, the data suggest that the regulation of the hexose carrier is an important "post-receptor step" in insulin-stimulated hexose transport

REFERENCES

(1) Germinario, R.J., Ozaki, S. and Kalant, N. (1984) Arch. Biochem. Biophys. 234, 559-566.
(2) Van Patten, J.P.M. and Krans, H.M.J. (1985) J. Biol. Chem. 260, 7996-8001.
(3) Germinario, R.J., Oliveira, M. and Leung, H. (1978) Can. J. Biochem. 56, 80-88.
(4) Germinario, R.J. and Oliveira, M. (1979) J. Cell. Physiol. 99, 313-318.
(5) Christopher, C.W., Colby, W.W. and Ullrey, D. (1976) J. Cell. Physiol. 89, 683-692.

CHARACTERIZATION OF AN α-AMIDATING ENZYME FROM RAT CA-77 CELLS: ITS USE FOR THE PRODUCTION OF RECOMBINANT HUMAN CALCITONIN AND GHRF

J.P. Gilligan, S.J. Lovato, S.D. Young, B.N. Jones, J.A. Koehn, L.F. LeSueur, A.M. Sturmer, A.H. Bertelsen, T.G. Warren, R.S. Birnbaum,* and B.A. Roos*

Unigene Laboratories, Fairfield, NJ; Medical Research Service, VA *Medical Center, Tacoma, WA; and Department of Medicine University of Washington, Seattle, WA.

INTRODUCTION

Many small peptide hormones require an amidated carboxyl terminus for full biological activity. Amidation is a post-translational processing event responsible for converting larger precursor polypeptides to mature secretory products. The reaction is catalyzed by an amidating enzyme, peptidyl glycine α-amidating monooxygenase, which requires a substrate consisting of the sequence of the mature hormone with an additional glycine at the carboxyl terminus (1). The majority of the published information concerning this enzyme is based on observations obtained from pituitary or brain extracts (2). We have previously shown that the neoplastic rat C-cell line, CA-77, elaborates the amidated form of the hypocalcemic hormone calcitonin (3). Studies were undertaken to compare the amidating enzyme activity of this cell line to that of the pituitary enzymes.

MATERIALS AND METHODS

Enzyme activity was measured by monitoring the conversion of D-Tyr-Val-Gly or the fluorescently tagged tripeptide to the corresponding amidated molecule (4). The amidated product was separated from substrate by reversed-phase HPLC and the amount of product was quantitated by starting the absorbance at 280 nm or relative fluorescent intensity. The starting source of the enzyme was an ammonium sulfate precipitate of tissue culture medium from the CA-77 cell line. The conversion of Gly^{33} calcitonin and Gly^{45} GHRF to the amidated peptides was assessed by RP-HPLC and an enzyme-linked immunosorbent assay specific for the mature hormone, and amino acid analysis.

RESULTS

Assay conditions were first established which yielded a linear accumulation of product with time and protein concentration. As with other amidating enzymes, exogenous copper was required for optimum activity. Maximum rates of conversion were observed with 0.5-5 uM copper sulfate; higher concentrations were inhibitory. Exogenous ascorbic acid was stimulatory, with maximum activity observed at 3-8 mM. A concentration of 3 mM ascorbate was used routinely. Addition of catalase to the reaction mixture was found to preserve enzyme activity. In the absence of catalase, conversion of substrate to product plateaued at 20-30%, in the presence of catalase conversion was linear up to 60-70%. Under optimum assay conditions (300 uM substrate) the specific activity of the ammonium sulfate pellet was about 800 pmol/min/mg protein. The specific activity of partially purified preparations of the enzyme used in these studies was 20,000 pmol/min/mg protein. This partially purified preparation of amidating enzyme was also used to convert [Gly^{33}]-calcitonin to the amidated product (Fig. 1). The conversion was monitored by RP-HPLC and confirmed by an ELISA assay specific for the amidated peptide (5).

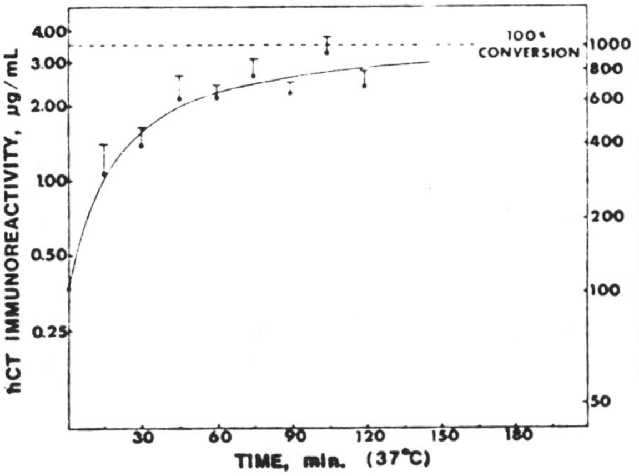

Figure 1. Immunochemical Determination of Amidated Calcitonin. Samples were taken at various time points during amidation. Samples were assayed using an ELISA-based assay specific for the amidated peptide. Data points represents the mean ± S.E. of five determinations.

DISCUSSION

The α-amidating enzyme activity secreted by the rat neoplastic C-cell line appears qualitatively similar to amidating enzyme from pituitary and brain (2). In contrast to primary pituitary cultures; however, the CA-77 cell line continues to secrete both amidated products and the α-amidating enzyme in an ascorbate independent manner. The levels of α-amidating enzyme secreted into the media make possible the α-amidation of relatively large amounts of glycine-extended calcitonin and GHRF. These products have been shown to be the mature, biologically active peptides. Finally, this enzyme may prove useful for the commercial scale synthesis of numerous amidated peptide hormones.

REFERENCES

(1) Bradbury, A.F., Finnie, M.D.A., and Smyth, D.G. (1982) Nature (Lond.) 298, 686-688.

(2) Eipper, B.A., Myers, A.C., and Mains, R.E. (1985) Endocrinology 116, 2505-2515.

(3) Birnbaum, R.S., Mahoney, W.C., and Roos, B.A. (1986) J. Biol. Chem., in press.

(4) Gilligan J.P., Jones B.N., Birnbaum R.S., and Scott R.W. Fourth International Symposium on HPLC of Proteins, Peptides and Polynucleotides 1984.

(5) Jones B.N., Warren T.G., Gilligan J.P., Sturmer A.M., Lovato S.J., Koehn J.A., Young S.D., Ray M.L., and Bertelsen A.H. Symposium of American Protein Chemists 1985.

REFEEDING INDUCES A GROWTH STIMULATING ACTIVITY IN THE PROXIMAL SMALL INTESTINE IN RATS AFTER 24 HOUR STARVATION

V.L. Grey, and C.L. Morin
Centre de Recherche Pédiatrique, Hôpital Sainte-Justine, Montreal, Quebec, Canada H3T 1C5

Luminal nutrition influences normal small intestine structure and function (1). Starvation generally results in mucosal hypoplasia and on refeeding the intestine returns to the normal steady state. These events are accompanied by a diminished proliferative activity (as measured by tritiated thymidine incorporation) after fasting and on refeeding with a normal diet, this proliferative activity is restored to normal levels (2). The mechanism by which food influences this activity is largely unknown. Small bowel resection also alters the equilibrium that exists between crypt cell production rate and villous cell loss, the result being mucosal hyperplasia (3). An important stimulus for the adaptive response is the oral intake of food (4). In a previous study (5) we reported the presence of a growth stimulatory activity in the proximal small intestine that could be responsible for the adaptive hyperplasia observed after small bowel resection. The growth stimulating activity was detected 48 hours after surgery and persisted for 96 hours. By 8 days the activity was undetectable. The activity present in the resected animals at 96 hours and due to 2 peptides of approx mol wt 4,500 and 1,500, could play a role in promoting the observed hyperplasia after resection. In this report we describe the presence of a similar activity in animals that have been starved for 24 hours then refed. This activity is detectable only at 24 hours after feeding. Animals that are fed ad libitum do not demonstrate this growth stimulating activity.

DETECTION OF THE GROWTH STIMULATING ACTIVITY. Male Sprague-Dawley rats were starved for 24 hours then refed. 24 hours after refeeding 13 cm of the proximal intestine, distal to the ligament of Treitz, was removed. An acidic extract of the mucosal scraping was prepared and tested for the growth stimulating activity as previously described (3). The stimulation index was quantitated by measuring the rate of thymidine incorporation into DNA in an organ culture system after preincubation with the acidic extract for 10 hours (5). Table 1 shows that the stimulating activity is only detected 24 hours after refeeding. No activity is detectable in normal animals that were not starved.

Table 1. Stimulation index in 24 hours starved animals.

	Hours after refeeding		Ad libitum
Stimulation index	24	48	
	160	112	110

The stimulation index was determined from the proximal intestine of 6 animals. 100 μg protein in the acidic extract was used for the preincubation. The results represent the mean of 6 determinations.

CHARACTERIZATION OF THE STIMULATING ACTIVITY. Sephadex G-25 filtration. The acidic extract was prepared as previously described (4) and applied to a Sephadex G-25 column. 2.5 ml fractions were collected and three fractions pooled and tested for stimulating activity. The stimulation index of the pooled fractions was quantitated by measuring the rate of thymidine incorporation into DNA in an organ culture system after preincubation with the designated fraction as previously described (4). The results are shown in Fig. 1. The bar graph represents the mitogenic activity in the extract and two distinct peaks of stimulation activity, one just after the void volume with a molecular weight 4,500 daltons and the other at 1,500.

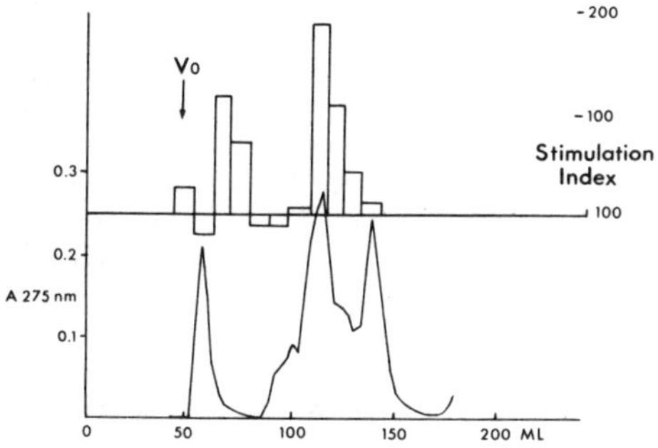

Fig. 1. Sephadex G-25 gel filtration of acidic extract of proximal intestine from a pool of 8 animals that were starved for 24 hours then refed. The conditions were column size 1.5 x 87 cm; eluant 0.01 N HCl 0.15 NaCl; and flow rate 3.3 ml/h. The column fractions were tested for mitogenic activity in quadriplicate.

The specific activity per mg of protein is 8,358 and it represents a 200-fold increase in the activity of the acidic extract prior to gel filtration.

CONCLUSION. The results indicate that the molecules responsible for the growth stimulating activity in response to refeeding after starvation are of the same molecular size as those obtained after a small bowel resection. The difference between the extent of the response of the intestine after resection and after refeeding could therefore be due to the longer duration of the molecules in the intestine after the resection. Further work is in progress on the identification of the peptides.

ACKNOWLEDGEMENTS. The authors would like to thank Mrs C. Garofalo, A. Duhaime and T. Rouleau for technical help.

REFERENCES

(1) Morin, C.L., Ling, V., Bourassa, D. (1980) Dig. Dis. Sci. 25, 123-128.
(2) Al-Dewachi, H.S., Wright, N.A., Appleton, D.R., Watson, A.J. (1975) J. Anat. 119, 105.
(3) Hanson, W.R., Osborne, J.W., Sharp, J.G. (1977) Gastroenterology, 72, 692-700.
(4) Morin, C.L., Ling, V., Van Caillie, M. (1978) Pediatr. Res. 12, 268-271.
(5) Grey, V.L., Morin, C.L. (1985) Gastroenterology, in press.

CLONING OF A HORMONE-REGULATED ISOFORM OF THE REGULATORY SUBUNIT OF TYPE II cAMP-DEPENDENT PROTEIN KINASE

T. Jahnsen[ab], L. Hedin[a], S.M. Lohmann[c], U. Walter[c], V.J. Kidd[a], W.G. Beattie[a], T.Z. Schulz[a] and J.S. Richards[a]

[a]Department of Cell Biology, Baylor College of Medicine, Houston, Texas 77030; [b]Institute of Pathology, Rikshospitalet, Oslo 1, Norway; [c]Department of Physiological Chemistry and Medicine, University of Wurzburg, West Germany

ABSTRACT. We constructed a λgt11 cDNA expression library from poly(A)$^+$ RNA of estradiol and FSH-primed rat granulosa cells. A polyclonal antibody raised against bovine heart R-II (the regulatory subunit of type II cAMP-dependent protein kinase) was purified by affinity chromatography and used for screening the cDNA library. A 1.6 kb cDNA insert was isolated from a plaque purified bacteriophage clone and subcloned into M13mp18 vector for DNA sequencing. The cDNA contained a nucleotide sequence coding for amino acids which were homologues to amino acids around the autophosphorylation site of bovine brain R-II, but which were slightly different from bovine heart R-II. These results document that we have cloned a cDNA for the isoform of R-II which is present in rat brain and ovary and which is distinct from the other isoform of R-II characteristic of rat heart.

INTRODUCTION. The regulatory subunit of type II cAMP-dependent protein kinase, R-II, is present in high concentrations in rat granulosa cells of preovulatory follicles and is induced by the synergistic actions of estradiol and FSH (1) or cAMP (2,3). To gain further insight into the molecular events regulating the action of FSH (and cAMP) on R-II content we have recently purified and characterized the ovarian R-II subunits (4,5). Rat ovarian $R\text{-}II_{52/51}$ (Mr=52-51,000) is structurally and immunologically similar to rat brain (neural) $R\text{-}II_{52}$ (Mr=52,000), but is distinct from $R\text{-}II_{54}$ (Mr=54,000) present in rat heart and also in rat brain and ovary. $R\text{-}II_{52/51}$ but not $R\text{-}II_{54}$ is hormonally regulated in the rat ovarian follicle. In the present work we have cloned the cDNA for rat $R\text{-}II_{52/51}$.

MATERIALS AND METHODS.

Construction of a λgt11 cDNA library from rat granulosa cells. Double-stranded cDNA (ds cDNA) from estradiol-FSH primed rat granulosa cells was synthesized as described by Gubler and Hoffman (6). From 100 μg of poly(A)$^+$ RNA, 10 μg of ds cDNA with an average size of 1.5 kb was recovered. The ds cDNA was sized on a 5-20% sucrose density gradient and fractions containing cDNA greater than 1.0 kb (5 μg) were combined and used to construct a λgt11 cDNA expression library (7). One hundred ng of ds cDNA was ligated to 1 μg λgt11 vector arms to generate 4×10^6 independent clones, of which 99% were recombinant. The cDNA library was subsequently amplified to 4×10^{12} phage.

Screening of the λgt11 rat granulosa cell cDNA library. One million recombinant phage plaques were screened (50,000 plaques per 150 mm plate) as described by Young and Davis (7).

RESULTS AND DISCUSSION. The strategy used to clone the rat $R\text{-}II_{52/51}$ cDNA involved constructing and screening an expression λgt11 cDNA library with polyclonal antibodies against R-II (7). The polyclonal antibodies used for screening the library (anti-bovine heart R-II)

was affinity-purified using purified ovarian R subunits coupled to Sepharose 4B. The affinity-purified bovine heart R-II antibodies recognized $R\text{-}II_{52/51}$ in soluble cell extracts of hormone-primed rat ovaries, purified ovarian $R\text{-}II_{52/51}$ and purified rat heart $R\text{-}II_{54}$. The sensitivity of the antibody was 1 ng of pure ovarian $R\text{-}II_{52/51}$ based on a dot blot assay. We constructed a λgt11 cDNA library from estradiol-FSH primed rat granulosa cell $poly(A)^+$ RNA and screened one million recombinant clones using the affinity-purified polyclonal antibody. One clone, found positive in the primary screening, was rescreened and plaque-purified. From the plaque-purified clone, a 1.6 kb cDNA insert was isolated, subcloned into M13mp18 vector and used for DNA sequence analysis. A restriction map and partial DNA sequence analysis were generated. As shown in Fig. 1, the 1.6 kb fragment revealed an open reading frame of nucleotide sequences coding for amino acids homologous to bovine brain R-II.

P

1. Arg Arg Val Ser Val Cys Ala Glu Thr Tyr Asn Pro Asp Glu Glu Glu
2. Arg Arg Ala Ser Val Cys Ala Glu Ala Tyr Asn Pro Asp Glu Glu Glu
3. Arg Arg Ala Ser Val Cys Ala Glu Ala Tyr Asn Pro Asp Glu Glu Glu

Fig. 1. Comparison of amino acid sequences around the autophosphorylation site of R-II. Lines 1 and 2: Amino acid sequences for bovine heart R-II(8) and bovine brain R-II(9,10), respectively. Line 3: Amino acid sequence deduced from a partial nucleotide sequence of the rat granulosa cell 1.6 kb R-II cDNA. Differences between the rat ovary $R\text{-}II_{52/51}$ bovine brain R-II and bovine heart R-II are underlined. The autophosphorylation site is marked with a P.

Based on these observations, we conclude that a cDNA for the $R\text{-}II_{52/51}$ isoform of cAMP-dependent protein kinase type II present in rat ovary and brain has been cloned. This clone will be used to analyze the mechanisms by which estradiol and FSH regulate $R\text{-}II_{52/51}$ mRNA expression in rat granulosa cells.

ACKNOWLEDGMENTS. This work was supported by NIH-HD-16272 (JSR), Deutsche Forschungsgemeinschaft (SFB 176 A-5; UW), a Fulbright Fellowship (TJ) and the Norwegian Society for Fighting Cancer (TJ).

REFERENCES.

1. Richards, J.S. & A.I. Rolfes. 1980. J. Biol. Chem. 225:5481-5489.
2. Darbon, F.-M., M. Knecht, T. Ranta, M.L. Dufau & K.J. Catt. 1984. J. Biol. Chem. 259:14778-14782.
3. Ratoosh, S.L. & J.S. Richards. 1985. Endocrinology 117:917-927.
4. Jahnsen, T., S.M. Lohmann, U. Walter, L. Hedin & J.S. Richards. 1985. J. Biol. Chem. In press.
5. Jahnsen, T., L. Hedin, S.M. Lohmann, U. Walter & J.S.Richards. 1985.Submitted publication.
6. Gubler, U. & Hoffman, B.J. (1983) Gene 25., 263-269.
7. Young, R.A. & Davis, R.W. (1983) Science 222, 778-782.
8. Takio, K., S.B. Smith, E.G. Krebs, K.A. Walsch & K. Titani. 1982. Proc. Natl. Acad. Sci. USA. 79:2544-2548.
9. Weldon, S.L., M.C. Mumby & S.S. Taylor. 1985. J. Biol. Chem. 260:6440-6448.
10. Stein, J.C. & C.S. Rubin. 1985. J. Biol. Chem. 260:10991-10995.

ANTIGENIC REGIONS OF BOVINE SOMATOTROPIN DEFINED BY MONOCLONAL ANTIBODIES

Gwen G. Krivi and Edwin Rowold, Jr., Biological Sciences, Monsanto Co., Chesterfield, MO 63198

Antibodies to somatotropin (growth hormone) have been used to analyze structure/function relationships of this important protein. Early work focused on the cross-reactions of somatotropins from different species with polyclonal anti-somatotropin antisera (for review see 1). Recently, using monoclonal antibodies to study the antigenic structure of human somatotropin (hST), various groups have described either 3 or 4 distinct epitopes on the hST protein (2-4). This report describes the use of monoclonal antibodies to bovine somatotropin (bST,5) as probes of the immunological structure of this molecule.

Western blot analysis of antibody binding to deletion derivatives of bST

Genes coding for derivatives of bovine somatotropin deleted for the amino acids indicated in Fig. 1 were prepared by oligonucleotide site-directed mutagenesis of the bST gene described previously (6). The proteins were produced in *E. coli* W3110 as described and extracts run on reducing SDS-PAGE gels. The proteins were transferred to filter paper and incubated with monoclonal antibodies to bST. Antibodies bound to the filter were detected with ^{125}I-protein A. Figure 1 indicates that three distinct patterns of binding were seen with six monoclonal antibodies. Three of the monoclonal antibodies, as well as anti-bST polyclonal antibodies (rabbit 609), bind to all deletion forms of the protein studied as well as to the intact molecule. One antibody, F10A2D2, binds to bST only if the sequence of amino acids from 134-150 is present. Two other antibodies, F13A3C3 and F14G11, require the sequence of amino acids from 181-190 (the small disulfide loop of bST) to bind to the protein in the Western blot analysis. The results of this study indicate at least 3 distinct epitopes are present on the bST molecule.

FIGURE 1. Figure 1-I shows the Coomassie Brilliant Blue-stained SDS-PAGE gel analysis of *E. Coli* W3110 cell extracts containing recombinant bovine somatotropin (rbST) or engineered molecules with deletions of amino acids as described for lanes A, B, C, D and E. Figures 1-II through 1-IV are Western blot analyses of duplicate gels which are probed with mouse monoclonal antibodies or rabbit serum as indicated below each figure. The molecular weight markers are BSA (66K), ovalbumin (45K), trypsinogen, PMSF treated (24K), bovine somatotropin (22K), beta-lactoglobin (18.4K), and lysozyme (14.3K).

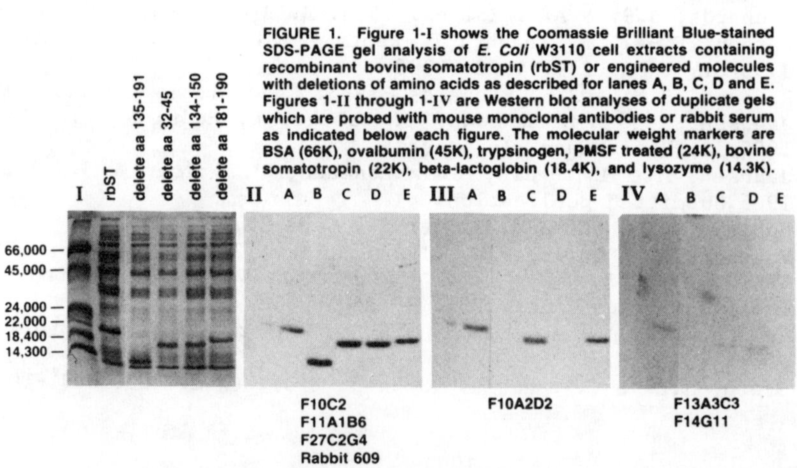

The interaction of bST monoclonal antibodies with somatotropins of other mammalian species

In order to further define the binding patterns of the bST monoclonal antibodies, somatotropins from human, rat (rST), chicken (cST), and pig (pST) were tested for their ability to compete with ^{125}I-recombinant bST (rbST) for binding to monoclonal antibodies immobilized in wells of microtiter plates. Table 1 gives potency of each somatotropin in the assay relative to the potency (1.0) of pituitary bovine somatotropin purchased from A. L. Parlow (UCLA).

Table 1. Relative potency[1] of somatotropins as competitors in solid-phase RIA.

	Protein Tested As Competitor				
Antibody	rbST	rST	pST	hST	cST
F11A1B6	1.2	0.02	0.08	0.06	0.04
F10A2D2	0.7	0.4	0.01	0.01	0.4
F10C2	0.1	0.8	0.4	0.01	0.2
F27C2G4	0.1	1.6	0.4	0.005	0.3
F14G11	1.1	<0.001	<0.001	<0.001	0.4

[1] Relative potency was calculated as the ratio of the concentration of the indicated somatotropin needed to compete 50% of the labeled rbST off the solid-phase antibody to the concentration of pituitary bovine somatotropin necessary to give the same competition.

The results shown in Table 1 indicate 4 patterns of cross-reactivity with the tested somatotropins, suggesting at least 4 distinct epitopes on the bovine somatotropin molecule. F14G11 reacts well with rbST, slightly with cST, and not at all in this assay with rST, hST, or pST. F10A2D2 recognizes all the somatotropins, although it binds pST and hST poorly. The F11A1B6 antibody reacts with all the somatotropins, although the potencies of non-bovine somatotropins are 2% to 10% the activity of bovine somatotropin. The other 2 antibodies differentiate between recombinant bST and pituitary bST, with rbST only 1/10 as potent as the pituitary material.

SUMMARY

Three distinct antigenic regions of bovine somatotropin were identified on the basis of the ability of a set of monoclonal antibodies to bind to deletion variants of rbST in Western blot analyses. One of the regions is further subdivided into two epitopes on the basis of the cross reaction of somatotropins from several species with the same set of antibodies. The total of 4 antigenic regions on the bST molecule parallels the results described for human somatotropin. Furthermore the results suggest that amino acids 134-150, 181-190, and the amino terminus may all be involved in the binding specificity of antibodies to the bovine somatotropin molecule.

REFERENCES

(1) Wallis, M. 1975. Biol. Rev. **50**:35-98.
(2) Ivanyi, J. 1982. Mol. Immunol. **19**:1611-1618.
(3) Jonsdottir, I. *et al*. 1983. Mol. Immunol. **20**:871-876.
(4) Surowy, T. K. *et al*. 1984. Mol. Immunol. **21**:345-352.
(5) Krivi., G. G. and Rowold, E. 1984. Hybridoma **3**:151-161.
(6) Seeburg, P. H. *et.al*. 1983. DNA **2**:37-45.

MOLECULAR CLONING OF HUMAN ANGIOTENSINOGEN cDNA AND EVIDENCE FOR THE PRESENCE OF TWO mRNAs IN RAT BRAIN.

Satya P. Kunapuli and Ashok Kumar
Department of Human Biological Chemistry & Genetics, Division of Cell Biology, The University of Texas Medical Branch, Galveston, Tx. 77550.

INTRODUCTION. Renin-angiotensin system plays an important role in the control of blood pressure and in the regulation of thirst. Angiotensin is synthesized by the cleavage of a larger precursor molecule called angiotensinogen. It is mainly synthesized in liver but has also been shown to be present in brain. We have isolated and sequenced the cDNA clone for human angiotensinogen. Using the nick translated cDNA clone as a hybridization probe, we provide evidence for the presence of two mRNAs in rat brain, whereas, rat liver has only one mRNA species.

RESULTS. A radio-labelled synthetic oligonucleotide (Fig. 1) prepared by phosphoroamidate approach, was used to isolate the cDNA clone from human liver library. The nucleotide sequence of the cDNA clone was determined by Sanger's dideoxy chain termination method after subcloning in M13. The partial nucleotide sequence is shown in Fig. 2. The nucleotide sequence was found to be identical with the sequence published earlier (1). Total RNA was prepared from rat liver and brain by the procedure of Chirgwin, et al. and separated on 1.5% formaldehyde-agarose gel electrophoresis. The RNA was Northern blotted to nitrocellulose and hybridized with nick translated human angiotensinogen cDNA. The autoradiograph revealed two positive bands indicating the presence of two angiotensinogen mRNAs in rat brain while rat liver showed only one band (Fig. 3).

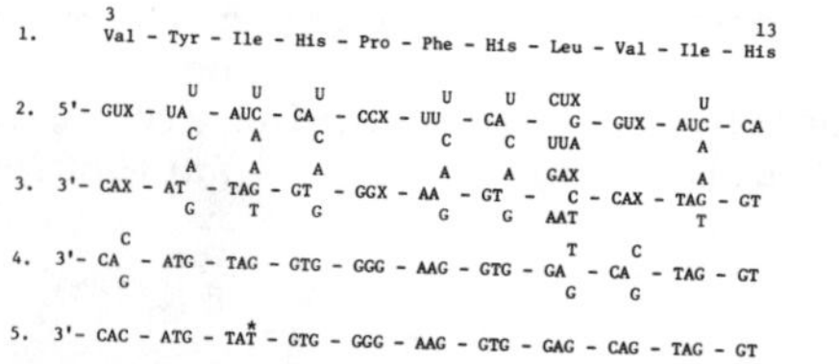

FIG. 1. SEQUENCE OF THE SYNTHETIC OLIGONUCLEOTIDE. 1)THE PEPTIDE SEQUENCE OF ANGIOTENSINOGEN, 2) THE NUCLEOTIDE SEQUENCE OF THE PUTATIVE MRNA, 3) THE NUCLEOTIDE SEQUENCE OF THE COMPLEMENTARY OLIGONUCLEOTIDE, 4)THE SEQUENCE OF THE SYNTHETIC OLIGONUCLEOTIDE USED IN THE ISOLATION OF THE cDNA CLONE AND 5)THE ACTUAL SEQUENCE FOUND IN THE cDNA.

DISCUSSION. Several workers (3 and ref. therein) have provided evidence for the presence of angiotensinogen in brain. But evidence for its local synthesis in the brain is only indirect. By *in vitro* translation experiments, Campbell, et al. (3) showed the presence of two proteins (55.7 and 52.5 KD) immuno reactive to anti-angiotensinogen antibodies in rat brain and liver. The difference in their size was attributed to the lack of pro-sequence (2) in the 52.5 KD protein and hence due to post-translational modification. Cleavage of these two precursors by renin to 47.5 KD (des-(AI)-angiotensinogen) and the abundance of the 52.5 KD protein in both brain and liver suggested that mature angiotensinogen is the obligatory product of a single angiotensinogen mRNA in rat liver. However, presence of two closely related angiotensinogen mRNAs was demonstrated recently in human liver (1), whereas rat liver had only one mRNA species (2). These two mRNAs are suggested to have originated from different polyadenylation sites.

```
                10              20              30              40              50              60
                *               *               *               *               *               *
GCA GGT GAC CGG GTG TAC ATA CAC CCC TTC CAC CTC GTC ATC CAC AAT GAG AGT ACC TGT
Ala Gly Asp Arg Val Tyr Ile His Pro Phe His Leu Val Ile His Asn Glu Ser Thr Cys

                70              80              90             100             110             120
                *               *               *               *               *               *
GAG CAG CTG GCA AAG GCC AAT GCC GGG AAG CCC AAA GAC CCC ACC TTC ATA CCT GCT CCA
Glu Gln Leu Ala Lys Ala Asn Ala Gly Lys Pro Lys Asp Pro Thr Phe Ile Pro Ala Pro

               130             140             150             160             170             180
                *               *               *               *               *               *
ATT CAG GCC AAG ACA TCC CCT GTG GAT GAA AAG GCC CTA CAG GAC CAG CTG GTG CTA GTC
Ile Gln Ala Lys Thr Ser Pro Val Asp Glu Lys Ala Leu Gln Asp Gln Leu Val Leu Val

               190             200             210             220             230             240
                *               *               *               *               *               *
GCT GCA AAA CTT GAC ACC GAA GAC AAG TTG AGG GCC GCA ATG GTC CGG ATG CTG GCC A
Ala Ala Lys Leu Asp Thr Glu Asp Lys Leu Arg Ala Ala Met Val Arg Met Leu Ala
```

FIG. 2. PARTIAL NUCLEOTIDE SEQUENCE AND THE DERIVED AMINO ACID SEQUENCE OF HUMAN ANGIOTENSINOGEN cDNA CLONE. THE AMINO ACID SEQUENCE OF ANGIOTENSIN-II (OCTAPEPTIDE) IS UNDERLINED.

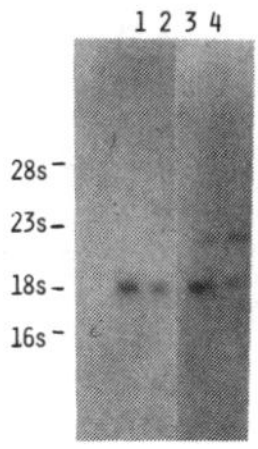

FIG. 3. NORTHERN HYBRIDIZATION OF TOTAL RNA. TOTAL RNA FROM 1)HUMAN LIVER, 2)RAT LIVER AND 3 & 4) RAT BRAIN WAS ELECTROPHORESSED ON 1.4% AGAROSE-FORMALDEHYDE GEL, BLOTTED TO NITROCELLULOSE PAPER AND HYBRIDIZED WITH NICKTRANSLATED ANGIOTENSINOGEN cDNA CLONE AT 65°C FOR 18 H IN 6 X SSC AND 5 X DENHARTS BUFFER. THE FILTER WAS WASHED AT 52°C IN 1 XSSC AND 0.1% SDS.

Experiments reported here suggest the presence of two mRNAs for angiotensinogen in rat brain. The two species are well separated from each other unlike two very closely related mRNAs shown to be present in human liver. Our experiments suggest an alternate processing of angiotensinogen gene transcript in rat brain. A high molecular weight angiotensin (1250-1500 daltons) has been reported to be present in brain, although its structure has not been established. The mechanism of synthesis of two mRNAs in brain, as well as the structural differences between the two species remains to be studied. Experiments are now in progress to determine the nucleotide sequence of the brain angiotensinogen mRNAs so as to understand their biological functions.

REFERENCES

1. Kageyama, R., Ohkubo, H. and Nakanishi, S. (1984) Biochemistry 23:3603-3609.

2. Ohkubo, H., Kageyama, R., Ujihara, M., Hirose, T., Inayama, S., and Nakanishi, S. (1983). Proc. Natl. Acad. Sci. U.S.A. 80:2196-2200.

3. Campbell, D.J., Bouhnick, J., Menard, J. and Corvol, P. (1984) Nature 308:206-208.

4. Inagami, T. (1982) Neuroendocrinology 35:475-482.

IMMUNOREACTIVE β-ENDORPHIN IN THE GONADOTROPIN-PRIMED IMMATURE RAT OVARY

Edith Lovegren, Stephen Zimniski and David Puett

Department of Biochemistry and the REPSCEND Laboratories, University of Miami School of Medicine, Miami, FL 33101

β-Endorphin (β-EP) is a 31-residue opiate peptide synthesized in the pituitary and brain as a larger precursor, proopiomelanocortin (POMC). Recent reports have suggested that POMC mRNA and immunoreactive (ir) β-EP are also localized within animal ovaries, including follicular fluid (FF), and may be under hormonal regulation (1-8). The objective of the present study was to determine the amount of irβ-EP in ovaries of immature rats before and after hormonal treatment.

Experimental Methods: Sprague-Dawley female rats (27 days old) were injected with 50 IU PMSG to stimulate follicular proliferation, and, after 48-50 hr, some animals were sacrificed while others were injected with 25 IU hCG to induce ovulation. To determine the ovarian irβ-EP content, tissues were removed and homogenized in cold PBS. In other experiments granulosa cells and FF were removed 48-50 hr after 20 IU PMSG priming. Portions of the supernatant (FF) were partially purified using Sep-Pak columns and subsequently analyzed by reverse phase HPLC. Granulosa cells were cultured in a serum-free medium for 2-96 hr. The carboxy terminal-specific β-EP antiserum used in all RIAs was kindly provided by Dr. N. Ling. The sensitivity of the RIA was about 25 pg, and assays were performed on pooled homogenates and fluids.

Results: Table I summarizes the irβ-EP contents of ovaries from control and gonadotropin-primed immature rats. It can be seen that, expressed per ovary, the amount of irβ-EP increases with PMSG and hCG treatment. However, when the data are referred to ovarian weight or ovarian protein, the amount of irβ-EP is relatively constant or may decrease somewhat with treatment (data not shown). Several independent preparations of FF from PMSG-primed animals yielded irβ-EP levels between 0.5-1.5 ng/ovary, and most of this co-chromatographs with standard β-EP on HPLC (Fig. 1). Granulosa cells from PMSG-primed animals were cultured with different hormonal and other additions, and in all cases the media from the cells gave undetectable levels of irβ-EP.

Discussion: These results confirm and extend earlier reports of ovarian irβ-EP (1-5). Comparing our results on FF with the ovarian levels given in Table I, it appears that a significant portion of the irβ-EP in PMSG-primed immature rats is located in FF. Interestingly, since we know that POMC mRNA is present in granulosa cells under the conditions used (6,8), any secreted irβ-EP must either accumulate in the medium at levels less than 0.25 ng/ml or be proteolytically degraded. It should be emphasized that some proteolysis of β-EP appeared to occur during tissue extractions since when protease inhibitors or acidic acetone was used the level of irβ-EP was elevated several fold. In summary, these studies demonstrate the validity of the PMSG-primed immature rat for further investigations into the regulation and processing of ovarian opiate peptides. Supported by NIH AM33973.

REFERENCES

1. Tsong, S.D., Phillips, D.M., Halmi, N., Krieger, D. and Bardin, C.W. (1982) Biol. Reprod. 27, 755-764.
2. Lim, A.T., Lolait, S., Barlow, J.W., O, W.S., Zois, I., Toh, B.H. and Funder, J.W. (1983) Nature 303, 709-711.
3. Shaha, C., Margioris, A., Liotta, A.S., Krieger, D.T. and Bardin, C.W. (1984) Endocrinology 115, 378-384.
4. Lolait, S.J., Autelitano, D.J., Lim, A.T.W., Smith, A.I., Toh, B.H. and Funder, J.W. (1984) Endocrinology 117, 161-168.
5. Zimniski, S., Osteen, K. and Puett, D. (1985) Abstracts of the 67th Endocrine Society Meeting, abstr. no. 516 (Baltimore, MD).
6. Melner, M. H., Luo, Y., Koos, R.D., Clark, M.R., Roberts, J.L. and Puett, D. (1984) 7th International Congress of Endocrinology, Excerpta Medica, 952 (Quebec, CANADA).
7. Chen, C.L.C. and Chang, C.C. (1985) Abstracts of the 67th Endocrine Society Meeting, abstr. no. 515 (Baltimore, MD).
8. Melner, M.H., Czerwiec, F., Roberts, J.L., Puett, D. and Koos, R.D. (1985) J. Cell Biol. 101, abstr. no. 1713 (Atlanta, GA).

TABLE I. Ovarian Content of irβ-EP in Immature Rats

Treatment (n[a])	irβ-EP[b]	Treatment (n[a])	irβ-EP[b]	
Effect of PMSG:		Effect of hCG post-PMSG:		
			10 hr	24 hr
Control (13)	0.6	Control (6)	2.4(2.5)[c]	3.2(3.1)[c]
PMSG (6)	2.0	hCG(6)	2.5(3.4)[c]	3.9(4.5)[c]

[a]Number of animals per group. [b]The values are the average content in ng/ovary. [c]The number in parentheses denotes the mean of two experiments with 20 IU PMSG and 10 IU hCG and a combined n of 7.

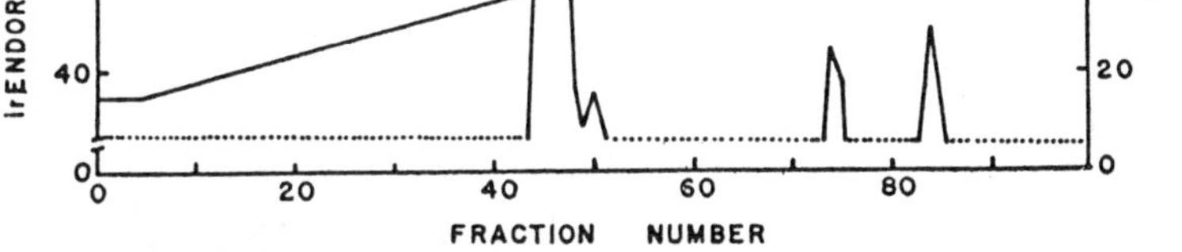

FIG. 1. RIA following HPLC of a partially purified FF fraction from PMSG-primed immature rats. The limit of detection is indicated (...).

POSSIBLE ROLE OF INSULIN-LIKE GROWTH FACTORS IN THE REGULATION OF THYROID GROWTH

W.W. Mak[1], B. Bhaumick[2], R.M. Bala[2], J.E. Kudlow[1], M.C. Eggo[1] and G.N. Burrow[1]. [1]Dept. of Medicine, University of Toronto, Toronto, and [2]Dept. of Medicine, University of Saskatchewan, Saskatoon, Canada.

Thyrotropin (TSH) has been considered a major stimulus for the growth of the thyroid gland (1). In vitro studies produced variable effects of TSH on growth in different thyroid cell culture systems. Ovine thyroid cells in primary culture have been shown to display TSH-dependent differentiated functions including follicle formation, uptake and organification of iodide, production of cAMP, synthesis of thyroglobulin, and production of thyroid hormones and plasminogen activator (2), but not TSH-dependent growth. We have investigated the possibility that in the ovine thyroid cells, growth may be mediated by growth factors as a measure of differentiation. In this communication, we report the production of insulin-like growth factors and their binding proteins by ovine thyroid cells.

Results and Discussion

The ability of conditioned media from primary cultures of ovine thyroid cells to stimulate growth was measured by the incorporation of ^{3}H-thymidine into TCA-precipitable material in the cells used for assay. The standard culture medium was used as control for the conditioned medium. Growth of NRK cells in the absence of serum was reduced to about 17% but was restored to about 42% of optimal growth on the addition of conditioned media. The production of this growth promoting activity by the ovine thyroid cells was further shown to remain constant over a period of 3 weeks. Growth of the rat thyroid cell line, FRTL5, which requires TSH for growth, was almost completely suppressed in the absence of TSH and serum, but again could be restored to about 42% of the optimal growth with the addition of conditioned media.

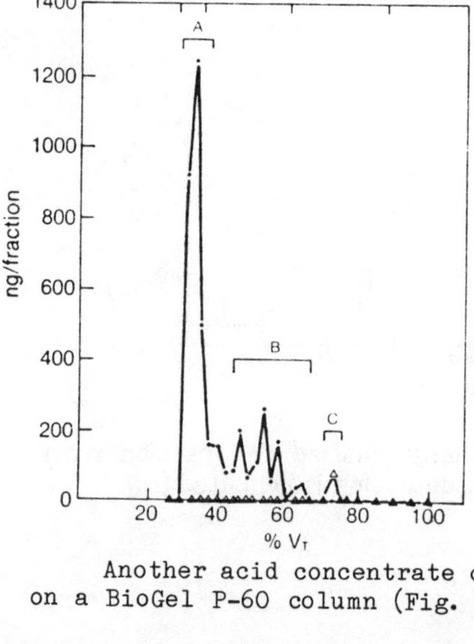

Fig. 1. Chromatography of an acid concentrate of conditioned media on a Bio-Gel P-60 column. Fractions were collected and assayed for IGF-I and -II by RIA and RRA. (▵ IGF-I; • IGF-II)

By the use of a radioimmunoassay (RIA) for IGF-I (3) which has very little or no reactivity with IGF-II and insulin, and a radioreceptor assay (RRA) using rat placental membranes (4) which is more specific for IGF-II, we found different levels of both IGF-I and IGF-II (15.2 ± 3.4 and 42.0 ± 8.2 ng/ml, respectively) in an acid concentrate of conditioned media from ovine thyroid cells. The acid concentrate of standard medium did not contain any detectable levels of IGF.

Another acid concentrate of conditioned media was chromatographed on a BioGel P-60 column (Fig. 1). Assay of the fractions for IGF-I by

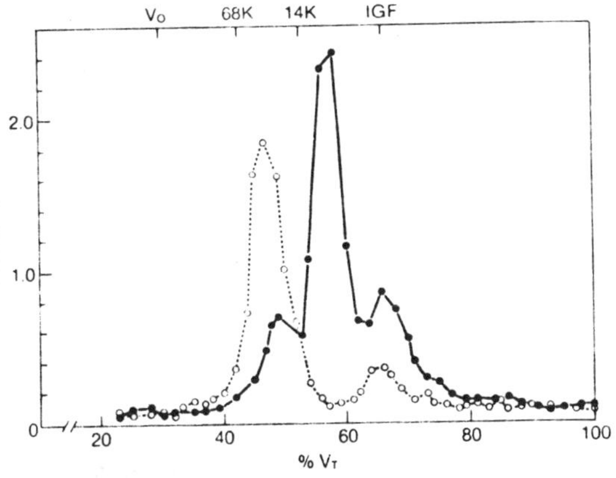

Fig. 2. Chromatography of Peak A material incubated with ^{125}-I labeled IGF-I in the absence (o--o) and presence (●—●) of a crude preparation of unlabeled IGF-I. Fractions were collected and counted in a gamma counter.

RIA revealed one peak (Peak C) between the markers of ribonuclease (14K) and insulin (6K). Several peaks of IGF-II were identified by RRA (Peak B) which may suggest the presence of mature and precursor forms of IGF-II. A large peak of apparent IGF-II reactivity was also found (Peak A) which co-chromatographed with carbonic anhydrase (30K). To investigate the possibility that Peak A contained IGF binding proteins which have been shown to complex with IGFs in vivo (5), the Peak A material was added to ^{125}I-labeled IGF-I or -II and analyzed on a Sephacryl S-200 column in phosphate buffer at pH 7.4 (Fig. 2). Addition of Peak A material resulted in a shift of the radioactivity peak (~7K) to a higher molecular weight peak (close to 68K), but the addition of Peak A material together with a crude preparation of unlabeled IGF in a separate run resulted in the appearance of a major peak of radioactivity with lower molecular weight (<14K) than that of ~68K. These data suggest that Peak A contains IGF binding proteins.

Preliminary studies on the TSH-regulation of IGF production showed a two-fold increase in the levels of IGF-I and -II when TSH (100 μU/ml) was added to an ovine thyroid cell culture maintained in the regular culture medium without TSH. Regulation of the production of IGF binding proteins however remains to be investigated.

Since IGF receptors are widely distributed in various tissues and cultured cells (5), their presence on thyroid cells was demonstrated by binding studies. Preliminary studies of the binding of ^{125}I-labeled IGF-I and IGF-II was carried out on the ovine thyroid cells and the rat thyroid cell line, FRTL5. There was binding of both IGFs on both cell types and the binding could be displaced with the acid concentrate of conditioned media from ovine thyroid cells. The acid concentrate of the standard media did not contain any significant displacing activity on the binding. Insulin by itself at 2 μM could not displace any of the binding either. Finally, the binding of IGF to ovine thyroid cells was elevated two-fold in the cells maintained in the presence of TSH as compared to those without.

References

1. Dumont,J.E. (1971) in Vitamins and Hormones (Harris, R.S., Manson, P.L., Diczfalusy, E. and Glove, J. eds.) vol. 29, pp.287, Academic Press, New York.
2. Eggo, M.C. et al. (1985) in Thyroglobulin-The Prothyroid Hormone. (Eggo, M.C. and Burrow, G.N. eds.) p.201. Raven Press, New York.
3. Bala, R.M. and Bhaumick, B.(1979) J Clin Endocrinol Metab 49:770
4. Daughaday, W.H. et al.(1981) J Clin Endocrinol Metab 53:282
5. Nissley, S.P. and Rechler, M.M.(1984) Horm Prot Peptides 12:127

AN INSULIN-MEDIATED DIFFERENTIAL INDUCTION OF SPECIFIC HEPATIC mRNAs

K.M. McHugh, C.G. Mucenski, and R.L. Drake
Department of Anatomy and Cell Biology, University of Cincinnati College of Medicine, Cincinnati, OH 45267 U.S.A.

INTRODUCTION

Insulin alters the synthesis of numerous hepatic proteins by effecting an increase in the amount of each of their respective mRNAs. However, it has not been determined whether these increases represent a coordinate regulation of mRNAs or a differential induction of specific mRNAs. Initial studies in our laboratory have shown that insulin mediates an asynchronous accumulation of hepatic albumin and malic enzyme mRNAs in insulin-treated diabetic rats (1). To further investigate the basic question of synchronous versus asynchronous accumulation of mRNAs encoding insulin-inducible proteins, we examined the accumulation of albumin and malic enzyme mRNAs in insulin-treated normal rats.

MATERIALS AND METHODS

Insulin treatment of normal male Sprague-Dawley rats consisted of subcutaneous injections of 4 units of regular insulin and 4 units of NPH insulin every 12 h for 12, 24 or 36 h. All rats receiving insulin treatment were also placed on a high carbohydrate, fat-free diet. Total cellular RNA was extracted from pools of at least 5 livers in each experimental group. The livers were homogenized in buffer and extracted with phenol-chloroform. The aqueous phase was re-extracted with a mixture of phenol-chloroform-isoamyl alcohol, ethanol precipitated, and washed to remove DNA. Poly(A^+)RNA was prepared by affinity chromatography on oligo(dt)cellulose. Specific quantities of poly(A^+)RNA were denatured and applied to nitrocellulose using a Hybrid-Dot manifold. The nitrocellulose was baked and probed (1) with either the radiolabeled plasmid prME, containing the 1250 bp rat hepatic malic enzyme cDNA, or the plasmid pmalb2, containing the 700 bp mouse albumin cDNA.

RESULTS AND DISCUSSION

Dot blot hybridization of total hepatic poly(A^+)RNA with radiolabeled cDNA probes was used to quantitate albumin and malic enzyme mRNA levels. As reported previously (1), albumin mRNA is present in relatively large amounts in normal rats while malic enzyme mRNA is present in levels barely detectable. Diabetes causes a significant drop in both mRNAs. Following insulin treatment, the accumulation of albumin mRNA occurs steadily throughout the entire treatment period of 60 h returning to approximately normal levels. The rate of accumulation of malic enzyme mRNA is similar to albumin mRNA in the first 12 h of insulin treatment. However, by 24 h post insulin malic enzyme mRNA shows an enhanced accumulation which results in a 500% increase over normal malic enzyme mRNA levels by 60 h of insulin treatment.

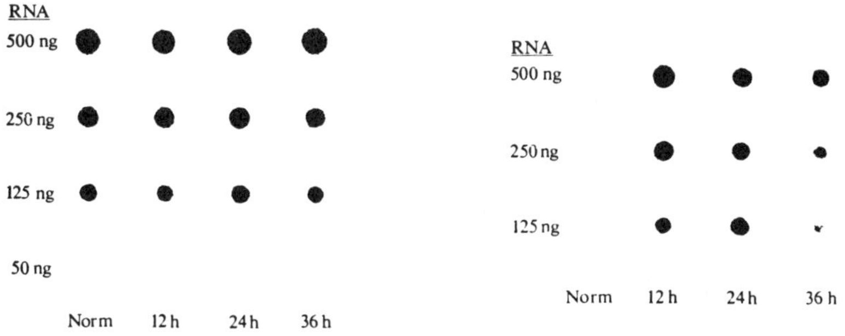

<u>Fig. 1.</u> **Estimation of hepatic albumin (left) and malic enzyme (right) mRNA levels by dot blot hydridization.** Varying amounts of hepatic total cellular poly(A^+)RNA isolated from normal rats treated with insulin for 12 h, 24 h, 36 h were spotted onto nitrocellulose membranes and hybridized with radiolabeled pmalb2 (left) and prMe (right).

By comparison, albumin mRNA levels are unchanged in insulin-treated normal rats over the entire treatment period, while malic enzyme mRNA levels are dramatically altered (Fig. 1). For this specific mRNA, the initial low levels observed in normal rats are increased 140% by 12 h of insulin treatment. These results demonstrate that insulin's influence on hepatic mRNA synthesis varies depending on the initial physiological condition of the experimental animal.

In summary, these results further support our supposition that insulin regulates the accumulation of these two hepatic mRNAs in an asynchronous manner. In insulin-treated diabetic rats it appears that insulin first initiates a general increase in mRNA transcription, as evidenced by the increase in albumin mRNA, followed by a specific induction of mRNAs encoding metabolic enzymes. This specific induction is determined by the physiological condition of the experimental animal. In insulin-treated normal rats, mRNA transcription is generally unaltered, as indicated by unchanged albumin mRNA levels. However, insulin still maintains its ability to stimulate the accumulation of malic enzyme mRNA as required by the metabolic needs of the animal. Thus, insulin's influence on the accumulation of mRNAs encoding insulin-inducible proteins involves additional regulatory processes which occur at the level of transcription.

REFERENCES

(1) Drake, R.L. and Mucenski, C.G. (1985) Biochem. Biophys. Res. Comm. 130, 317-324.

Receptors for β-MSH in synchronized Cloudman melanoma cells exhibit positive cooperativity in the late S and G2 phases of the cell cycle.

J. McLane and J. Pawelek, Department of Dermatology, Yale University School of Medicine, New Haven, CT.

Cloudman S91 mouse melanoma cells respond in culture to β-MSH with changes in morphology, growth rates, tyrosinase activity, and melanin production. These effects appear to be mediated through a stimulation of the cAMP system. Several years ago it was reported that at least some of the responses to MSH (increased cAMP production and tyrosinase activity) occur in the G2 phase of the cell cycle (1) and the apparent reason for this cell cycle restriction in that receptors for MSH are most active in the G2 phase (2). However, in the earlier work, the mechanism(s) for increased receptor activity were not studied (i.e. increased number? increased affinity?). In this report we examined these phenomena in detail. We found that by 3 separate methods of obtaining populations of cells in the G2 phase of their cycle — centrifugal elutriation, or synchronization with either colchicine or thymidine -- we observed increased binding of MSH by cells in the G2- and possibly late S-phases of their cycle. However, cultures of cells passing through their cycle in synchrony were quite different from non-synchronized (random) cultures. Both synchronized and random cultures expressed receptors for MSH in the G2-phase of their cycle, but synchronized cultures bound 15-20 times more MSH per cell than random cultures. This increased binding of MSH by synchronized cells was accompanied by an increase in tyrosinase activity and melanin content, providing direct proof of a relationship between cellular binding of MSH and cellular responsiveness to MSH. Analyses by Scatchard and Hill methods indicated that receptors from synchronized cells exhibited positive cooperativity, while receptors from random cells exhibited no cooperativity. Figure 1 shows a Scatchard plot demonstrating this phenomenon. From 5 combined experiments, the average Hill coefficient for random cells was n = 0.82 and for synchronized cells n = 1.42 (Figure 2). Understanding the nature of these differences in receptor populations should be of fundamental value in understanding the mechanism of action of the MSH-receptor complex in regulating proliferation and pigmentation.

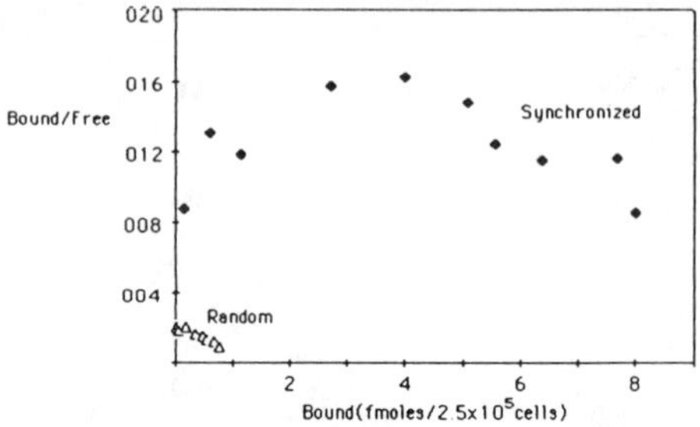

Figure 1

References

(1) Wong,G. et al. Nature 248:351-354,1974.

(2) Varga,J.M. et al. PNAS 71:1590-1593, 1974.

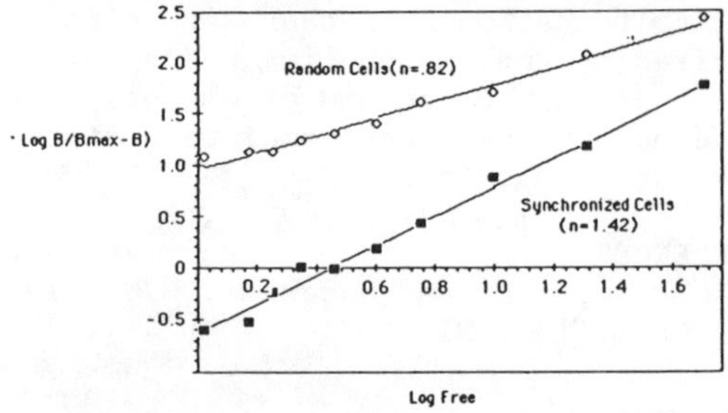

Figure 2

Phosphorylation of a protein of approximately 90K daltons is a factor in the regulation of melanoma cell growth by insulin and the expression of high affinity receptors for insulin.

T. McNeely, A. Słominski, A. Bomirski and J. Pawelek, Department of Dermatology, Yale University School of Medicine, New Haven, CT., and University of Gdansk Medical School, Gdansk, Poland.

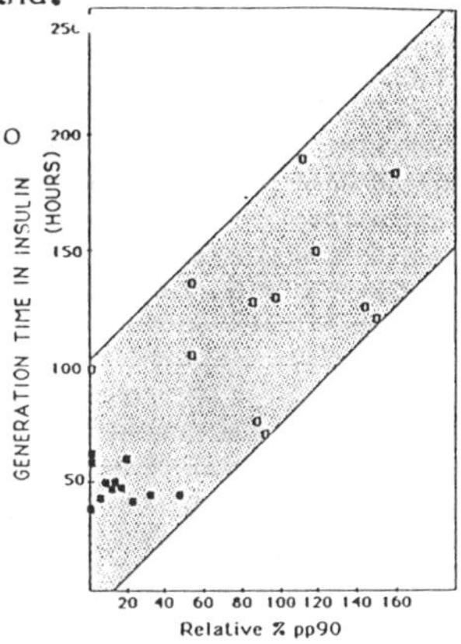

Figure 1

Growth of Cloudman S91 melanoma cells can be either inhibited or stimulated by physiological concentrations of insulin, and the effects appear to be mediated through the binding of insulin to specific, high affinity receptors on the outer cell surface (1). It was recently reported that three variant cell lines which were resistant to the effects of insulin on growth were unable to phosphorylate a protein of somewhat less than 90K daltons (pp90), but that the ability to phosphorylate this protein was restored in complementing, insulin-responsive hybrids between these mutants (2). The phosphoprotein differs by a number of criteria from the β-subunit of the insulin receptor. It was also observed that the protein was phosphorylated on both tyrosine and serine residues and that a specific phosphatase activity toward this protein could be detected in extracts of Cloudman cells (2). In this report we present some further results on this protein. A survey of 24 cell lines showed that the relative density of labelling of pp90 detected on SDS-PAGE gels by autoradiography correlated strongly with the generation time of each of these lines in insulin (Fig 1). (Note that the closed circles (●) indicate lines where selective pressure was applied for insulin resistance). Furthermore, Scatchard analyses indicated that whereas insulin-responsive (wild-type) lines display high-affinity receptors for insulin (Fig 2 left), 5 out of 6 lines that were selected for insulin-resistance displayed greatly reduced or absent high affinity receptors (Fig 2 right). Thus, we have demonstrated a relationship between growth in insulin, the ability to phosphorylate a particular protein, and the ability to express high affinity receptors for insulin. We have also shown recently that another cell line, the Bomirski melanoma, can be either stimulated or inhibited in growth by insulin, and that cells from this line responsive to insulin have the ability to phosphorylate pp90. We do not yet know if non-melanoma cell lines which are responsive to insulin express the ability to phosphorylate pp90.

References

(1) Kahn, R. et al. J. Cell. Physiol. 103:109-120, 1980.
(2) Fleischmann R. and Pawelek, J. PNAS 82:1007-1011, 1985.

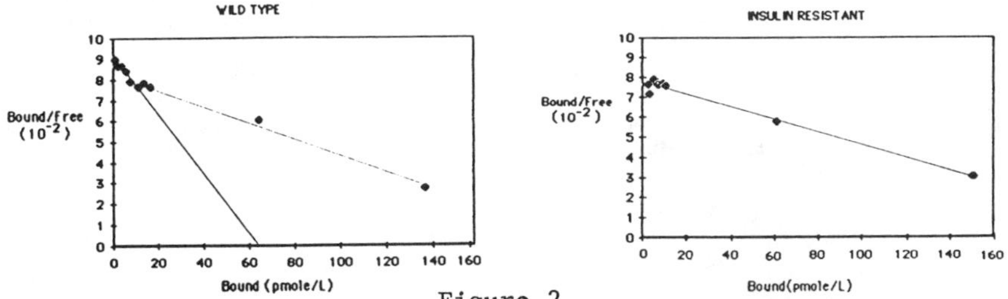

Figure 2

EFFECTS OF PEPTIDES AND OTHER FACTORS ON IN VITRO GROWTH AND DIFFERENTIATION OF NORMAL AND MALIGNANT HUMAN COLON CELLS

M.P. Moyer, P.S. Dixon, D. Escobar, A. Culpepper and J.B. Aust. Dept. of Surgery, The Univ. of Texas Health Science Center at San Antonio, San Antonio, TX 78284

INTRODUCTION. Peptides, nutrients and other factors which regulate colonic mucosa growth and differentiation at the cell and tissue levels are poorly understood. However, improved methods for in vitro culture of normal and malignant colon and other gastrointestinal (GI) cells have recently been developed (1-4). These better permitted the purpose of this work to directly test individual factors and compare their effects on normal and malignant human colon cells in vitro.

METHODS. Human normal colonic mucosa (NCM) and colon cancer (HCC) cells were initiated and propagated as described elsewhere (1-4). The cells were shifted down to base medium supplemented only with 1% fetal bovine serum, antibiotics and the test growth factor. A range of concentrations was tested. Relative cell numbers were the measure of growth. The index of differentiation was the proportion of mucin-producing and columnar epithelial cells based on morphology and histological staining.

RESULTS. Tables I, II and III show the many individual factors tested and their effects on growth of NCM and HCC cells. NCM cells generally had greater growth factor requirements than HCC cells. Although there were some unique factors for each, other factors crossed categories when tested in separate experiments. The peptides NGF, FGF and PDGF had no effect on growth of either the NCM or HCC cells. Many factors which stimulated growth (e.g., glucagon, prolactin, amino acids,

TABLE I

NCM and HCC cells generally prefer or require similar concentrations

Oxaloacetate	Butyrate
CCK	Acetoacetate
Tolbutamide	B-hydroxybutyrate

NCM cells generally prefer or require higher concentrations than HCC cells

Acetate	Pyruvate	Aldosterone
Lactate	Calcitonin	TPA
Glucosamine	CCK	Bile salts/acids
Glycylglycine	ECGS	Bombesin
Selenium	Transferrin	Glucagon
	O-phosphorylethanolamine	

NCM cells generally prefer or require much higher concentrations

Glutamine	Prolactin
Amino Acids	Gastrin/Pentagastrin
Sugars	Pituitary extract
Insulin	Yeast extract (L Broth)
EGF	Bile salts/acids

HCC cells stimulated or not inhibited at higher concentrations than NCM cells

Somatostatin	FBS
GIP	CCK
GRP	VIP
Calcium	

TABLE II

FACTORS THAT CAN STIMULATE NCM CELLS BUT HCC CELLS MAY BE NONRESPONSIVE OR INHIBITED

Prolactin	Yeast Extract
Pyruvate	Bile salts/acids
Calcitonin	Pituitary Extract
GIP	VIP
O-phosphorylethanolamine	

TABLE III

FACTORS THAT CAN EXERT VARIABLE EFFECTS ON GROWTH OF NCM AND/OR HCC CELLS

Bombesin	Mercaptopropionylglycine
Somatostatin	Mercaptoethylamine
VIP	Hydra Peptide
GIP	GH_3 Cell Supernatants (GH, Prolactin)
Vitamins	

aldosterone, CCK, butyrate, VIP, pyruvate, oxaloacetate) also caused differentiation of normal and/or malignant cells. Enhanced differentiation also was seen with some factors which generally did not stimulate growth (e.g., glucosamine, amiloride, ouabain). However, there was great heterogeneity of responsiveness in the NCM and HCC cells tested.

DISCUSSION. In concert with previous work (1-7), these data are a prelude to better understanding the potential role of peptides and other factors in colon homeostasis at the cellular level, and defining differences between growth factor responsiveness of normal and malignant human colon cells. As with other tumor systems, colon cancer cells frequently had reduced growth factor requirements. This was possibly due to autocrine stimulation, but the system is very complex, and other mechanisms can be envisioned. Further work will be necessary to define mechanisms of responsiveness and whether or not features distinguishing the normal and malignant cells will prove potentially useful for prevention, diagnosis, and/or treatment of colon cancer and other GI diseases.

ACKNOWLEDGMENTS. Partial support by NIH R23 CA35933, NIH R01 CA32722 and the Morrison Trust is acknowledged.

REFERENCES

(1) Moyer, M.P. (1983) Proc. Soc. Exp. Biol. Med. 174, 12-15.
(2) Moyer, M.P. (1983) J. Tiss. Cult. Meth. 8, 63-68.
(3) Moyer, M.P., and Aust, J.B. (1984) Science 224, 1445-1447.
(4) Moyer, M.P., Page, C.P., and Moyer, R.C. (1985) **in:** In Vitro Models for Cancer Research Vol. 1 (Webber, M.M. and Sekely, L.I., eds.) pp. 183-205, CRC Press Inc., Boca Raton, Fla.
(5) Moyer, M.P., Dixon, P., Escobar, D., Aust, J.B. (1984) **in:** Growth, Cancer and the Cell Cycle (Skehan, P. and Friedman, S.J., eds.) pp. 297-305, The Humana Press, Clifton, NJ.
(6) Sirinek, K.R., Levine, B.A. and Moyer, M.P. (1985) Am. J. Surg. 149, 35-39.
(7) Moyer, M.P., Aust, J.B., Dixon, P.S., Levine, B.A., and Sirinek, K.R. (1985) Am. J. Surg. 150, 676-679.

CLONING OF cDNA FOR A PROLACTIN-INDUCIBLE PROTEIN (PIP) AND STUDIES ON THE HORMONAL CONTROL OF PIP GENE EXPRESSION IN T47D HUMAN BREAST CANCER CELLS

Leigh Murphy, Yvonne Myal, Deborah Tsuyuki and Robert Shiu. Department of Physiology, University of Manitoba, Winnipeg, Manitoba, Canada

Recently in this laboratory it was shown that in the human breast cancer cell line T47D, human prolactin or human growth hormone in the presence of hydrocortisone induced the synthesis and secretion of PIP's, a family of proteins which differed only in their degree of glycosylation (1). This finding represented the first demonstration of an induction of specific proteins by prolactin in human target cells and has provided us with a unique model in which to study the molecular mechanism of multihormonal actions as well as the possible significance of prolactin in human breast cancer.

In order to facilitate our studies we have cloned PIP cDNA. The strategy chosen was the preparation of a lambda GT11 expression cDNA library (2) from poly A^+ RNA isolated from 5 day prolactin (1 ug/ml) and hydrocortisone (1 ug/ml) treated T47D human breast cancer cells. A recombinant library of approximately 5×10^5 individual members was obtained and subsequently amplified. The amplified library was screened using polyclonal antibodies prepared to highly purified PIP (1). Plaques expressing a fusion protein were detected by anti-PIP antibodies and visualised by autoradiography following incubation with I^{125}-protein A. Positive signals were plaque purified, lambda phage DNA isolated and the size of the cDNA insert estimated after Eco R1 digestion and electrophoresis on 1% agarose gel. The longest insert isolated in this way was approx. 600 base pairs (bp). This insert was subcloned into pBR 322 (pBR-PIP) and subsequently characterized by a) hybrid-selection translation and b) restriction mapping.

a) pBR-PIP hybrid selected (3) a transcript from 5 day prolactin/hydrocortisone treated T47D mRNA which when translated in vitro produced a 12500 dalton protein which was immunoprecipitable by anti-PIP antibody. The hybrid-select translation product corresponds to the precursor form of PIP as previously described (1).

b) Restriction map analysis of the PIP cDNA approx. 600 bp insert revealed two Pst 1 sites and a unique Acc 1 site. Pst 1 digested the insert into fragments of approx. 395, 150 and 50 bp in length. Acc 1 digested the insert into fragments of approx. 310 and 275 bp in length. These fragments have been subcloned into phage vector M13 for sequencing.

Nick-translated pBR-PIP when incubated under stringent conditions (50% formamide/42°C or aqueous/68°C) with a Northern blot of either total RNA or poly A^+ RNA isolated from 3 or 5 day prolactin/hydrocortisone treated T47D cells, hybridised to a single transcript of approx. 900 bases in length. Northern analysis revealed that prolactin/hydrocortisone treated cells contained 10-20 fold more PIP-mRNA than untreated cells. However, cells treated with either hormone alone contained 5-7 fold more PIP-mRNA than untreated cells. This is in contrast to the situation where the production of significant levels of the PIP-protein requires the presence of both hormones (1).

In summary a PIP-cDNA has been cloned which has allowed us to follow changes in PIP gene expression. Preliminary studies indicated that the accumulation of PIP mRNA is under hormonal control although the precise mechanisms by which prolactin and hydrocortisone interact to result in PIP expression remain to be elucidated.

REFERENCES

(1) Shiu, R.P.C. and Iwasiow, B. (1985) J. Biol. Chem. 260, 11307.

(2) Young, R.A. and Davis, P.W. (1983) Proc. Natl. Acad. Sci. 80, 1194.

(3) Riccardi, P.P., Miller, J.S. and Roberts, B.E. (1979) Proc. Natl. Acad. Sci. 76, 4927.

REGULATION OF ATRIOPEPTIGEN GENE EXPRESSION ATRIUM AND VENTRICLE OF RAT HEART

H. E. Tolunay, E. I. Harding, R. C. Wiegand Department of Biological Sciences, Monsanto Company St. Louis, Missouri 63198

Atriopeptigen, precursor to natriuretic, diuretic and vasorelaxant peptides known as atriopeptins or atrial natriuretic factor (1,2), is expressed primarily in the atria of the heart. Small amounts of atriopeptigen have also been found in hypothalamus and various regions of brain (3,4). Even though the atrium and ventricle of the heart are closely related tissues there is a striking difference in the level of atriopeptigen expression. In atrium atriopeptigen mRNA makes up about 2% of polyA RNA, whereas in ventricle this number is less than 0.1%. Atrium and ventricle thus provide an excellent system to study the tissue specific regulation of atriopeptigen gene expression.

Using mixed synthetic oligonucleotide probes we isolated a cDNA clone from a rat atrial cDNA library prepared in λgt10. This cDNA was fully sequenced and was shown to be a full-length clone encoding pre-pro-atriopeptin. The cloned cDNA was the probe used in the experiments described below.

Atrium of the heart behaves like an endocrine organ; in response to physiological changes induced by endogenous or exogenous stimuli it releases atriopeptins into plasma. A bolus IV injection of 1-desamine-8-arginine vasopressin (dAVP), an analog of vasoconstrictor 8-arginine vasopressin, transiently increases the circulating atriopeptin (28 amino acid atriopeptide, AP28) level by 7- to 10-fold in a dose dependent manner (5,6). AP28 is released primarily from the right atrium and the amount stored in granules is depleted by about 30% (7). Thus a transcriptional and/or translational response is suggested to the large release induced by dAVP.

Studies have been initiated to examine the transcriptional and translational state of atriopeptigen in normal and dAVP stimulated rat atrium and normal rat ventricle. A procedure for isolation of polysomes from these tissues has been established. Polysomes have been separated into membrane-bound and free fractions and relative distribution of atriopeptigen mRNA have been determined. The examination of the translational state of atriopeptigen mRNA is in progress.

REFERENCES

1. Currie, M. G., Geller, D. M., Cole, B. R., Boylan, J. G., Wu, Y. S. Holmberg, S. W. and Needleman, P. (1983) Science **221**, 71-73.
2. DeBold, A. J., Borenstein, H. B., Veress, A. T. and Sonenberg, H. (1981) Life Sci. **28**, 89-94.
3. Saper, C. B., Standaert, D. G., Currie, M. G., Schwartz, D., Geller, D. M. and Needleman, P. (1985) Science **227**, 1047-1049.

4. Samson, W. K. (1985) Endocrinology **117**, 1279-1281.

5. Manning, P. T., Schwartz, D. and Katsube, N. C., Homberg, S. W., Needleman, P. (1985) Science **229**, 395-397.

6. Schwartz, D., Geller, D. M., Manning, P. T., Siegel, N. R., Fok, K. F., Smith, C. E. and Needleman, P. (1985) Science **229**, 397-400.

7. Katsube, N. C., personal communication.

VARIANT CDNA FOR CANINE PANCREATIC POLYPEPTIDE

P.J. Toothman and T.L. Paquette, Diabetes Research Center, Dept of Medicine, ZB34, U. of Washington, Seattle, WA 98195, USA

INTRODUCTION. Pancreatic polypeptide (PP) is a major pancreatic islet secretory product(1). PP cells are more prevalent in the developmentally distinct region of the pancreas which forms the uncinate process (UP) compared to the splenic lobe (SL)(2). PP cDNA clones have been isolated from a library of canine polyA+ RNA from UP pancreatic endocrine cells in primary culture. The sequence of one cDNA is homologous to the published sequences of human PP cDNAs isolated from pancreatic tumours (3,4,5). The sequence of a variant cDNA differs from the first at its 5' end. While polyA+ RNA homologous to the PP coding region showed the predicted lobe specificity, i.e. more PP mRNA in the UP compared to the SL, RNA homologous to the variant portion of the PP cDNA was not lobe specific. Under stringent conditions of hybridization the coding region probe detected a single pancreas specific RNA 500bp long while probes to the variant region detected additional RNA species which were present in both lobes of the pancreas and liver.

MATERIALS AND METHODS. PolyA+ RNA was isolated from UP pseudo islet cultures from 15 dogs (6). First strand synthesis by reverse transcriptase was followed by addition of polyC tails, priming of the second strand with oligodG and Klenow extension. The double stranded cDNA was again tailed and ligated to PstI cleaved PBR322. DNA sequence determination was by the method of Maxam and Gilbert.

```
                                                 TC CGC CCC
  * *** *** *** *** *** *** *** *** *** *** *** *** *** ***
  A GCC TCG GTC AGG TAG GGT AAG TCC TGG GGG TGG GGT GGG GGG
--- --- --- --- --- AMB Gly Lys Ser Trp Gly Trp Gly Gly Gly

TTA GGA CTC GGG AUG>
***  *  ***  *  *** *         **  *         *
CAA GCA GGT CTG GAT CCT GCC GCC TGC CGC TGC CTC TTC CTG CTG
Gln Ala Gly Leu Asp Ala Ala Ala Cys Arg Cys Leu Phe Leu Leu
                -30
          * *     *       *       *   *       *  **
CTC CTG TCA GCC TGT GTG GCT CTG TTG CTG CAG CCG CCA CTG GGT
Leu Leu Ser Ala Cys Val Ala Leu Leu Leu Gln Pro Pro Leu Gly
**   **   *       *                   * ***
ACC CGG GGG GCC CCG CTG GAG CCA GTG TAT CCG GGG GAC GAT GCC
Thr Arg Gly Ala Pro Leu Glu Pro Val Tyr Pro Gly Asp Asp Ala
         -1 1
                              *           *         *
ACA CCA GAG CAG ATG GCC CAG TAC GCG GCT GAG CTC CGC AGA TAC
Thr Pro Glu Gln Met Ala Gln Tyr Ala Ala Asp Leu Arg Arg Tyr
                                                *    *   **
ATC AAC ATG CTG ACC AGG CCT AGG TAT GGG AAA AGA GAC AGA GGA
Ile Asn Met Leu Thr Arg Pro Arg Tyr Gly Lys Arg Asp Arg Gly
                                  36             40
  *  *   *   *  *   **      *       *       *       *   *  **
GAA ATG CGG GAC ATC CTG GAA TGG GGC TCC CCC CAT GCA GCC GCC
Glu Met Arg Asp Ile Leu Glu Trp Gly Ser Pro His Ala Ala Ala

              *  ** *** ***             ***************  **
CCC AGG GAG CTG ATG GAC GAG TAA TGCCACCTCCAAGTAATGCCACCTCTG
Pro Arg Glu Leu Met Asp Glu OCH
      59
******* *** ****** *** ** **** *  **  *** *****
CCTCTCTCAGGCCAATGCCAGCCTACCTCTCCCCTCTGCACCCCTGG
```

FIG. 1. PP cDNA Sequences
*= Nucleotides differing in variant canine and human PP cDNA
_= PP and icosapeptide sequences
<>= Nucleotides of normal PP clone

RESULTS. Tetracycline resistant colonies were screened in duplicate for homology to a 17 base pair, 256 fold degenerate probe which codes for the PP amino acid sequence GluProValTyrProGly. Positive clones were rescreened with a second probe 11 base pairs long coding for the PP amino acids GluGlnMetAla. The single positive clone obtained was used to rescreen the library. Four positive clones were obtained out of 4360 screened. The three longest clones were sequenced. The two independently isolated cDNAs coding for the variant form of PP have been sequenced entirely on both strands and are identical (Fig. 1).

The variant form does not have a methionine initiator codon at the position corresponding to the intiator in the human PP cDNA and in addition has a chain termination codon in the reading frame further upstream. The sequence of the third cDNA has only been completed on both strands at the end corresponding to the 5' of the PP mRNA. Further sequencing will determine whether a few sequence differences

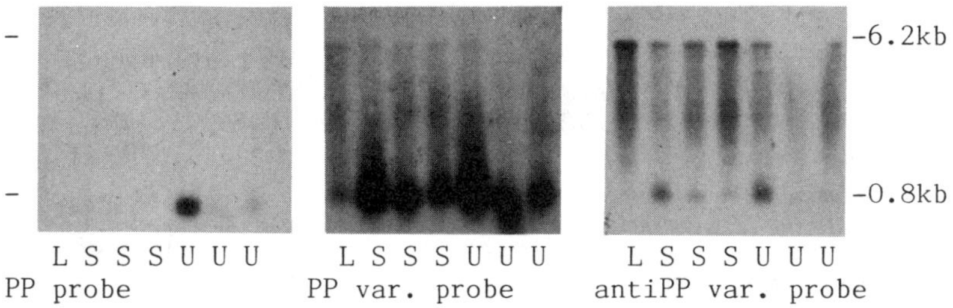

Figure 2 Northern blot analysis of pancreas poly A+ RNAs S=SL, U=UP, L=liver

in the PP "coding region" between the variant and normal clones are actually real. Sequencing gels indicated that this clone includes the poly A+ tail unlike the variant PP cDNAs. This third clone also contained the methionine initiator codon at the same position as that found for human. The sequence of this 5' untranslated region bears no homology to the 5'end of the variant cDNA clone.

Sequences homologous to the PP coding region and the 5'end of the variant PP were detected on Northern blots after labeling the appropriate restriction fragments with P32 by random priming (Fig. 2). Hybridization to the PP coding region probe indicated a single uncinate process specific band in three separate isolates of pancreas RNA. The variant specific probe showed intense cross reactivity to a slightly larger sized RNA in both lobes of the pancreas in addition to a high molecular weight species. If instead of a double stranded probe, a single stranded probe homologous to the anti sense strand of the variant PP cDNA was used to probe the Northerns, the same variant specific bands were seen. This implies that the variant sequence may be part of an inverted repeat that is present in transcripts other than the PP variant transript. Hybridization to Southern blots of genomic digests is consistent with the variant and the PP coding sequences being present in more than one copy in the dog genome (data to be presented).

DISCUSSION. A variant cDNA containing sequences identical to PP prepro mRNA but differing in 5' untranslated regions has been isolated from a canine UP pseudo islet library. The origin and complete sequence of the variant region are of interest since homologous sequences are apparently present in other RNA transcripts.

REFERENCES 1. Floyd, J.C., Fajans, S.S., Pek, S., and Chance, R. (1977) Rec. Prog. in Hormone Research 33, 519-569.

2. Orci, L., Malaisse-Lagae, F., Baetens, D., and A. Perrelet (1978), Lancet, December 2, 1200-1201

3. Boel, E., Schwartz, T.W., Norris, K.E., and Fiil, N.P. (1984) EMBO Journal 3, 909-912

4. Leiter, A.B., Keutman, H.T., and Goodman, H. (1984) J. Biol. Chem. 259,14702-14705

5. Takeuchi, T. and Yamada, T. (1985) Proc. Natl. Acad. Sci. 82 1536-1539

6. Paquette, T.L., Gingerich, R. and Scharp, D.W., (1981) Biochemistry 20 7403-7408

REGULATION OF PROLACTIN PRODUCTION BY PROGESTIN, ESTROGEN AND RELAXIN IN HUMAN ENDOMETRIAL STROMAL CELLS

L. Tseng and P. Bischof, Dept. of OB/GYN, State University of New York at Stony Brook, Stony Brook, NY 11794 U.S.A. and Dept. of OB/GYN, University of Geneva, Geneva, Switzerland.

INTRODUCTION Human endometrial stromal cells synthesize and secrete prolactin (Prl). Endometrial Prl is identical to pituitary Prl based on several criteria: immune response, electrophorectic mobility, bioactivity and ability of endometrial Prl mRNA to hybridize pituitary Prl cDNA (1). Prolactin production from both organs is regulated by steroids (2,3) while TRH and dopamine, known modulators of pituitary Prl synthesis, have no effect on endometrial Prl production. This study was undertaken to investigate the mode of actions of steroids, peptide hormone, and the adenylate cyclase stimulator on endometrial Prl production. We have investigated the stimulatory effects of progestin, estrogen, relaxin (RLX) and forskolin (Fk) and the inhibitory effect of antiprogestin, Ru 486, on endometrial Prl production. These substances were previously found to regulate the endometrial aromatase activity and production of pregnancy associated plasma protein (Tseng and Mazella, Bischof and Tseng, unpublished observations).

METHODS Human endometrial stromal cells were isolated from nine proliferative and secretory endometria by digesting the tissue fragments in 0.1% collagenase solution (4). Stromal cells were cultured in medium RPMI 1640 containing 10% fetal calf serum, 0.2 U/ml insulin and antibiotics. Various types of hormones or Fk were added to the culture medium after stromal cells were > 90% confluent, approximately 1-3 days after plating. Culture medium in control and hormone treated cells were collected every day. Prolactin content was measured in 5 fold concentrated media by RIA (IRE PROL-100, Bedlgium). Intraassay coefficient variation was less than 6%. Medium not exposed to cells were used as assay blank (< 3 ng/5 ml). Results were expressed in ng Prl/d x mg cell protein.

RESULTS AND DISCUSSION Prolactin productions in cultured endometrial stromal cells without hormones ranged from 4 to 12 ng/d x mg protein in nine specimens. Medroxyprogesterone acetate (MPA) caused 2-6 fold increase over the control in various specimens. Estradiol (E_2) or RLX alone did not appreciably change the production rate but they enhanced the effect of MPA to increase Prl production up to 15 fold over the control. Forskolin increased intracellular cAMP content (>10 fold over the control) in stromal cells and enhanced Prl production in the presence of MPA. These results were confirmed in at least 2 different specimens.

Modulation of Prl production by various hormones is shown in fig. A and B. In secretory endometrial stromal cells, fig. A, Prl production was increased after the 1st day of hormonal treatment, while proliferative endometrial stromal cells, fig. B, showed a lag period of induction indicating that hormonal milieu in vivo influences the Prl production pattern in vitro. Prolactin production in stromal cells treated with MPA + E_2 was double of that of MPA alone. Addition of Ru 486 blocked the Prl productions in MPA and MPA+ E_2 treated stromal cells, suggesting that the action of progestin on Prl production is mediated by a receptor mechanism and the effect of E_2 depends on the binding of progestin to its receptor. Relaxin, fig. B, is able to increase Prl production in MPA pretreated cells after 24 h of incubation. Concerted effect of MPA and RLX on Prl production was noted when stromal cells were continuously treated with these two hormones.

In summary, endometrial Prl production, distinct from pituitary Prl, is initiated and sustained by progestin through a receptor mediated mechanism and enhanced by estrogen, RLX, and intracellular cAMP. This study also provides the evidence that endometrium is a target organ of relaxin, a peptide hormone, which exerts a concerted effect with steroids to regulate the production of endometrial proteins.

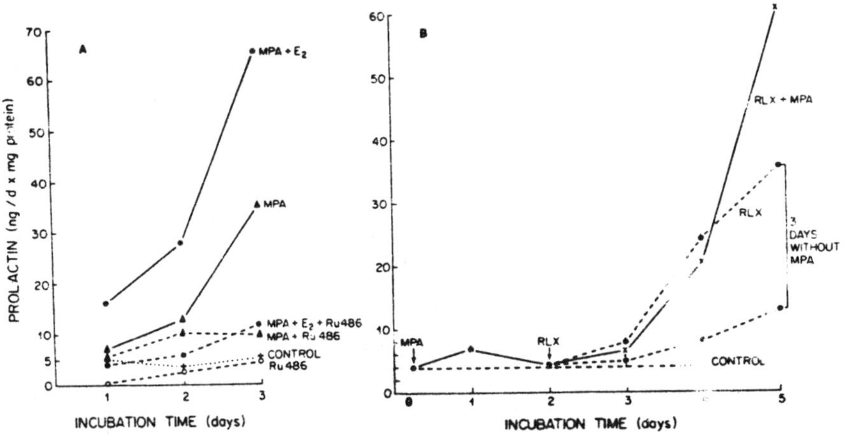

Fig. A AND B Modulation of PRL production by hormones and Ru 486 in stromal cells from a secretory endometrium (A) and a proliferative endometrium (B). In fig. A, stromal cells were treated with 1 uM MPA, MPA +36 uM E_2, 1 uM Ru 486 and Ru 486+ hormones. In fig. B, stromal cells were treated with MPA for 2 days, MPA was then removed from two sets of dishes (dashed lines). Porcine RLX (10 ng/ml, NIADDK) was added to dishes with MPA (solid line), without MPA (dashed line) after two days MPA treatment.

1. Clements, J. Whitefeld, P., Cooke, N., Healey, D.L., Matheson, B., Shine, J. and Funder, J. (1983) Endocrinology 112:1133-1134.
2. Shull, J.D. and Gorski, J. (1985) Endocrinology 116:2456-2462.
3. Daly, D.C., Maslar, I.A. and Riddick, D.H. (1983) Am. J. Obstet. Gynecol. 145:672-678.
4. Tseng, L. (1984) Endocrinology 137:833-835.

ANALYSIS OF THE PROLIFERIN GENE FAMILY IN MOUSE CELLS

Elizabeth L. Wilder and Daniel I. H. Linzer
Department of Biochemistry, Molecular Biology and Cell Biology
Northwestern University, Evanston, IL 60201

Proliferin is a growth-related member of the prolactin - growth hormone family (1,2). In quiescent mouse cells in culture, proliferin mRNA is absent, but this mRNA increases dramatically in amount following stimulation with serum or with purified platelet-derived growth factor (1, 3). In vivo, proliferin mRNA is synthesized specifically in the placenta, and peak levels of proliferin mRNA are detected at mid-gestation (4). As shown in Figure 1, proliferin cDNA clones prepared from BALB/c 3T3 tissue culture cell RNA and BALB/c placental RNA differ by five single base substitutions, resulting in four amino acid changes (4).

```
PLF-2                                                GGCTTCCAACTCCAGTAAAGCATCTTCCCGGAATCCACAGCTAAGCCTGGGTAGGACTCTGC
            1                                                                                                    26
            Met Leu Pro Ser Leu Ile Gln Pro Cys Ser Trp Ile Leu Leu Leu Leu Leu Val Asn Ser Ser Leu Leu Trp Lys Asn
PLF-1   AGAGATG CTC CCT TCT TTG ATT CAA CCA TGC TCC TGG ATA CTG CTC CTA CTA CTG GTG AAC AGC TCG TTA TTG TGG AAG AAT
PLF-2   ------- --- --- --- -C- --- --- --- --- --- --- --- --- --- --- --- --- --- --- --- --- --- --- --- --- ---
                            Ser
        27                                                                                                       53
        Val Ala Ser Phe Pro Met Cys Ala Met Arg Asn Gly Arg Cys Phe Met Ser Phe Glu Asp Thr Phe Glu Leu Ala Gly Ser
PLF-1   GTT GCC TCA TTT CCC ATG TGT GCA ATG AGG AAT GGT CGT TGC TTT ATG TCC TTT GAA GAC ACA TTT GAA TTA GCC GGC AGT
PLF-2   --- --- --- --- --- --- --- --- --- --- --- --- --- --- --- --- --- --- --- --- --- --- --- --- --- --- ---
        54                                                                                                       80
        Leu Ser His Asn Ile Ser Ile Glu Val Ser Glu Leu Phe Thr Glu Phe Glu Lys His Tyr Ser Asn Val Ser Gly Leu Arg
PLF-1   TTG TCT CAT AAT ATC AGT ATA GAA GTT TCA GAA CTG TTC ACT GAA TTT GAA AAA CAT TAT TCT AAC GTG TCT GGG CTC AGA
PLF-2   --- --- --- --- --- --- --- --- --- --G --- --- --- -A- --- --- --- --- --- --- --- --- --- --- --- --- ---
                                            Ser             Asn
        81                                                                                                      107
        Asp Lys Ser Pro Met Arg Cys Asn Thr Ser Phe Leu Pro Thr Pro Glu Asn Lys Glu Gln Ala Arg Leu Thr His Tyr Ser
PLF-1   GAC AAA AGC CCC ATG AGA TGC AAT ACT TCT TTC CTT CCA ACT CCA GAA AAC AAG GAA CAA GCC AGG CTC ACA CAC TAT TCA
PLF-2   --- --- --- --- --- --- --- --- --- --- --- --- --- --- --- --- --- --- --- --- --- --- --- --- --- --- G--
                                                                                                                Ala
        108                                                                                                     134
        Ala Leu Leu Lys Ser Gly Ala Met Ile Leu Asp Ala Trp Glu Ser Pro Leu Asp Asp Leu Val Ser Glu Leu Ser Thr Ile
PLF-1   GCT CTT CTG AAA TCA GGA GCC ATG ATT TTG GAT GCC TGG GAA AGC CCT CTG GAC GAT CTA GTG AGT GAA TTA TCT ACC ATA
PLF-2   --- --- --- --- --- --- --- --- --- -C- --- --- --- --- --- --- --- --- --- --- --- --- --- --- --- --- ---
                                            Ser
        135                                                                                                     161
        Lys Asn Val Pro Asp Ile Ile Ile Ser Lys Ala Thr Asp Ile Lys Lys Lys Ile Asn Ala Val Arg Asn Gly Val Asn Ala
PLF-1   AAA AAT GTC CCT GAT ATA ATC ATC TCC AAA GCC ACA GAC ATA AAG AAA AAG ATC AAC GCA GTC CGG AAC GGG GTT AAT GCC
PLF-2   --- --- --- --- --- --- --- --- --- --- --- --- --- --- --- --- --- --- --- --- --- --- --- --- --- --- ---
        162                                                                                                     188
        Leu Met Ser Thr Met Leu Gln Asn Gly Asp Glu Glu Lys Lys Asn Pro Ala Trp Phe Leu Gln Ser Asp Asn Glu Asp Ala
PLF-1   CTC ATG AGC ACC ATG CTT CAG AAT GGA GAT GAA GAA AAG AAG AAC CCT GCC TGG TTC TTG CAA TCT GAC AAT GAA GAT GCT
PLF-2   --- --- --- --- --- --- --- --- --- --- --- --- --- --- --- --- --- --- --- --- --- --- --- --- --- --- ---
        189                                                                                                     215
        Arg Ile His Ser Leu Tyr Gly Met Ile Ser Cys Leu Asp Asn Asp Phe Lys Lys Val Asp Ile Tyr Leu Asn Val Leu Lys
PLF-1   CGC ATT CAT TCT TTA TAT GGC ATG ATC AGC TGC CTA GAC AAT GAC TTT AAG AAG GTT GAT ATT TAT CTC AAC GTC CTG AAG
PLF-2   --- --- --- --- --- --- --- --- --- --- --- --- --- --- --- --- --- --- --- --- --- --- --- --- --- --- ---
        216                             224
        Cys Tyr Met Leu Lys Ile Asp Asn Cys STOP
PLF-1   TGT TAC ATG TTA AAA ATA GAT AAC TGC TGA  TATTTCTTTCATGTGCTCTGCTTCTGAAATATCATGTAATATCCTTTCAATTTGTATCTTTTGAAT
PLF-2   --- --- --- --- --- --- --- --- --- ---  ------------------------------------------------------------------

PLF-1   TTGTTGTTGACTCATTTAAAAATAAAAAGTAGCTCTCAGAAATATA
PLF-2   ------------------------------------------
```

Figure 1. Comparison of the nucleotide sequences of proliferin cDNA clones derived from BALB/c 3T3 tissue culture cells (PLF-1) and from BALB/c placenta (PLF-2).

It is of interest that all five of these differences occur at residues encoding serine or threonine in one or both of the cDNAs. Proliferin is secreted in a glycosylated form (4), and the proliferin sequence includes three copies of the N-linked glycosylation signal Asn-X-(Ser or Thr). However, these five single base differences between the two forms of proliferin do not affect these glycosylation sites. Whether these particular amino acid residues play some other important role in the structure or function of proliferin is at present unknown.

Several possible explanations can account for the nucleotide sequence differences found between the two forms of proliferin. It is possible that reverse transcription errors could have contributed to the observed differences, or that cultured BALB/c 3T3 cells and current BALB/c stocks have diverged. Another possibility is that multiple proliferin genes exist and that they encode nearly identical, but distinguishable, forms of proliferin. Hybridization analysis reveals the presence of several copies of the proliferin gene in the mouse genome. We have isolated a number of proliferin genomic clones, and have analyzed whether they contain the PLF-1 or PLF-2 sequence. Oligonucleotides corresponding to PLF-1 or PLF-2 hybridize to distinct subsets of this group of genomic clones, indicating that the mouse genome harbors both PLF-1 and PLF-2 genes. We have also used these oligonucleotide probes to investigate the cell- and tissue-specific expression of these genes. Surprisingly, both PLF-1 and PLF-2 mRNAs are detected in all proliferin-expressing cell types that we have examined.

REFERENCES

(1) Linzer, D. I. H. and Nathans, D. (1983) Proc. Natl. Acad. Sci. USA 80, 4271-4275.

(2) Linzer, D. I. H. and Nathans, D. (1984) Proc. Natl. Acad. Sci. USA 81, 4255-4259.

(3) Linzer, D. I. H. and Nathans, D. (1984) in Cancer Cells: The Transformed Phenotype (Cold Spring Harbor Laboratory, Cold Spring Harbor, New York) 1, 111-115.

(4) Linzer, D. I. H., Lee, S.-J., Ogren, L., Talamantes, F. and Nathans, D. (1985) Proc. Natl. Acad. Sci. USA 82, 4356-4359.

Growth Factors and Oncogenes

CHANGES IN GENE EXPRESSION FOLLOWING GROWTH STIMULATION OF CULTURED CELLS

D. Nathans, L. F. Lau, S-J. Lee and D. I. H. Linzer[1], Howard Hughes Medical Institute Laboratory, Department of Molecular Biology & Genetics, Johns Hopkins University School of Medicine, Baltimore, MD USA 21205, and [1]Department of Biochemistry, Molecular Biology and Cell Biology, Northwestern University, Evanston, IL USA 60201.

To identify genes that may be part of a genetic program for the growth of mammalian cells, we are characterizing cDNA clones derived from mRNAs that appear at various times after stimulation of resting BALB/c 3T3 cells with serum or growth factors. cDNA libraries were prepared from polyA$^+$ RNA from cells stimulated with serum for various periods of time, and the libraries were differentially screened with ^{32}P-cDNA probes made from stimulated or resting cell mRNA. One cDNA library was prepared from cells that were stimulated with serum for 3 hrs in the presence of cycloheximide. Our purpose in inhibiting protein synthesis was two-fold: first to limit new mRNAs to those that do not require _de novo_ protein synthesis for their accumulation (analagous to "immediate early" viral RNAs); and second, to amplify mRNAs that are superinduced by serum in the absence of protein synthesis, thus enriching both the library and probe for cDNAs derived from such mRNAs. Of approximately 50,000 recombinant phage plaques screened, 357 clones hybridized to probes derived from stimulated-cell RNA but not to probes from resting-cell RNA. Cross hybridization analysis showed that 4 RNA sequence families accounted for over 95% of the clones; other sequences were found only once. One of the clones hybridized to an actin probe; none hybridized to any of 13 oncogene probes tested, including _fos_ and _myc_. The mRNAs corresponding to five members of this set that were investigated further (see Table 1) appeared within 10 to 20 minutes following addition of serum, PDGF, FGF, or TPA, reached maximal levels by 40 to 90 minutes, and rapidly decayed. This is similar to the time course of c-_fos_ mRNA reported previously. One of the mRNAs (3CH61) showed a secondary rise thereafter. The estimated maximal level of mRNA varied from about 2 copies per cell to about 50 copies per cell (see Table 1). Nuclear run-off experiments indicated that in each case serum treatment of quiescent cells led within 5 minutes to increased transcription of the corresponding gene. Our results indicate that a considerable number of genes are activated very rapidly during the G0 to G1 transition of 3T3 cells and they presumably play a role in the cellular growth response to mitogenic stimulation.

Another cDNA library was prepared from mRNA of cells stimulated by serum for 12 hrs, the time of onset of DNA synthesis. From this library clones were isolated that correspond to mRNAs that appear several hours after stimulation. One of these clones was derived from an mRNA that appeared about 3 hrs post-stimulation and reached a maximal level at 12 to 18 hrs. This mRNA encoded a protein of 25 kd with 39% sequence similarity to preprolactin. (The processed protein has been named "proliferin".) Preproliferin has a hydrophobic leader, 6 cysteine and 2 tryptophan residues in positions nearly identical to those in prolactins, and 3 potential N-glycosylation sites. Proliferin cDNA was fused to a plasmid gene for bacterial transposon $\gamma\delta$-encoded resolvase and the resulting fusion protein was used to raise anti-proliferin serum. The antiserum precipitated a heterogeneous set of glycoproteins of approximately 25-35 kd secreted by cells infected with an SV40/proliferin recombinant virus and by BALB/c 3T3 cells. In each case tunicamycin produced a marked reduction in the amount of the 25-35 kd protein and the appearance of an immunoprecipitable 22 kd protein, the size predicted for unmodified proliferin. In a survey of mouse tissues proliferin mRNA was found only in placenta after day 8 of pregnancy. Minced placenta secreted proliferin in glycosylated form. By reaction with anti-proliferin and anti-placental lactogen sera (kindly provided by Frank Talamantes and Peter Colosi) proliferin and the placental lactogens were shown to differ. Comparison of the sequence of a placental proliferin cDNA (from BALB/c mice) with that derived from BALB/c 3T3 cell mRNA revealed 4 codon differences. Since restriction analysis of mouse genomic DNA revealed the presence of 3 to 5 proliferin genes per haploid amount of DNA, these sequence differences may reflect the presence of a functional family of proliferin genes.

During the isolation of placental proliferin cDNA, a second set of cDNA clones was detected that partially hybridized to the proliferin probe. These cDNAs encode a proliferin-related protein (PRP) with homology to proliferin, prolactin, and growth hormone. PRP mRNA appears in mouse placenta somewhat later than proliferin mRNA. Although PRP is also different from the 23 kd mouse placental lactogen described by Talamantes and his colleagues, its relationship to the higher molecular weight, mid-placental lactogen described by these authors is not yet known. Thus mouse placenta produces at least three different prolactin-related proteins.

In summary, our results and those from other laboratories indicate that following stimulation of resting 3T3 cells with serum or growth factors, specific mRNAs appear sequentially, regulated in part at the level of gene transcription. These growth-responsive genes, which include _fos_, _myc_, r-_fos_, p53, ornithine decarboxylase, proliferin, and others yet to be defined, appear to make up a complex genetic program for the growth of mammalian cells. The proliferin gene encodes a prolactin-like protein that is secreted by proliferating mouse cells and by mouse placenta. We hypothesize that proliferin acts as a growth factor both in cultured cells and in pregnant animals.

Table 1.

Clone	Number of Cross-Hybridizing Clones	Size of mRNA	Estimated maximal level of mRNA
C3H61	226	2.7 kb	50 copies/cell
C3H134	75	2.8	25
C3H77	14	3.6	35
C3H92	5	2.2	15
C3H96	1	1.6	2

REFERENCES

1. Linzer, D. I. H., and Nathans, D. Nucleotide Sequence of a Growth-Related mRNA Encoding a Member of the Prolactin-Growth Hormone Family. Proc. Natl. Acad. Sci. USA, 81:4255-4259, 1984.
2. Linzer, D. I. H., Lee, S-J., Nathans, D., Ogren, L., and Talamantes, F. Identification of Proliferin mRNA in Mouse Placenta, Proc. Natl. Acad. Sci. USA, 82:4356-4359, 1985.
3. Linzer, D. I. H. and Nathans. D. A New Member of the Prolactin-Growth Hormone Gene Family Expressed in Mouse Placenta. EMBO Journal 4:1419-1423, 1985
4. Lau, L. F. and Nathans, D. Identification of a Set of Genes Expressed During the GO/Gl Transition of Cultured Mouse Cells. EMBO Journal, 1985, in press.

EXPRESSION OF GROWTH FACTOR GENES IN TRANSGENIC MICE

B.L. Davison[1], L.S. Mathews[1], G. Norstedt[2], R.E. Hammer[3], G.I. Bell[4]
R.L. Brinster[3] and R.D. Palmiter[1]

1- Howard Hughes Medical Institute, Dept. of Biochemistry, Univ. of Washington, Seattle, Washington 98195.
2- Center for Biotechnology, Huddinge Hospital F82, Karolinska Inst., Stockholm, Sweden.
3- School of Veterinary Medicine, Univ. of Pennsylvania, Philadelphia, Pennsylvania 19104.
4- Chiron corporation, 4560 Horton St., Emeryville, Calif. 94608.

INTRODUCTION

Growth factor cascade. Coordinated body growth in vertebrates is the result of a complex, multigene hormonal control mechanism. The growth hormone (GH) cascade plays a primary role in this mechanism (Fig. 1). The best characterized elements in this cascade are: the hypothalamic peptides, growth hormone releasing factor (GHRF) and somatostatin; the pituitary hormone, GH; insulin and the somatomedins, insulin-like growth factors I (IGF-I) and II (IGF-II). GH is synthesized in the pituitary under the control of GHRF and somatostatin (1). According to the somatomedin hypothesis (2), GH has no direct growth-promoting activity but acts to stimulate hepatic IGF-I synthesis. IGF-I in turn directs growth of cartilage, skeletal muscle and other peripheral tissues in the adult. In contrast, IGF-II levels are not responsive to GH and are believed to regulate fetal growth and development (3). The IGFs are structurally very similar to proinsulin and can act as mitogens for a variety of cell types. While the bulk of circulating IGF-I in the adult is derived from the liver, IGF-I and IGF-II synthesis also occurs in a variety of peripheral tissues indicating that autocrine as well as endocrine modes of growth regulation may be involved (4). Circulating IGFs are bound to specific carrier proteins which are hormonally regulated. These carriers may act to increase serum IGF half-lives or to enhance cell surface receptor discrimination or both (5). The situation is further complicated in that IGF receptors may be regulated by insulin action (6).

HYBRID GENE EXPRESSION IN TRANSGENIC MICE

Circumventing regulatory constraints. To understand more about how peptide growth factors participate in regulating vertebrate growth and development, we wanted to assess the consequences of elevated serum GH levels in mice. With the potential of expressing hybrid genes in a variety of cell types throughout development the transgenic mouse paradigm seemed particularly suited for this type of experiment (7). We therefore established transgenic mouse lines harboring rat or human GH gene constructions. In these constructions, GH structural gene sequences were fused to mouse metallothionein-I (MT) promoter sequences (8,9). In transgenic animals expressing these hybrid genes, GH production occurred in a variety of tissues, notably liver, heart, intestine and kidney, under the transcriptional control of the inducible MT promoters. This scheme circumvents regulatory constraints normally affecting the endogenous GH promoters in pituitary somatotrophs (see shunt in Fig. 1). Mice containing MT-GH fusion genes have higher than normal serum GH levels (up to 1,000-fold higher) and grow to be twice normal size (8,9). Such animals also contain elevated IGF-I levels (Table 1). A similar scheme involving MT-GHRF fusion genes has also resulted in elevated GH levels and enhanced growth (10).

Fig. 1

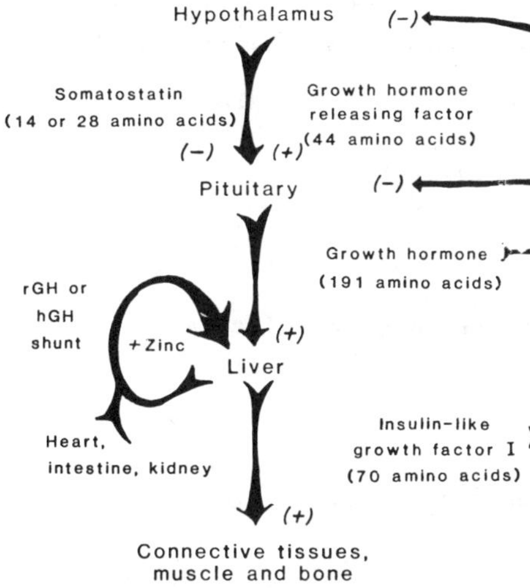

Table 1

Animal	hGH (μg/ml)	IGF-I (μg/ml)
Hyb-182-3♂	14.6 ± 1.4*	1.48 ± 0.13
Hyb-184-1♀	11.9 ± 0.7	1.73 ± 0.06
Hyb-184-5♂	18.0 ± 1.5	1.21 ± 0.08
Hyb-186-4♀	143.0 ± 6.5	1.04 ± 0.12
Controls	0	0.55 ± 0.04

*Standard error of the mean. $N = 4$ (samples per animal collected about 1 week apart).

Expression of IGFs in transgenic mice. We are also using the gene fusion approach to assess the consequences of expressing human IGF-I and -II in mice. If the somatomedin hypothesis is correct, it should then be possible to observe enhanced growth in transgenic animals expressing IGF-I genes under control of heterologous promoters. Effects of hIGF-II expression on fetal growth and development might also be revealed using this approach. Accordingly, we have fused human IGF-I and IGF-II cDNAs (11,12) to MT promoter sequences and hGH poly·A addition sites (Fig. 2). When transfected into cultured cells, the hIGF-I construct gives rise to production of biologically active peptides. These constructions have recently been introduced into fertilized mouse ova and serum hIGF-I has been detected in the resulting transgenic animals.

Fig. 2

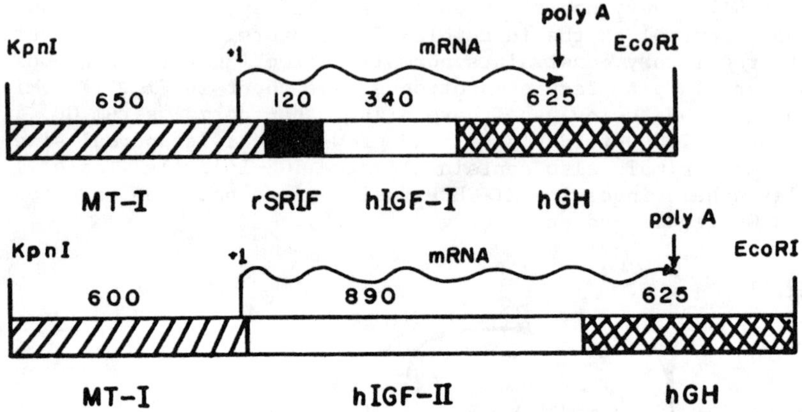

MT-I - mouse metallothionein I promoter
rSRIF - rat somatostatin signal peptide
hIGF - human insulin-like growth factor (I or II)
hGH - human growth hormone poly A addition site
(numbers above maps refer to size in base pairs)
(wavy lines above maps represent mature mRNA molecules)

REFERENCES

(1) Brazeau, p., et al. (1973) Science 179, 77.
(2) Daughaday, W.H., et al. (1972) Nature 235, 107.
(3) Moses, A.C., et al. (1980) Proc. Natl. Acad. Sci. USA 77, 3649
(4) D'Ercole, A.J., Stiles, A.D. and Underwood, L.E. (1984) Proc. Natl. Acad. Sci. USA 81, 4028.
(5) Moses, A.C., et al. (1976) Nature 263, 137.
(6) Oka, Y., et al. (1984) Proc. Natl. Acad. Sci. USA 81, 935.
(7) Palmiter, R.D. and Brinster, R.L. (1985) Cell 41, 343.
(8) Palmiter, R.D., et al. (1982) Nature 300, 611.
(9) Palmiter, R.D., et al. (1983) Science 222, 809.
(10) Hammer, R.E., et al. (1985) Nature 315, 413.
(11) Jansen, M., et al. (1983) Nature 306, 609.
(12) Bell, G.I., et al. (1984) Nature 310, 775.

REGULATION OF INSULIN-LIKE GROWTH FACTOR GENE EXPRESSION

M. M. Rechler, C. B. Bruni[*], Y. W.-H. Yang, H. J. Whitfield, D. E. Graham, R. Frunzio[*], A. L. Brown and S. P. Nissley.

National Institutes of Health, Bethesda, MD 20892 and [*]University of Naples, 80131 Napoli, Italy

Definitions, Structure and Actions.

Insulin-like growth factor I and II (IGF-I and II) are mitogenic polypeptides in plasma. They are single chain molecules of Mr 7500 with 4 structural domains: NH_2-B-C-A-D-COOH (1). IGF-I and IGF-II are chemically related; the B- and A-domains of both peptides are ∿ 40% identical to insulin.

The IGFs are mitogenic for many cultured cells. For example, serum-free media containing IGFs, epidermal growth factor (EGF), and platelet derived growth factor (PDGF) support the growth of Balb/c 3T3 fibroblasts (2). The IGFs act via one or both IGF receptor subtypes (3). Type I IGF receptors contain intrinsic tyrosine-specific protein kinase activity (4), like the transforming genes of many retroviruses and growth factor receptors (e.g., EGF, PDGF, insulin).

Although IGF-I and IGF-II are similar _in vitro_, they appear to have distinct _in vivo_ biological roles. IGF-I is growth hormone-dependent, and appears to mediate the action of growth hormone on cartilage to promote skeletal growth (5). The role of IGF-II is less clearcut: it is present at high levels in fetal serum in rats (6) and other species, suggesting a possible role in fetal growth, and also in extracts of brain (7), suggesting a possible role in nervous system function.

Biosynthesis of rat IGF-II

Dulak and Temin (8) observed that a permanent cell line established from normal rat liver, BRL-3A, grew in serum-free media and secreted growth factors with properties similar to the IGFs. Our laboratories have purified this growth factor, multiplication stimulating activity (MSA), studied its biological properties, and established radioligand assays for it (9, 10). MSA behaved quite similarly to IGF-II purified from human plasma. Its amino acid sequence is identical to human IGF-II at 62 of 67 residues, indicating that MSA represented rat IGF-II (11).

Biosynthetic labeling of intact BRL-3A cells identified a Mr ∿ 20,000 biosynthetic precursor, pro-rIGF-II, in immunoprecipitates of cell lysates (12). Pro-rIGF-II was rapidly labeled, converted to smaller forms, and did not appear in media. Amino acid sequence analysis of biosynthetically labeled Mr ∿ 20,000 pro-rIGF-II confirmed that mature 67 residue rIGF-II is present at the amino-terminus of the precursor (13).

Poly A-containing RNA from BRL-3A cells directs the synthesis of Mr ∿ 22,000 pre-pro-rIGF-II in a reticulocyte lysate cell-free translation system (14). Inclusion of microsomal membranes in the translation incubation converted pre-pro-rIGF-II to Mr ∿ 20,000 pro-rIGF-II by removal of the signal peptide (12).

Deduced structure of rIGF-II mRNA

A 12S fraction of BRL-3A RNA was enriched in mRNA that directed translation of pre-pro-rIGF-II (15). From a cDNA library established from this RNA fraction, Whitfield et al. (16) isolated a clone that contained a long open reading frame encoding the C, A, and D-domains of rIGF-II and an E-domain propeptide of 89 amino acids, followed by a 3'-noncoding region (Figure 1). The deduced 156 amino acid pro-rIGF-II confirmed the structure of the precursor indicated in biosynthetic studies (12, 13). Dull et al. (17) and Soares et al. (18) reported nearly identical sequence information for this region, as well as the nucleotide sequence of the prepeptide and B-domain. The structure of human IGF-II mRNA is similar (19, 20).

To determine the size of IGF-II RNA, we next performed primer extension experiments using a fragment of our cDNA clone (15, 16) or synthetic oligonucleotides (Figure 1). End-labeled single-strand DNA fragments were hybridized to BRL-3A RNA and extended with reverse transcriptase. From the size of the extended fragments, it was deduced that IGF-II RNA was ∿ 1030 bases long and contained a 5'-noncoding region of ∿ 100 nucleotides. This is consistent with the size of the functional 12S RNA used to generate the cDNA library from which our cDNA clone was isolated.

Size of IGF-II RNA by Northern blot analysis

The size of rIGF-II RNA also was determined by hybridization to Northern blots. When Northern blots prepared from BRL-3A RNA were hybridized to the rIGF-II probe, the predominant hybridizing species was ∿ 4 kilobases (kb), 3-4 times larger than expected. Weaker signals were present at 2.2 and 1.2 kb (21). Similar results were obtained with poly A+ RNA and with RNA from neonatal rat liver, indicating that this was not limited to the BRL-3A cell line. The 4 kb RNA is located almost exclusively in the cytoplasm. It is co-linear with a 551 base restriction fragment of the 1.2 kb IGF-II RNA that covers the C-A-D-E domains and part of the 3'-noncoding region. This supports the possibility that the 4 kb and 1.2 kb RNAs arise from a single transcript of the same gene by alternative processing. Indeed, preliminary evidence suggests that the rat genome contains only a single IGF-II gene (unpublished results).

Coordinate developmental regulation of 4 kb and 1.2 kb IGF RNAs in rat liver

If the 4 kb and 1.2 kb RNAs arise from a single primary RNA transcript, we reasoned that they should exhibit similar regulation. The most profound regulation of IGF-II levels in plasma occurs with development: IGF-II levels are 20-100-fold higher in the fetus and early neonate, and decrease abruptly by the third week of life (6). Slot-blot (15) and Northern blot analysis (21) of rat liver RNA indicate that the abundance of IGF-II RNA shows the same developmental pattern. Moreover, the 4 kb RNA as well as 1.2 kb and intermediate forms show identical regulation. We conclude that all IGF-II

RNAs probably arise from a single transcript by alternative processing.

IGF-II RNA levels in different tissues and in human tumors

Although it was initially thought that IGF-II might be principally synthesized in the liver, it appears that IGF-II RNA is present in multiple fetal rat tissues (22). In addition, the same multiple size forms of IGF-II RNA were detected. In each of 11 tissues, IGF-II RNA levels are increased in the fetus and decrease postnatally, similar to the developmental regulation observed in the liver. Similar results (fetal > adult IGF-II RNA) recently were reported in rat liver and muscle (18) and human liver and kidney (23).

Recently, Scott *et al*. (24) reported that IGF-II RNA levels were increased in a specific group of tumors frequently associated with each other and with genetic syndromes involving chromosomal defects in the short arm of chromosome 11, the location of the human IGF-II gene. These tumors include Wilm's nephroblastoma, rhabdomyosarcoma, and hepatoblastoma. Whether overexpression of the IGF-II gene is causally related to tumor growth or is a marker/epiphenomenon remains to be established.

Translatability of high molecular weight IGF-II RNA: implications for autocrine growth

BRL-3A RNA has been size fractionated, and fractions containing 4 kb IGF-II RNA used to direct protein synthesis in a cell-free translation system (21). Although S1 nuclease protection experiments and oligonucleotide hybridization experiments are consistent with the 4 kb RNA containing an intact protein-coding region, no Mr ∿ 22,000 pre-pro-rIGF-II was identified in total translation products or after immunoprecipitation. Either the 4 kb IGF-II RNA cannot be translated efficiently or it encodes an altered protein product that goes unrecognized. The former possibility might arise if the structure of the 4 kb RNA prevents its translation without an independent activation event. A similar mechanism has been proposed to account for the lack of transformation of cells that contain c-fos rather than v-fos, and the lack of translation of c-fos RNA *in vitro* (25).

At the present time, there is little evidence that the high molecular weight IGF-II RNAs in fetal tissues or in human tumors are functional. Synthesis of rIGF-II or its protein precursors has been demonstrated only in fetal liver (26), fibroblasts (27) and muscle (28). A subclone of BRL-3A cells, BRL-3A2, contains appreciable 4 kb IGF-II RNA by hybridization, but does not synthesize IGF-II or its precursor forms (15). Thus, although the presence of IGF-II RNA in various cell types and tumors suggests that IGF-II may be involved in the growth of these cells, it remains to be demonstrated that this RNA is processed to translationally active forms, that biosynthetic protein precursors are processed to mature active IGF-II, and that the cells possess appropriate receptor and effector pathways to respond to IGF-II.

REFERENCES:

1. Humbel, R.E.: In Li, C.H. (Ed.): Hormonal Proteins and Peptides, Vol. XII, Academic Press, 1984, pp. 57-79
2. Leof, E.B., Wharton, W., Van Wyk, J.J., and Pledger, W.J. Exp. Cell Res. 141, 107-115, 1982
3. Rechler, M.M., and Nissley, S.P. Ann. Rev. Physiol. 47, 425-442, 1985
4. Sasaki, N., Rees-Jones, R.W., Zick, Y., Nissley, S.P., and Rechler, M.M. J. Biol. Chem. 260, 9793-9804, 1985
5. Zapf, J., Schmid, C., and Froesch, E.R. Clinics Endocrinol. Metab. 13, 3-30, 1984
6. Moses, A.C., et al., Proc. Natl. Acad. Sci. U.S.A. 77, 3649-3653, 1980
7. Haselbacher, G.K., Schwab, M.E., Pasi, A., and Humbel, R.E. Proc. Natl. Acad. Sci. U.S.A. 82, 2153-2157, 1985
8. Dulak, N.C., and Temin, H.M. J. Cell. Physiol. 81, 153-160, 1973
9. Rechler, M.M., et al., J. Supramol. Struct. Cell. Biochem. 15, 253-286, 1981
10. Nissley, S.P., et al., In Spencer, E.M. (Ed.): Insulin-like Growth Factors/Somatomedins: Basic Chemistry, Biology, and Clinical Importance. Walter de Gruyter Co., 1983, pp. 31-48
11. Marquardt, H., Todaro, G.J., Henderson, L.E., and Oroszlan, S. J. Biol. Chem. 256, 6859-6865, 1981
12. Yang, Y.W.-H., Romanus, J.A., Liu, T.-Y., Nissley, S.P., and Rechler, M.M. J. Biol. Chem. 260, 2570-2577, 1985
13. Yang, Y.W.-H., Rechler, M.M., Nissley, S.P., and Coligan, J. E. J. Biol. Chem. 260, 2578-2582, 1985
14. Acquaviva, A.M., Bruni, C.B., Nissley, S.P., and Rechler, M. M. Diabetes, 31, 656-658, 1982
15. Rechler, M.M., et al., Cancer Cells 3, 131-138, 1985
16. Whitfield, H.J., Bruni, C.B., Frunzio, R., Terrell, J.E., Nissley, S.P., and Rechler, M.M. Nature 312, 277-280, 1984
17. Dull, T.J., Gray, A., Hayflick, J.S., and Ullrich, A. Nature 310, 777-781, 1984
18. Soares, M.B., Ishii, D.N., and Efstratiadis, A. Nucl Acids Res. 13, 1119-1134, 1985
19. Bell, G.I., et al., Nature, 310, 775-777, 1984
20. Jansen, M., et al., FEBS Letts. 179, 243-246, 1985
21. Graham, D.E. et al. (in preparation)
22. Brown A.L. et al., this volume
23. Bell, G. I., Gerhard, D.S., Fong, N.M., Sanchez-Pescador, R., and Rall, L.B. Proc. Natl. Acad. Sci. U.S.A. 82, 6450-6454, 1985
24. Scott, J., et al., Nature 317, 260-262, 1985
25. Miller, A. D., Curran, T., and Verma, I. M. Cell 36, 51-60, 1984
26. Rechler, M.M., et al., J. Biol. Chem. 254, 7942-7950, 1979
27. Adams, S.O., Nissley, S.P., Handwerger, S., and Rechler, M.M. Nature 302, 150-153, 1983
28. Hill, D.J., et al., Endocrinology 117, 2061-2072, 1985

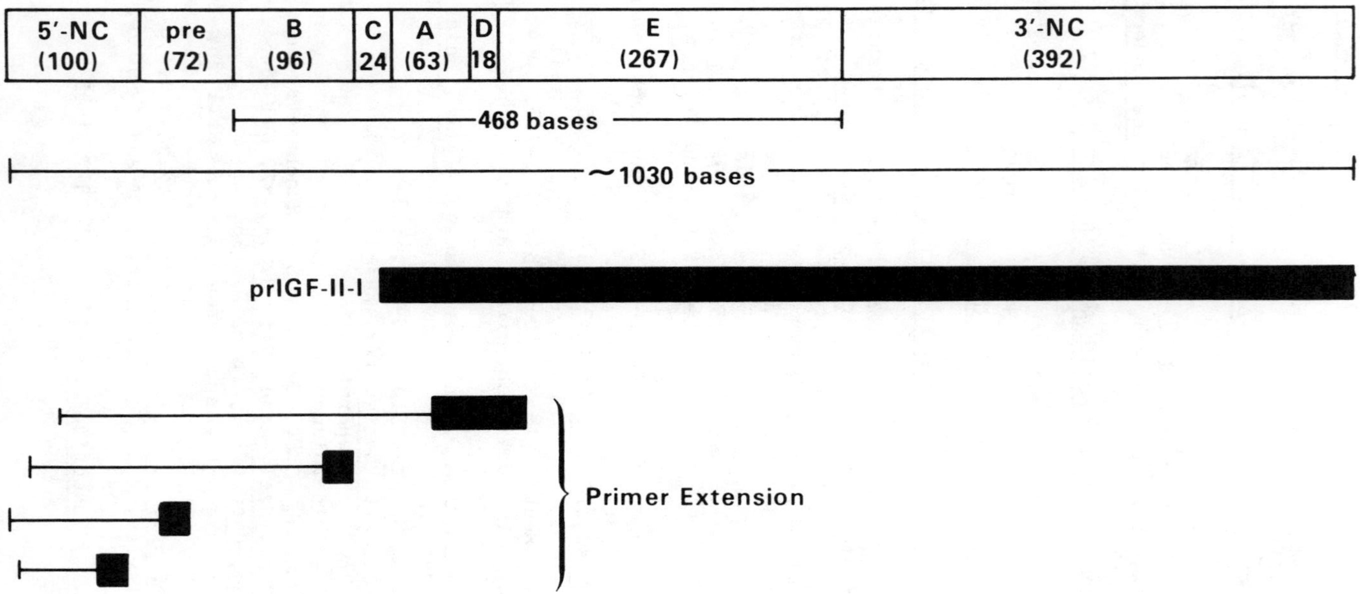

FIGURE 1. Structure of functional 12S rIGF-II mRNA deduced from the nucleotide sequence of the prIGF-II-I recombinant plasmid insert (15, 16) and extension with reverse transcriptase of oligonucleotide fragments (native or synthetic) hybridized to BRL-3A RNA. The position and relative size in nucleotides (in parentheses) of the 5'- and 3'-noncoding regions (NC), the prepeptide (pre), the B-C-A-D domains of mature IGF-II, and the E-propeptide are indicated.

REGULATION OF GENE EXPRESSION BY PLATELET-DERIVED GROWTH FACTOR

C.D. Stiles
Department of Microbiology and Molecular Genetics, Harvard Medical School and the Dana-Farber Cancer Institute, Boston, MA

SUMMARY

Platelet-derived growth factor (PDGF) regulates gene expression in Balb/c-3T3 cells. Expression of the c-*myc* gene, the c-*fos* gene and several other genes is stimulated promptly and dramatically by PDGF. The translation product of these rapidly inducible genes may function to initiate a round of cell division. At later times, PDGF stimulates the expression of beta-fibroblast interferon and of (2'-5')-oligoadenylate synthetase. It is possible that these late gene products function as feedback inhibitors of the mitogenic response to PDGF.

INTRODUCTION

At any given time, the majority of cells in the body are in a quiescent, growth arrested state (1). Transition from growth arrest to exponential growth requires mRNA synthesis (2). The requirement for *de novo* RNA synthesis during early stages of the mitogenic response is something of a paradox. Comparative analysis of rapidly growing vs. quiescent cells indicates little difference in the absolute rate of mRNA synthesis (3); moreover there is little qualitative difference in the kinds of mRNA transcribed in quiescent and actively proliferating cell cultures (4). This paradox is reconciled by a variety of recent observations indicating that mitogens stimulate the expression of rare, low abundance mRNAs during the G1 phase of the cell cycle (5-7). We have documented and detailed this phenomena in Balb/c-3T3 cells stimulated to proliferate with platelet-derived growth factor (PDGF).

THE PDGF INDUCIBLE "COMPETENCE GENE FAMILY"

Normal fibroblast cells in culture probably express between 10,000 to 12,000 individual genes (8). In 1983, we demonstrated that platelet-derived growth factor (PDGF) stimulates expression of between 0.1 to 0.3% of these genes within hours after addition to the culture medium (5). Using differential colony hybridization, we isolated representative members of a PDGF-inducible gene family from a cDNA library directed to PDGF-treated 3T3 cells. We designated this PDGF-inducible gene family "competence" after the term coined originally to describe the response of Balb/c-3T3 cells to PDGF (9). Together with Kathy Kelly and Philip Leder from Harvard Medical School, we demonstrated that the c-myc proto-oncogene was a member of the competence gene family (10). Subsequently, we and others showed that c-fos was also contained within the competence gene family (11-14).

THE C-MYC GENE PRODUCT FUNCTIONS AS AN INTRACELLULAR MEDIATOR OF THE GROWTH RESPONSE TO PDGF

In subsequent studies, a chimeric myc gene was constructed wherein the normal transcription initiation elements of the mouse germ line c-myc gene were replaced with the steroid inducible promoter from mouse mammary tumor virus (15). This MMTV:c-myc chimeric was stably integrated into Balb/c-3T3 cells by transfection with a selectable drug resistance marker. When the transfected 3T3 cells were exposed to hydrocortisone (in the absence of PDGF) expression of the exogeneous myc gene was induced and the cells began to proliferate. From these results, we concluded that the c-myc gene product functions as an intracellular mediator of the growth response to PDGF. We noted however that the mitogenic response to the gratitutiously-induced exogeneous myc gene was not as great as the response to PDGF itself. We speculated, therefore that other intracellular molecules function together with the myc gene protein to induce the full cellular response to PDGF (15).

PDGF AND DOUBLE STRANDED RIBONUCLEIC ACID STIMULATE EXPRESSION OF THE SAME GENES IN BALB/c-3T3 CELLS

Over the past several years, we have searched for other agents that would function as analogues of PDGF to stimulate expression of the competence genes in Balb/c-3T3 cells. A variety of hormones, growth factors, drugs and ionophores were screened with negative results. We found that fibroblast growth factor, epidermal growth factor and certain tumor promoters are weak users of this gene family; however, we have found one agent which induces the genes as promptly and as dramatically as PDGF itself. That agent, surprisingly enough, is double stranded ribonucleic acid (16).

Synthetic double stranded ribonucleic acids such as poly(I):poly(C) are well known gratuitous inducers of beta-fibroblast interferon in fibroblast cell cultures.

For this reason, we wished to determine whether PDGF stimulates expression of genes which are normally induced by double stranded RNA. Our experiments show that PDGF stimulates expression of the beta-fibroblast interferon gene and of the (2'-5')-oligoadenylate synthetase gene; however, induction of these genes occurs over a much slower time course than observed previously for genes such as c-*myc* and c-*fos*.

CONCLUSIONS

PDGF stimulates prompt and dramatic expression of a "competence" gene family in Balb/c-3T3 cells. The c-*myc* gene and the c-*fos* gene are contained within the competence gene family. Expression of the c-*myc* gene has functional consequences. In Balb/c-3T3 cells and in other cell systems, it would appear that expression of *myc* gene protein sensitizes cells to the mitogenic action of other growth factors in the culture medium (15, 17-19).

More recently we have shown that PDGF stimulates expression of interferon and of (2'-5')-oligoadenylate synthetase. Induction of these late genes occurs over a much slower time course than previously described for the competence gene family. To date, functional consequences of interferon gene induction and (2'-5')-oligoadenylate gene induction have not been demonstrated; however it is tempting to speculate that these slowly inducible genes may function as feedback inhibitors of the mitogenic response to PDGF.

1 Baserga, R. (1985) The Biology of Cell Reproduction. Harvard Univesity Press.
2. Baserga, R., Waechter, D.E., Soprano, K.J. and Galanti, N. (1982) Ann. N.Y. Acad. Sci. 397, 110-120.
3. Rossini, M. and Baserga, R. (1978) Biochemistry 17, 858-863.
4. Williams, J.G. and Penman, S. (1975) Cell 6, 197-206.
5. Cochran, B.H., Reffel, A.C., and Stiles, C.D. (1983) Cell 33, 939-947.
6. Linzer, D.I.H. and Nathans D. (1983) Proc. Natl. Acad. Sci. USA 80, 4271-4275.
7. Hirschhorn, R.R., Aller, P., Yuan Z-A., Gibson, C.W. and Baserga, R. (1984) Proc. Natl. Acad. Sci. USA 81, 6004-6008.

8. Lewin, B. (1980) Gene Expression 2. 2nd ed. John Wiley & Sons, Inc. N.Y.
9. Pledger, W.J., Stiles, C.D., Antoniades, H.N. and Scher, C.D. (1977) Proc. Natl. Acad. Sci. USA 74, 4481-4485.
10. Kelly, K., Cochran, B.H., Stiles, C.D. and Leder, P. (1983) Cell 35, 603-610.
11. Greenberg, M.E. and Ziff, E.B. (1984) Nature 311, 433-442.
12. Cohran, B.H., Zullo, J., Verma, I.M. and Stiles, C.D. (1984) Science 226, 1080-1082.
13. Kruijer, W., Cooper, A.J., Hunter, T. and Verma, I.M. (1984) Nature 312, 711-716.
14. Muller, R., Bravo, R., Burckhardt, J. and Curran, T. (1984) Nature 312, 716-720.
15. Armelin, H.A., Armelin, M.C.S., Kelly, K., Stewart, T., Leder, P., Cochran, B.H. and Stiles, C.D. (1984) Nature 310, 655-660.
16. Zullo, J., Cochran, B.H., Huang, A. and Stiles, C.D. (1985) Cell, in press.
17. Mougneau E., Lemieux, L., Rassoulzadegan, M. and Cuzin, F. (1984) Proc. Natl. Acad. Sci. USA 81, 5758-5762.
18. Keath, E.J., Caimi, P.G. and Cole, M.D. (1984) Cell 39, 339-348.
19. Kaczmarek, L., Hyland, J.K., Watt, R., Rosenberg, M. and Baserga, R. (1985) Science 228, 1313-1315.

ACKNOWLEDGEMENTS

The research conducted in this work was supported by grants from the NIH and the Ajinomoto Co., Inc. of Tokyo, Japan.

PROTO-ONCOGENE FOS: STRUCTURE, EXPRESSION AND REGULATION

Inder M. Verma
Molecular Biology Laboratory, The Salk Institute, P.O. Box 85800, San Diego, CA 92138

Proto-oncogene fos is the cellular cognate of the resident transforming gene (v-fos) of FBJ murine osteosarcoma virus which causes bone tumors in vivo and transforms fibroblasts in vitro. The complete molecular architecture of the fos gene has been elucidated and illustrated in Figure 1. The salient features can be summarized as follows:

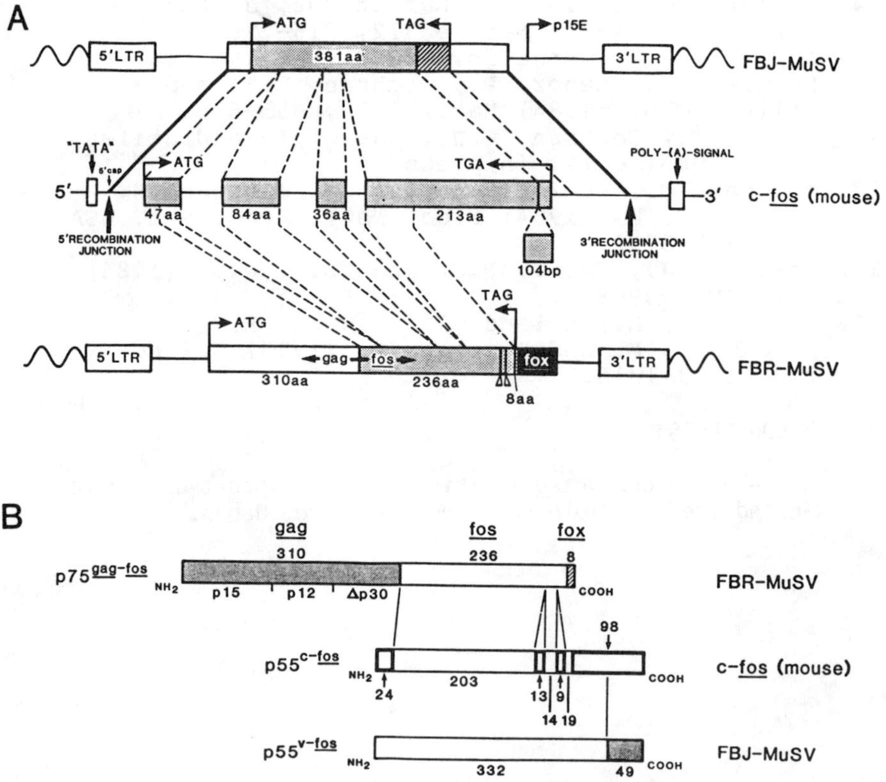

Fig. 1. Schematic drawings of FBJ-MSV and FBR-MSV. (A) Comparison of the genome organizations of FBJ-MSV and FBR-MSV to the organization of the mouse c-fos gene. (B) Comparison of the gene product of the mouse c-fos gene to those of FBJ-MSV and FBR-MSV.

(1) FBJ-MSV proviral DNA contains 4,026 nucleotides, including two long terminal repeats (LTRs) of 617 nucleotides each, 1,639 nucleotides of acquired cellular sequences (v-fos), and a portion of the viral envelope (env) gene. Both the initiation and termination codons of the v-fos protein are within the acquired sequences that encode a protein of 381 amino acids, having a molecular weight of 49,601 (Van Beveren et al., 1983).

(2) In cells transformed by FBJ-MSV, a phosphoprotein with an apparent M_r of 55,000 (p55) on SDS polyacrylamide gel electroporesis (SDS-PAGE) has been identified as the transforming protein (Curran and Teich, 1982; Curran et al., 1985).

(3) The sequences in the c-fos gene that are homologous to those in the v-fos gene are interrupted by four regions of nonhomology, three of which represent bona fide introns. The 104 nucleotide long fourth region, which is present in both mouse and human c-fos genes, represents sequences that have been deleted during the biogenesis of the v-fos gene. (The additional 104 nucleotides in the c-fos gene transcripts do not increase the predicted size of the c-fos proteins, because of a switch to a different reading frame.) Thus the c-fos protein has 280 amino acids, which is remarkably similar to the size of the v-fos protein (381 amino acids) (Van Beveren et al., 1983; van Straaten et al., 1983).

(4) In the first 332 amino acids, the v-fos and mouse c-fos proteins differ at only 5 residues, while the remaining 48 amino acids of the c-fos protein are encoded in a different reading frame from that in the v-fos protein. Thus the v-fos and c-fos proteins, though largely similar, have different carboxyl termini (Fig. 1B).

(5) Despite their different carboxyl termini, both the v-fos and c-fos proteins are located in the nucleus. The c-fos protein undergoes more extensive modifications than the v-fos protein (Curran et al., 1984).

(6) FBR-MSV proviral DNA contains 3,791 nucleotides (specifying a genome of 3,284 bases) and encodes a single gag-fos fusion product of 554 amino acids. The fos portion of the gene lacks sequences that encode the first 24 and the last 98 amino acids of the 380 amino acid mouse c-fos gene product (Fig. 1B). In addition, the coding region has sustained three small in-frame deletions, one in the p^{30gag} portion and two in the fos region as compared with sequences of AKR-MLV and the c-fos gene, respectively (Van Beveren et al., 1984). The gene product terminates in sequences termed fox (Fig. 1A) which are present in normal mouse DNA at loci unrelated to the c-fos gene. The c-fox gene(s) is expressed as an abundant class of polyadenylated RNA in mouse tissue.

Proto-oncogene fos is expressed during prenatal development and the highest levels accumulate in amnion cells (Muller et al., 1982, 1983). The fos gene is a highly inducible gene; often the expression is very rapid and transient (Cochran et al., 1984; Greenburg and Ziff, 1984; Kruijer et al., 1984, 1985; Muller et al., 1984; Curran and Morgan, 1985; Mitchell et al., 1985). Figure 2 summarizes the number of cell types where fos gene is expressed upon induction with a variety of differentiation-specific agents or mitogens. Detailed analysis of fos expression in promonocyte differentiation will be discussed. The regulation of the fos gene at the transcriptional and post-transcriptional levels will also be discussed.

The work I will present was carried out by Drs. C. Van Beveren, R.L. Mitchell, W. Kruijer, J. Deschamps and F. Meijlink.

c-fos INDUCTION

1) PROMONOCYTE/MONOMYELOCYTE $\xrightarrow[\text{Vit } D_3]{\text{TPA}}$ MACROPHAGES

2) PC12 $\xrightarrow[\text{cAMP, } K^+]{\text{NGF}}$ NEURITES

3) PARTIAL HEPATECTOMY

4) SPLEEN CELLS STIMULATED WITH ConA OR LPS

5) RESTING BALB/C OR NIH 3T3 CELLS STIMULATED WITH PDGF, SERUM OR TPA

6) HEPATOCYTES STIMULATED WITH GROWTH FACTORS

NO c-fos INDUCTION

1) MONOMYELOCYTE $\xrightarrow{\text{DMSO}}$ GRANULOCYTES

2) PC12 $\xrightarrow{\text{DEX}}$ CHROMAFFIN CELLS

Fig. 2. Summary of conditions under which induction of c-fos gene expression has been demonstrated.

References

(1) Cochran, B.H., Zullo, J., Verma, I.M., and Stiles, C.D. (1984). Science 226:1080-1082.

(2) Curran, T., and Morgan, J.I. (1985). Science 119:1265-1268.

(3) Curran, T., and Teich, N.M. (1982). J. Virol. 42:114-122.

(4) Curran, T., Miller, A.D., Zokas, L., and Verma, I.M. (1984). Cell 36:259-268.

(5) Curran, T., Van Beveren, C., Ling, N., and Verma, I.M. (1985). Mol. Cell. Biol. 5:167-172.

(6) Greenburg, M.E., and Ziff, E.B. (1984). Nature (London) 311:433-438.

(7) Kruijer, W., Cooper, J., Hunter, T., and Verma, I.M. (1984). Nature (LOndon) 312:711-716.

(8) Kruijer, W., Schubert, D., and Verma, I.M. (1985). Proc. Natl. Acad. Sci. USA 82:7330-7334.

(9) Mitchell, R.L., Zokas, L., Schreiber, R.D., and Verma, I.M. (1985). Cell 40:209-217.

(10) Muller, R., Bravo, R., Buckhardt, J., and Curran, T. (1984). Nature (London) 312:716-720.

(11) Muller, R., Slamon, D.J., Tremblay, J.M., Cline, M.J., and Verma, I.M. (1982). Nature (London) 299:640-644.

(12) Muller, R., Verma, I.M., and Adamson, E.D. (1983). EMBO J. 2:679-684.

(13) Van Beveren, C., van Straaten, F., Curran, T., Muller, R., and Verma, I.M. (1983). Cell 32:1241-1255.

(14) Van Straaten, F., Muller, R., Curran, T., Van Beveren, C., and Verma, I.M. (1983). Proc. Natl. Acad. Sci. USA 80:3183-3187.

REGULATION OF PROTEIN KINASES AND CELL PROLIFERATION BY TRANSFORMING GENE PRODUCTS

R.L. Erikson, J. Blenis and A. Bedard

Biological Laboratories, Harvard University, Cambridge MA 02138

INTRODUCTION. Several transforming gene products and growth factor receptors have tyrosine-specific protein kinase activity (1-3). Little is known, however, about the physiologically important cellular substrates of these enzymes despite prolonged investigations. The identification of such substrates is crucial for additional descriptions of the biochemistry of the cancer cell and of the regulatory events in normal cell divison. As an alternative to direct identification of cellular proteins containing phosphotyrosine, we have investigated cellular enzymes that, because of their increased activity in transformed cells, are potential physiological substrates of transforming gene products or growth factor receptors. Alterations in transformed cells provide some information concerning enzymes of interest. For example, normal cells in culture cease division and become quiescent when growth factors in serum are reduced or absent whereas, under similar conditions, their transformed counterparts continue to divide. A biochemical marker for such quiescent cells is the unphosphorylated 40S ribosomal subunit protein S6. Following the expression of $pp60^{v-src}$ or the addition of serum or tumor promoting phorbol ester, S6 is rapidly phosphorylated on serine residues (4). Thus the study of protein kinases and/or phosphoprotein phosphatases acting on S6 and their regulation by transforming gene products and growth factor receptors offers the possibility of identifying additional tyrosine-specific protein kinase substrates.

As a first step in our studies we have identified and carried out preliminary characterization of a protein kinase that phosphorylates S6 in 40S ribosomal subunits. We found that serum-deprived cells stimulated by $pp60^{v-src}$ expression, or by serum or phorbol ester addition yield a chromatographically similar enzyme activity (5). Because PMA is known to bind to and activate protein kinase C (for review see 6), these results suggest that the S6 kinase activation in PMA-treated cells may be mediated by protein kinase C. Because our results show the PMA-stimulated S6 kinase in CEF resembles the serum- and $pp60^{v-src}$-stimulated S6 kinases, protein kinase C may mediate both growth factor receptor and <u>src</u> gene product S6 kinase activation.

Quiescent cells stimulated by $pp60^{v-src}$ expression, by serum or by phorbol ester show altered gene expression. In an effort to identify potentially interesting changes we have identified proteins expressed uniquely in quiescent or proliferating cells and prepared cDNA clones of mRNAs expressed in the two populations. These studies are designed to gain information about cellular gene products that may contribute to the transformed cell phenotype.

RESULTS AND DISCUSSION. Activation of the ribosomal S6 protein kinase. Protein kinase activity capable of phosphorylating 40S ribosomal protein S6 on serine residues has been detected in chicken embryo fibroblasts (CEF). This activity appears to be regulated in direct response to expression of $pp60^{v-src}$ in CEF infected with a temperature-sensitive transformation mutant of Rous sarcoma virus. Partially purified S6 kinase activity was highly specific for S6 in 40S ribosomal subunits. The S6 kinase activity was not inhibited by calcium or by the heat-stable inhibitor of cAMP-dependent protein kinase, nor was it activated by phosphatidylserine, diacylglycerol and calcium. Thus it is distinct from protein kinase C and cAMP-dependent protein kinase which are capable of phosphorylating S6 *in vitro*.

The tumor-promoter, phorbol 12-myristate 13-acetate (PMA), also stimulated ribosomal protein S6 kinase activity in serum-starved CEF, whereas phorbol, the inactive analog of PMA, had no effect. S6 kinase activity stimulated by expression of $pp60^{v-src}$, by PMA, or by serum growth factors exhibited similar chromatographic properties upon ion-exchange chromatography. These results suggest that a common protein kinase may be activated by three diverse stimuli all involved in regulating cell proliferation.

The findings of Rozengurt and coworkers indicate that prolonged exposure of cells to phorbol ester results in down-regulation of protein kinase C activity and phorbol ester binding. Ribosomal protein S6 kinase activity was measured in lysates prepared from serum-deprived chicken embryo fibroblasts (CEF) treated for various times with phorbol 12-myristate 13-acetate (PMA). Maximal activity was observed within 15 min and it declined to the initial level by 4 hr. Incubation of these cells with PMA 4 to 60 hrs after the initial treatment did not result in an additional increase in S6 protein kinase activity. These results are consistent with down-regulation of the PMA receptor, protein kinase C, and the dependence of PMA-stimulated S6 kinase activity on this enzyme. Long-term pretreatment of CEF with PMA only partially attenuated the stimulation of the S6 protein kinase activity by serum or by expression of the Rous sarcoma virus transforming gene product, $pp60^{v-src}$. A similar protein kinase activity also is stimulated in cells treated with cycloheximide or sodium vanadate. Pretreatment with PMA had little effect on this response. These data indicate that it is likely there are at least two mechanisms through which S6 kinase activity can be regulated, one of which apparently utilizes protein kinase C whereas the other(s) does not.

Characterization of proteins and mRNAs expressed in quiescent or proliferating cell populations. An example of regulated protein expression is illustrated by a 20 kD protein synthesized and secreted by normal quiescent cells. Upon expression of $pp60^{v-src}$ or addition or growth factors quiescent cells cease synthesis of the 20 kD protein within a few hours. The functional role of the protein in the regulation of cellular proliferation is under investigation.

We also have examples of cDNA clones of mRNAs that are not expressed in quiescent cells, but are rapidly expressed after expression of $pp60^{v-src}$. The relationship of these mRNAs to known oncogenes will be discussed.

REFERENCES:

1. Erikson, R.L., Purchio, A.F., Erikson, E., Collett, M.S. and Brugge, J.S. (1980) J. Cell Biol. 87, 319-325.
2. Hunter, T. and Cooper, J.A. (1984) in Advances in Cyclic Nucleotide and Protein Phosphorylation Research 17 (eds. Greengard, P., Robison, G.A., Paoletti, R. and Nicosia, S.), pp.443-455, Raven, New York.
3. Heldin, C.-H. and Westermark, B. (1984) Cell 37, 9-20.
4. Blenis, J., Spivack, J.G. and Erikson, R.L. (1984) Proc. Natl. Acad. Sci. USA 81, 6408-6412.
5. Blenis, J. and Erikson, R.L. (1985) Proc. Natl. Acad. Sci. USA 82, 7621-7625.
6. Nishizuka, Y. (1984) Nature (London) 308, 693-698.

TYROSINE GLYCOSYLATION IS INVOLVED IN MUSCLE-GLYCOGEN SYNTHESIS

Ignacio R. Rodriguez, Juana S. Tandecarz, Brent R. Kirkman and William J. Whelan, Department of Biochemistry, University of Miami School of Medicine, P.O. Box 016129, Miami, FL 33101, U.S.A.

SUMMARY: 1. Rabbit-muscle glycogen contains a covalently bound protein having Mr 37,000 that we will henceforth refer to as glycogenin. It is completely insoluble in water at pH 5, and may be generated as a precipitate as a result of the combined actions on glycogen of α-amylase and glucoamylase, or by treatment with anhydrous hydrogen fluoride. In the former case the protein still carries some of the glucose residues of glycogen (10-30 per mole of glycogenin).

2. The linkage between glycogen and glycogenin has been identified as a novel glycosidic-amino acid bond. The amino acid is tyrosine, linked to glycogen via its hydroxyl group. The sugar in linkage to tyrosine appears to be glucose itself.

3. We have demonstrated glucosylation with UDP[^{14}C]glucose by a muscle extract of two rabbit-muscle proteins contained in the same extract. The relation of these proteins to glycogenin, and whether the amino acid undergoing glucosylation is tyrosine, remains to be explored.

4. The discovery of glycogenin is, we believe, an important clue to the mechanism of biogenesis of glycogen and may represent a previously unsuspected means of metabolic control of the glycogen content of the cell and the location of glycogen within the cell. The facts that the linkage between glycogen and glycogenin is via tyrosine, that insulin stimulates glycogen synthesis, and acts on its receptor by causing it to become an active tyrosine kinase, may be linked by a common thread.

BACKGROUND: The claim that glycogen contains protein goes back exactly 100 years (1). Because of the small amount of protein present (we find 0.35% in muscle glycogen) it has tended to be regarded as an impurity and the view that the protein is covalently bound to the glycogen has been the subject of controversy and scepticism. Only now is it possible to state definitively that in skeletal muscle glycogen, protein is present and covalently bound. There is much circumstantial evidence for the presence of protein in the glycogen of other tissues (for a review, see ref. 2), but skeletal muscle glycogenin is the first protein derived from glycogen for which a molecular weight, an amino acid analysis, and the amino acid involved in linkage to the glycogen have been reported. We also know that there is one mole of glycogenin per Mr 10^7 of glycogen, this being believed to be the limiting molecular weight of this macromolecule (3).

PREPARATION OF RABBIT-MUSCLE GLYCOGENIN: The preparation of muscle glycogen free from adventitious protein is described in ref. 2. Glycogenin is prepared from glycogen by hydrolysis with α-amylase/glucoamylase acting together. When the conversion into

This paper is dedicated to Luis F. Leloir in celebration of his forthcoming 80th birthday on September 6, 1986.

glucose passes 95%, glycogenin begins to precipitate (Fig. 1). Reductive methylation of the protein's amino groups with $H^{14}CHO$ (4), prior to glycogenolysis, permits the observation that the precipitation of radiolabel in the protein is essentially quantitative (2). The evidence that the protein has Mr 37,000 and contains bound glucose has been published elsewhere (2,5).

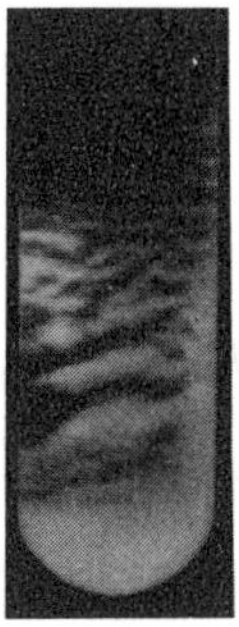

Fig. 1. Showing the precipitation of glycogenin on the side of the digest vessel when rabbit-muscle glycogen is hydrolyzed with α-amylase/glucoamylase (reproduced from ref. 2 with permission).

NATURE OF THE LINKAGE OF GLYCOGEN TO GLYCOGENIN: The amino acid involved in the linkage of glycogenin to glycogen is tyrosine (5). We were able to demonstrate this by degrading the protein contained in the glycogen with Pronase, finding that tyrosine was enriched in the material remaining attached to the carbohydrate and showing that the tyrosine hydroxyl was involved in covalent linkage, because of the inability to iodinate (^{125}I) or nitrate (tetranitromethane) the aromatic nucleus. Not previously reported is the retention of tyrosine by the glycogen, but not other amino acids, when the glycogen was treated with anhydrous hydrazine.

THE INITIATION OF GLYCOGEN BIOSYNTHESIS: Of the many questions opened up by the discovery of glycogenin, an important one is to learn the state of glycogenin in the cell. Is it all covalently bound to glycogen, or is there an excess of glycogenin, with a proportion of the molecules not bound to glycogen? Is there a family of intermediates - glycogenin molecules carrying growing glycogen molecules?

We have recently made an initial exploration of this question with intriguing positive results. We used an approach taken by Tandecarz et al. (9) when studying the initiation of starch synthesis in the potato. They were able to label a potato membrane protein with UDP[^{14}C]glucose as substrate and defined experimental conditions under which a single glucose residue, and no more, could be covalently attached such that on SDS gel electrophoresis a radiolabelled component was seen having Mr 38,000, strongly suggestive of the potato containing a protein similar to glycogenin.

Using the same experimental conditions and a high-speed pellet from rabbit skeletal muscle, we have now seen, by SDS gel electrophoresis of such an incubation mixture, that two radiolabelled proteins are formed (Fig. 2). We are now in process of learning whether either or both of these are related to native muscle glycogenin and whether the linkage of the [^{14}C]glucose unit(s) added in this _in vitro_ experiment is/are to tyrosine. We find it very interesting that a similar preparation from heart tissue also revealed a single radiolabelled protein, comigrating with the slower of the two radiolabelled protein species in skeletal muscle (Fig. 2). It should be noted that the high-speed pellet is acting both as the source of glucose-transferring enzyme and substrates.

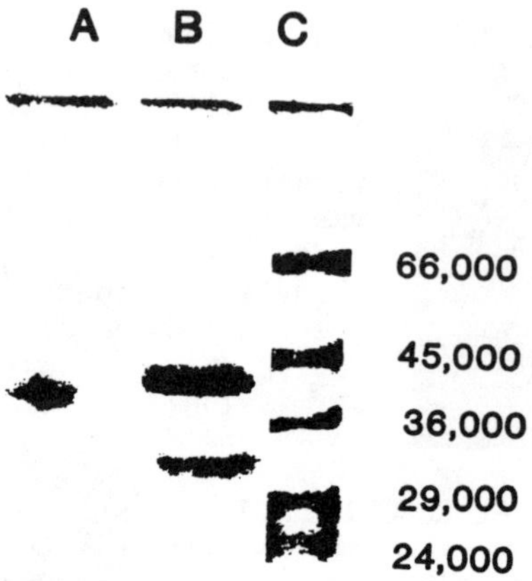

Fig. 2. [^{14}C]Glucosylation of endogenous muscle proteins by a 100,000g rabbit-heart (A) or -muscle (B) pellet with 5µM UDP[^{14}C]glucose. The product was electrophoresed in SDS in a 10% acrylamide slab gel. Lanes A and B are the radioautographs; lane C is the Coomassie blue stain of reference proteins.

SIGNIFICANCE OF THE PRESENCE OF GLYCOGENIN IN GLYCOGEN: That glycogen contains protein is a claim first made in 1886 (1), and one that we have only now finally settled. Although the topic has been worked on vigorously at various periods in the interim, notably in the 1930's and 1950's, the view finally prevailed in the 1960's that the protein was an artifact.

A physiological role for a protein component of glycogen was suggested by the pioneering work of Krisman in the early 1970's (6). She was able in _in vitro_ experiments with a high-speed pellet from liver, incubated with radiolabelled UDPglucose, to obtain labelled glycogen-like products that were precipitable with trichloroacetic acid, and therefore seemed to contain protein. In explanation of this finding, Krisman made the proposal shown in Fig. 3, that the biosynthesis of glycogen is preceded by the biosynthesis of a protein to which a putative enzyme, glycogen initiator synthase, adds glucose units from UDPglucose, building up short maltosaccharide chains, which, when they become long enough, act as the nuclei for the synthesis of glycogen molecules by glycogen

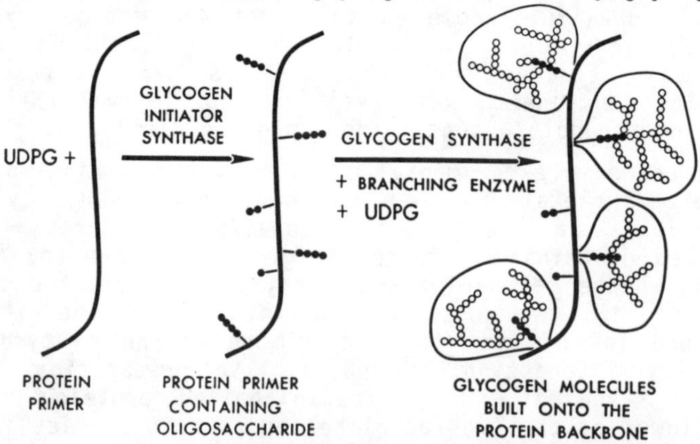

Fig. 3. Krisman's Hypothesis for Glycogen Biosynthesis

synthase and branching enzyme. This proposal by Krisman, originally based on *in vitro* experiments, has now been vindicated by our demonstration of a covalently bound protein in native muscle glycogen. We had earlier reported evidence for such a protein in liver glycogen (7), but did not, at that time, identify the amino acid involved, nor characterize the protein.

The discovery of glycogenin and the nature of its linkage to glycogen may throw some light on the still enigmatic process by which insulin promotes the synthesis of glycogen. The clue comes from the fact that tyrosine is the amino acid involved. Given that, as elaborated elsewhere in this Symposium (8), insulin is now known to transmit the hormonal message by causing its cell-surface receptor to become an active tyrosine kinase, the fact that glycogen is attached to glycogenin via tyrosine would seem to be more than coincidental. Naturally we analysed glycogenin (Fig. 1) for phosphate but found none. This does not rule out that the phosphorylation of glycogenin may precede the construction of glycogen on the protein. Glycogenin is to be seen as the biosynthetic origin of muscle glycogen. The genetic regulation of the amount of glycogenin and its location in the cell could represent another means of control of glycogen metabolism, this one linked to insulin action, with the covalent modification of tyrosine providing a clue as to how this might happen.

ACKNOWLEDGEMENT: This work was supported by the National Institutes of Health (grant no. AM 12532) and the Florida Affiliate of the American Heart Association.

REFERENCES:

(1) Kutz, R.Z. (1886) Z. Biol. 22, 161, cited by Stetten, D., Jr. and Stetten, M.R. (1960) Physiol. Rev. 60, 505-537.

(2) Kennedy, L.D., Kirkman, B.R., Lomako, J., Rodriguez, I.R. and Whelan, W.J. (1985) In "Membranes and Muscle", ed. by Berman, M.C., Gevers, W. and Opie, L.H. pp. 65-84, ICSU Press/IRL Press, Oxford.

(3) Goldsmith, E., Sprang, S. and Fletterick, R. (1982) J. Mol. Biol. 156, 411-427.

(4) Jentoft, N. and Dearborn, D.G. (1979) J. Biol. Chem. 245, 4359-4365.

(5) Rodriguez, I.R. and Whelan, W.J. (1985) Biochem. Biophys. Res. Commun. 132, 829-836.

(6) Krisman, C.R. and Barengo, R. (1975) Eur. J. Biochem. 52, 117-123.

(7) Butler, N.A., Lee, E.Y.C. and Whelan, W.J. (1977) Carb. Res. 55, 73-82.

(8) Advances in Gene Technology: Molecular Biology of the Endocrine System (1986) Ed. by Puett, D. et al. ICSU Short Reports, vol. 4, Cambridge University Press.

(9) Tandecarz, J.S., Moreno, S. and Cardini, C.E. (1984) Abstr. 4th PAABS Congress, Buenos Aires, p.70. See also Tandecarz, J.S., Szalai, E.N. and Cardini, C.E. (1982) FEBS Lett. 139, 313-316.

EXPRESSION AND ANALYSIS OF HUMAN TUMOR NECROSIS FACTOR

S.L. Berent, R.M. Torczynski, N.O. Hill, S. Pichyangkul, F. Jia, J.M. Hill, A. Kahn and A.P. Bollon
Wadley Institutes of Molecular Medicine, 9000 Harry Hines Blvd., Dallas, Texas 75235

Human tumor necrosis factor (TNF) is a protein which has been shown to be cytotoxic for various tumor cell lines and capable of killing solid tumors in mice (1). Human TNF cDNA has been isolated from mRNA from the HL-60 cell line (2,3) and the human TNF gene has been isolated from a human genomic library using a rabbit TNF cDNA probe (4). We have isolated human TNF cDNA made against mRNA from virus induced human peripheral blood leukocytes (PBLs) (5). The molecular weight of human recombinant TNF is 45,000 daltons by gel filtration and 17,000 daltons by SDS polyacrylamide gel electrophoresis (1-3). Mouse TNF has also been cloned and shown to have about 80% homology at the protein sequence level with human TNF (6,7).

(1) <u>High Level Transcription of TNF and IFN-α in Human PBLs.</u> Poly(A) RNA was isolated from uninduced and Sendai virus induced human PBLs. The poly(A) RNA of the induced cells was utilized for the construction of a cDNA library which contained over 30,000 <u>E. coli</u> clones. From this library at least 10 alpha interferon (IFN-α) clones were isolated. RNA dot hybridization with an IFN-α probe indicated high levels of IFN-α mRNA in induced poly(A) RNA compared to uninduced poly(A) RNA.

Surprisingly, RNA dot hybridization with a 17-base oligonucleotide TNF probe indicated that Sendai virus induced PBLs also contained a high level of TNF mRNA. The TNF mRNA levels peaked 3-5 hrs after the priming of the PBLs with IFN-α (1-3 hrs after induction with Sendai virus).

(2) <u>Cloning of Human TNF cDNA.</u> The cDNA library made against Sendai virus induced human PBLs was screened with the 17-base TNF probe. Four clones containing TNF cDNA were isolated from approximately 20,000 screened cDNA clones. In addition, one TNF cDNA clone constructed from the same Sendai virus induced mRNA contained a human TNF cDNA insert which encoded a full length mature protein sequence. Hybridization of the induced cDNA library filters with the TNF cDNA insert indicated that the frequency of TNF clones was at the surprisingly high level of 0.05%. These results suggest that the frequency of TNF mRNA in the PBLs was at least 10 fold higher than that found for HL-60 cells (2,3). In addition, these results suggest that the levels of TNF mRNA in the PBLs are similar to the levels of IFN-α mRNA. Comparison of the nucleotide sequence of the mature TNF cDNA isolated from human PBLs with the cDNA isolated from the HL-60 cell line (2,3) and a genomic TNF clone (4) indicates that the nucleotide sequences are identical.

Although the TNF and IFN-α mRNA levels are similiar in induced PBLs, the amount of IFN-α present in the media is about 200 fold higher than TNF. Possible explanations for these results are that the secreted TNF has a shorter half-life than the IFN-α, or the TNF mRNA is under some form of translational control.

(3) Expression of Human TNF in E. coli. For TNF expression, we have utilized an expression vector containing a consensus Shine-Dalgarno sequence, a P_L promoter, and a gene for a temperature sensitive cI repressor. The TNF cDNA contained in this vector is induced at 42°C and generates a 17,300 dalton polypeptide. TNF activity, based on L929 cell cytotoxicty, was at levels of up to 10^9 U/l (5).

(4) Analysis of Human TNF. Related and unrelated human tumor cell lines show varying degrees of sensitivity to recombinant TNF. The breast adenocarcinoma line BT-20 shows 50% kill with 250 U/ml of TNF, whereas the breast carcinoma cell line SKBR-3 requires 62,500 U/ml for 50% kill. Other human cell lines, such as cervix, melanoma, ovary and colon tumor cell lines, also show sensitivity to recombinant TNF. Potentiation of cytotoxic activity of TNF has been shown for sodium butyrate, IFN-α, and gamma interferon (IFN-γ) for cervix and melanoma cell lines. Recombinant TNF is effective in necrotizing sarcoma 180 tumors in female Balb/c mice. The LD_{50} of purified TNF in Balb/c mice was determined to be 6 X 10^7 U/kg. The therapeutic dose of TNF in sarcoma 180 bearing Balb/c mice was determined to be 3 X 10^5 U/kg.

Phase I clinical trials of recombinant TNF produced at the Wadley Institutes was initiated on September 25, 1985. The TNF has been administered intravenously and the doses escalated on alternate days by a modified Fibonacci scheme.

REFERENCES

(1) Old, L.J. (1985) Science 230, 630-632.

(2) Pennica, D., Nedwin, G.E., Hayflick, J.S., Seeburg, P.H., Derynck, R., Palladino, M.A., Kohr, W.J., Aggarwal, B.B. and Goeddel, D.V. (1984) Nature 312, 724-729.

(3) Wang, A.M., Creasey, A.A., Ladner, M.B., Lin, L.S., Strickler, J., Van Arsdell, J.N., Yamamoto, R. and Mark, D.F. (1985) Science 228, 149-154.

(4) Shirai, T., Yamaguchi, H., Ito, H., Todd, C.W. and Wallace, R.B. (1985) Nature 313, 803-806.

(5) Bollon, A.P., Torczynski, R.M., Hendrix, L.C., Sidhu, R.S. and Berent, S.L., "The Biology of the Interferon System," eds. Schellekens, H. and Stewart, W.E., Elsevier Science Publishers BV, Amsterdam, Netherlands, in press.

ACKNOWLEDGEMENTS

Some of this work was performed in the Oree Meadows Perryman Laboratory and supported by the Meadows Foundation, the Samuel Roberts Noble Foundation, Mary Kay Foundation, and in part a NIH grant to APB.

EXPRESSION OF c-myc, c-myb and c-fos mRNA DURING INDUCTION OF DIFFERENTIATION MYELOMONOCYTIC LEUKEMIC CELLS

F. Bettens, E. Schlick, W. L. Farrar and F. W. Ruscetti
Laboratory of Molecular Immunoregulation, BRMP, DCT, NCI-FCRF, Frederick, MD 21701-1013 USA

Two sublines, the WEHI-3B D^+ and the WEHI-3BD^- line have been derived from the murine myelomonocytic leukemic cell line WEHI-3B (1,2). The D^+ subline can terminally differentiate into granulocytes and/or macrophages in response to colony stimulating factor (G-CSF), whereas the D^- subline does not respond to G-CSF. This unresponsiveness was reported by Nicola et al (3) to be due to the alteration or loss of the G-CSF receptor. To determine whether the inability of the D^- line to respond to CSF was only due to absence of CSF receptor or whether other intracellular events involved in cell differentiation were intact in D^- as well as D^+ cells, phorbolester (PMA) and 1.25 dihydroxycholecalciferol (calciferol) were used as alternative inducing agents and the expression of oncogenes measured.

MATERIALS AND METHODS: Soft agar colony assay was performed according to Metcalf et al. (4). Briefly, 300 cells were plated in 0.3% agar and colonies counted after 7 days of incubation. For morphological studies cytospin preparation of cells were stained by Wright-Giemsa. For dot blot analyses polyribosomal RNA was extracted, blotted in increasing concentration of 5, 10, 20 ng/blot and hybridized with ^{32}P-labeled nick-translated c-oncogene plasmids.

RESULTS:

Effect of Calciferol and PMA on WEHI-3B Colony Formation and Morphological Differentiation. The WEHI-3BD^+ line which responds to G-CSF was induced to differentiate into monocyte-macrophages by PMA treatment but was unresponsive to calciferol. In contrast the subline WEHI-3BD^- which is unresponsive to G-CSF and PMA was induced to differentiate to granulocytes by low doses of calciferol. Both differentiation pathways were accompanied by increases in the number of differentiated colonies, a reduced number of cells per colony and cessation of cell proliferation (Table 1).

Effect of Calciferol and PMA on WEHI-Oncogene Expression. As seen in Table 2, the relative levels of c-myc, c-myb and c-fos induced in PMA or calciferol stimulated cells did not correlate with the ability of the cell to differentiate. Although not differentiated by PMA, the D^- line showed a greater increase in the expression of c-fos in response to PMA than the D^+ line. The G-CSF sensitive D^+ line, only showed small changes in c-myc and c-myb expression after PMA or calciferol induction. However the D^- line showed a decreased expression of c-myc and c-myb after PMA or calciferol induction.

DISCUSSION: Although unresponsive to the normal hematopoietic differentiation factor (G-CSF) or PMA, the D⁻ line still possesses the ability to differentiate in response to agents that bypass the plama membrane such as calciferol. The expression of oncogenes is also modulated in the D⁻ line, independent of morphological differentiation. Thus, although not differentiating into granulocytes or macrophages, the D⁻ line is still able to be stimulated to some extent to express c-fos by PMA. The results also suggest that regulation of oncogene expression in the WEHI-3B lines occurs independently of whether or not the inducing signals have concomitant antiproliferative and differentiative effects. Additionally, because of opposite effect of PMA or calciferol on c-myc and c-myb expression in the D⁻ versus the D⁺ line, the expression of oncogenes appears to be an attribute of the cell specific rather than an event linked to morphological cell differentiation.

Table 1: Soft Agar Colony Assay

Cell Line	Differentiation Agent	Total Number of Colonies	% Differentiated Colonies
WEHI-D⁺	-	147 ± 30	21 ± 6
	G-CSF	110 ± 19	95 ± 13
	PMA 40 ng/ml	73 ± 8	72 ± 2
	Calcif. 1.6 ng/ml	150 ± 29	27 ± 2
WEHI-D⁻	-	145 ± 15	5 ± 3
	G-CSF	134 ± 12	10 ± 3
	PMA 40 ng/ml	116 ± 24	4 ± 2
	Calcif. 1.6 ng/ml	106 ± 38	73 ± 15

Table 2: Changes in Oncogene Expression Levels

Cell Line	Hours of incubation	c-*fos*		c-*myc*		c-*myb*	
		PMA 40ng/ml	Calciferol 1.6/ml	PMA	Calciferol	PMA	Calciferol
WEHI-D⁺	24	+ 38	-10	+16	+28	-12	+30
WEHI-D⁻	24	+124	+30	-50	-42	-50	-20

a Densitometer scans of dot-blot analyses expressed as % of densities measured for RNA levels in unstimulated cells.

REFERENCES

1) Warner, N. L., Moore, M. A. S., and Metcalf, D. (1969) J. Natl. Cancer Inst. 43, 963-982.
2) Ralph, P., Moore, M. A. S., and Nilson, K. (1976) J. Exp. Med. 143, 1528-1533.
3) Nicola, N. A., and Metcalf, D. (1984) Proc. Natl. Acad. Sci. U.S.A. 81, 3765-3769.
4) Metcalf, D. (1980) Intl. J. Cancer 24, 616-623.

DEVELOPMENT-SPECIFIC EXPRESSION OF INSULIN-LIKE GROWTH FACTOR II mRNA IN DIFFERENT RAT TISSUES.

A. L. Brown, D. E. Graham, S. P. Nissley, D. J. Hill*, and M. M. Rechler

National Institutes of Health, Bethesda, MD 20892 and *University of Sheffield, Sheffield, S10 2TH, England

INTRODUCTION

Insulin-like growth factor II (IGF-II) is present at high levels in fetal and early neonatal rat serum, and decreases abruptly to 20-100-fold lower levels by 3 weeks after birth (1). Synthesis of IGF-II has been demonstrated *in vitro* in liver (2), fibroblasts (3), and muscle (4) from term gestation rats. Recently, using a cDNA probe for rat IGF-II (5, 6), several IGF-II RNA species have been demonstrated by Northern analysis in a rat liver cell line (BRL-3A) and in neonatal liver. These include a predominant 4 kilobase (kb) form, as well as 6, 2.2, 1.7, and 1.2 kb species (7). A coordinate decrease of all rIGF-II RNA species occurs in rat liver between 15 and 25 days after birth (8). We have proposed that they represent alternatively processed forms of a primary RNA transcript (8).

In the present study, we ask which fetal rat tissues express IGF-II RNA, whether the sizes of these RNAs are similar to those observed in rat liver, and whether IGF-II RNA levels in different tissues are regulated similarly.

METHODS

Total RNAs were isolated from rat tissues by the guanidinium thiocyanate-lithium chloride procedure (8). Slot blots or Northern blots were examined by hybridization with a rat IGF-II probe (5, 8). RNAs from all tissues were undegraded with the exception of pancreatic RNA, which was partially degraded but still hybridizable to a rat insulin probe in a slot-blot experiment.

RESULTS

(1) IGF-II RNA was detected in 11 of 13 fetal tissues (16 or 21 days gestation). These included liver, lung, muscle, heart, kidney, skin, thymus, intestine, hypothalamus, brain stem and cortex. No hybridization was observed to RNA from fetal spleen or pancreas.

(2) As many as 5 IGF-II RNA species (6, 4, 2.2, 1.7, and 1.2 kb) could be distinguished after short or long autoradiographic exposures of Northern blots of all fetal tissues that contained IGF-II RNA. In general, the 4 kb form was most prominent. Each RNA species corresponded to a form seen in BRL-3A cells and neonatal liver; no new RNA species were observed in any of the positive tissues.

(3) IGF-II mRNA levels were in general much higher in fetal tissues than in adult tissues (75 days of age). Preliminary results suggest a greater persistence of IGF-II RNA in adult hypothalamus and

cortex than in other tissues examined, possibly suggesting a special postnatal role for IGF-II in brain.

CONCLUSIONS

IGF-II mRNA is widely distributed in fetal rat tissues. The same five IGF-II RNA species previously observed in BRL-3A cells and neonatal rat liver, thought to arise by alternate processing of a single primary transport, were observed in all positive tissues. In all tissues, IGF-II RNA levels were high in the fetus and decreased after birth, suggesting that IGF-II may be a general growth factor in the fetus.

REFERENCES

1. Moses, A. C., Nissley, S. P., Short, P. A., Rechler, M. D., White R. M., Knight A. B., and Higa, O. Z. Proc. Natl. Acad. Sci. U.S.A. 77, 3649-3653, 1980.
2. Rechler, M. M., Eisen, H. J., Higa, O. Z., Nissley, S. P., Moses, A. C., Schilling, E. E., Fennoy, I., Bruni, C. B., Phillips, L. S., and Baird, K. L. J. Biol. Chem. 254, 7942-7950, 1979.
3. Adams, S. O., Nissley, S. P., Handwerger, S., and Rechler, M. M. Nature 302, 150-153, 1983
4. Hill, D. J., Crace, C. J., Nissley, S. P., Norrell, D., Holder, A. T., and Milner, R. D. G. Endocrinology 117, 2061-2072, 1985.
5. Whitfield, H. J., Bruni, C. B., Frunzio, R., Terrell, J. E., Nissley, S. P., and Rechler, M. M. Nature 312, 277-280, 1984.
6. Rechler, M. M., Bruni, C. B., Whitfield, H. J., Yang, Y. W.-H., Frunzio, R., Graham, D. E., Coligan, J. E., Terrell, J. E., Acquaviva, A. M., and Nissley, S. P. Cancer Cells 3, 131-138, 1985.
7. Rechler, M. M., Bruni, C. B., Yang, Y. W.-H., Whitfield, H. J., Graham, D. E., Frunzio, R., Brown, A. L., and Nissley, S. P. This volume.
8. Graham, D. E., Rechler, M. M., Brown, A. L., Frunzio, R., Romanus, J. A., Bruni, C. B., Whitfield, H. J., Nissley, S. P., Seelig, S., and Berry, S. Manuscript in preparation.

ACID PHOSPHATASES AS LOCAL MODULATORS OF PROSTATIC CELL GROWTH

S. Chevalier, C. Bourassa, G. Bleau, K. D. Roberts, A. Chapdelaine
Maisonneuve Hospital, 5415 L'Assomption, Montreal, Canada H1T2M4

In previous studies on acid phosphatase (AP), it was demonstrated that in canine and human prostatic epithelial cells, the AP content increases with the duration of the culture (1,2). In the canine model, the specific activity of the enzyme rises sharply by days 10-14, a period which coincides with the arrest of cell proliferation (3). The synthesis of AP also occurs and, after gel electrophoresis, the predominant form was similar to that present in freshly dissociated cells (3). The aim of the present investigation was first to determine whether this AP from cultured cells was similar to the prostatic acid phosphatases (PAP) secreted in seminal plasma, and secondly, to test the possibility that the enzyme may act as a phosphotyrosine protein phosphatase which could be involved in the regulation of cell proliferation. To this end, the immunoreactivity of the cellular and secreted AP was tested. The effect of phosphatase inhibitors and the activity of the enzyme towards substrates such as phosphoaminoacids were also evaluated.

(I) IMMUNOREACTIVITY. AP synthesis in canine prostatic epithelial cells is maximally induced after long term culture (3-4 weeks) in the presence of dog serum (4); extracts from cells cultured under these conditions were used for dot blotting on nitrocellulose. As shown in Fig 1, the following preparations gave a positive peroxidase reaction after incubation with a rabbit antiserum against purified human PAP: crude human seminal plasma (c) and its partially purified PAP (b), crude dog seminal plasma (d), and its PAP partially purified by gel filtration (e) and extracts from cultured cells (f). Bovine serum albumin did not react (a). All preparations gave a negative reaction when incubated with normal rabbit serum.

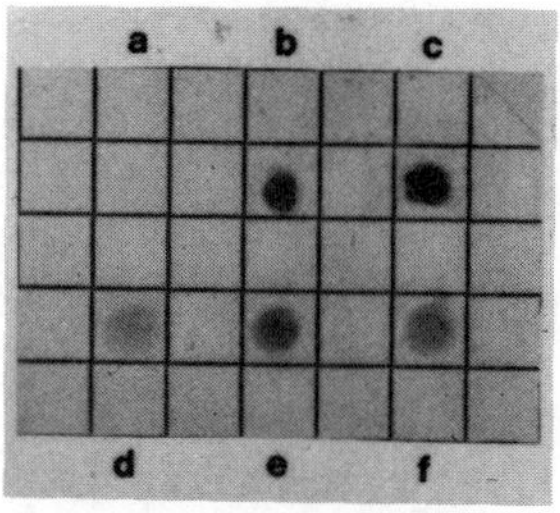

Fig.1. Immunodetection of PAP

(II) INHIBITORS. Canine seminal plasma was used as the source of PAP. The activity was assayed for 15 min as described (1). Phosphoaminoacids and known inhibitors of phosphatases were added along with 0.52 mM of p-nitrophenylphosphate (p-npp) as substrate. Fig. 2 shows that orthovanadate was the most potent inhibitor with a D_{50} (concentration which results in a 50% inhibition) of 43 uM. In decreasing order of potency were tartrate, molybdate and fluoride with D_{50} values of 0.19, 0.40 and 0.68 mM. o-p-tyrosine (p-tyr) also showed significant inhibitory activity (D_{50} of 5.0 mM) while $ZnCl_2$, o-p-threonine

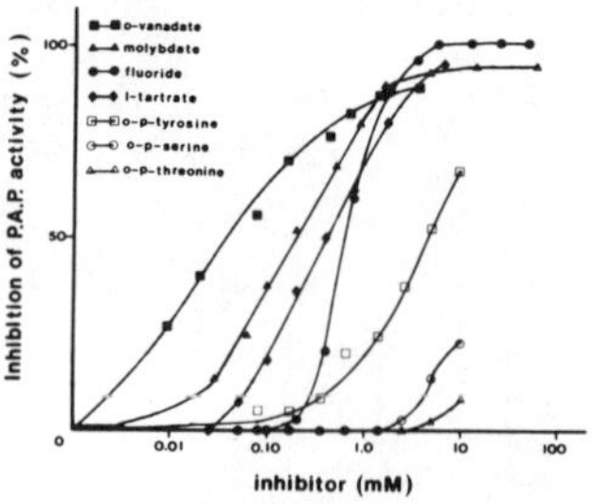

Fig. 2. Inhibition of PAP activity

(p-thre), o-p-serine(p-ser) and their dephosphorylated derivatives showed little or no inhibitory activity.

(III) PHOSPHOAMINOACIDS AS SUBSTRATES. Using phosphoaminoacids as substrates (at 5 mM), the activity of PAP was assayed as in (II); the reaction was followed by the determination of phosphate liberated (umole/h) (5). p-tyr was preferentially hydrolyzed (0.31) while minimal activity of PAP was observed towards p-thre (0.07) and p-ser (0.02). As shown in fig. 3, the K_m for p-tyr was 6.6 mM, a value similar to its D_{50} found in the inhibition of p-npp hydrolysis by PAP.

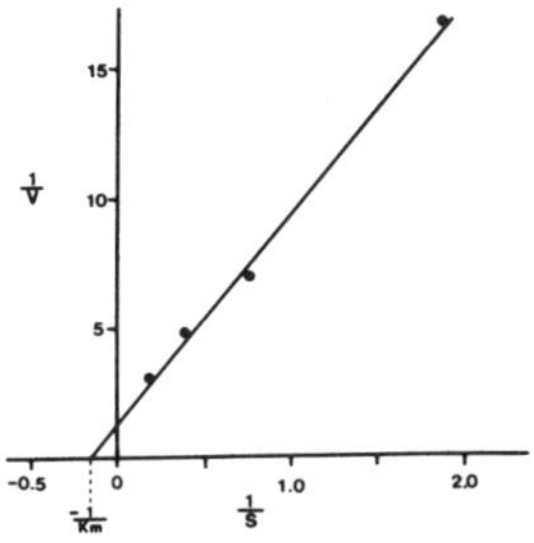

Fig.3.Lineweaver-Burk plot

The AP produced by cultured canine prostatic epithelial cells, like the PAP present in dog seminal plasma, was found to possess common antigenic determinants with secretory PAP of human seminal plasma. The fact that PAP from dog seminal plasma is strongly inhibited by orthovanadate, a specific inhibitor of phosphotyrosine protein phosphatase (6) and that it selectively hydrolyzes o-p-tyrosine, indicates that canine PAP, as reported for human PAP (7), may be a phosphotyrosine protein phosphatase. Interestingly, the arrest of cell proliferation coincides with a sharp increase in the specific activity of AP. Moreover, AP activity as well as the proliferation of canine and human prostatic cells in culture are reported to be regulated by non-steroidal factors, other than EGF and FGF, that are present in serum and prostatic tissue (4). From these data it is proposed that in vivo sex steroids may influence prostatic growth through non-steroidal intermediates and that within the cell, the level of PAP, acting as a phosphotyrosine protein phosphatase, may be an important factor in the modulation of cell growth.

Supported by MRC, FCAR, FRSQ, Univ of Montreal. The technical assistance of Ms D.Landry is acknowledged.

REFERENCES

1. Chevalier S., Bleau G., Roberts K.D., Chapdelaine A. (1981) Mol. Cell Endocrinol. 24, 195-208.
2. Chevalier S., Larochelle R., Dorais C., Bleau G., Roberts K.D. Chapdelaine A. (1980), Union Med. Can. (Suppl.) La Reproduction S29-33.
3. Dionne F.T., Chevalier S., Bleau G., Roberts K.D. Chapdelaine A. (1983) Mol. Cell Endocrinol. 33, 113-126.
4. Chapdelaine A., Chevalier S. (1985) In, "Regulation of Androgen Action". (Bruchovsky, N. et al., Eds.) pp 205-210, Congressdruck R. Bruckner, W. Berlin.
5. Ames B.N.,(1966) In, "Methods in Enzymology" (Neufeld E. F. and Ginsburg, V.,eds), vol 8, pp 115-118, Acad. Press Inc., NY.
6. Swarup G.,Cohen S., Garbers D.L., (1982) Biochem. Biophys. Res. Comm. 107, 1104-1109.
7. Li H.G., Chernoff J., Chen L.B., Kirschonbaum A. (1984). Eur. J. Biochem. 138, 45-51.

CONSTITUTIVE FORMATION OF MACROPHAGE-GRANULOCYTE (GM) AND MACROPHAGE (M) COLONY STIMULATING FACTORS BY MURINE LEUKEMIA X FIBROBLAST HYBRID CELLS

E.P. Cohen[1], H.S.Chow[2] and K. Hagen[1] [1]Department of Microbiology and Immunology, University of Illinois College of Medicine and [2]Department of Hematology, Rush Presbyterian St. Lukes Medical Center, Chicago. Box 6998 Chicago 60680

A leukemia x fibroblast hybrid cell line was found to form GM-CSF and M-CSF in the absence of granulocyte (G) CSF, without the deliberate addition of inducing agents. ASL-1 cells, a leukemia cell line maintained by serial transfer in histocompatible recipients ($H-2^a$), was fused with LM cells, an established mouse cell line of fibroblast origin. (1) (A thymidine kinase deficient varient was used to facilitate selection.) Selection of hybrid cells was accomplished in HAT-medium; they possessed a hybrid karyotype (65 ± 6 chromosomes) and expressed the histocompatibility antigens of both parental sources. (2) The cells were maintained under standard culture conditions in RPMI medium supplemented with 10 percent fetal calf serum and had been in continuous culture for a period of 10 months at the time the assays were performed.

Clonogenic assays for M, GM, granulocyte (G) and erythrocyte (E) precursors of rat or mouse marrow cells were performed in the presence of medium conditioned by the growth of 5×10^6 leukemia x fibroblast hybrid cells in 10 ml of medium for 24 hrs; the data were expressed as colony forming units (CFUs) per 10^5 mononuclear cells. In some experiments, antibody neutralization tests were carried out using goat antiserum against purified mouse M-CSF (3), (kindly provided by E.R. Stanley, Albert Einstein College of Medicine, N.Y.). As a known source of CSFs, media conditioned by WEHI-3 and rat spleen cells were substituted for conditioned medium (CM) from the hybrid cells.(4) The analysis revealed the presence of both GM and M (but not G) CFU in marrow cultures maintained in the presence of CM from hybrid cells (162 ± 10 total colonies per 10^5 cells) and from LM cells (65 ± 5). CM from ASL-1 cells did not lead to the formation of CFU.

The failure to detect G CFUs in the presence of GM and M CFUs was unexpected. This point was investigated further by preparing replicate cultures of marrow from C57Bl/6 mice and continuing the incubation for 14 days. G CFUs were not found at any point during the period.

Further experiments revealed that hybrid cell conditioned medium (CM) supported the development of M and GM (but not G) CFUs from the marrow of DBA, CAF_1, BDF_1 and $C3D2F_1$ as well as from C57Bl/6 mice. M and GM (but not G) CFUs were found in marrow cultures from Lewis, Brown Norway and Wistar Furth rats indicating that the activity in CM was not restricted to cells from mice alone.

Hybrid cell-CM supported the long-term cultivation of macrophage-like cells from mouse spleen, consistent with the presence of M-CSF. The cells were grown continuously for periods in excess of three months in RPMI medium supplemented with 10 percent fetal calf serum and 25 percent CM. Cells transfered to medium without CM ceased dividing and disintegrated within 10-14 days. Further confimation of the presence of M-CSF in the CM was obtained by radioimmunoassay, using purified M-CSF. (The analysis was performed by Dr. Stanley.)

The presence of M-CSF in hybrid cell-CM was also supported by the results of antibody neutralization studies. CM incubated with goat anti M-CSF before it was added to primary cultures of mouse marrow led to the reduction in both M as well as GM CFUs suggesting that these two CSFs express crossreactive antigenic determinants. Alternatively, the growth of GM CFUs might require the presence of both M as well as GM CSFs.

Attempts to detect each of several other previously defined growth factors were unsuccessful. Interleukins 1, 2 and 3, B cell growth factors, interferons α, β, and γ, erythopoietin and burst promoting factor were not detected in hybrid cell-CM.

REFERENCES.

1. Wang, D.-R., Slomski, R. and Cohen, E.P. Leukema x fibroblast hybrid cells prolong the lives of leukemic mice. Eur. J. Can. and Clin. Oncol. 21:637, 1985
2. Garber, S., Chang, I. and Cohen, E.P. Persistance of the immunoprotective effects of leukemia x fibroblast hybrid cells toward leukemia in histocompatible mice. Leuk. Res. 8:255, 1984
3. Stanley, E.R. and Guilbert, L.J. Methods for the purification, assay, characterization and target binding assay of a colony stimulating factor (CSF-1). J. Immunol. Methods 42:253, 1981.
4. Bowlin, T.L., Scott, A.N. and Ihle, J.N. Biological properties of interleukin-3. J. Immunol. 133:2001, 1984

HEPARINASE TREATMENT OF ENDOTHELIAL CELLS PREVENTS RESPONSE TO HEPATOMA-DERIVED GROWTH FACTOR

Daniel T. Connolly[1], Barry L. Stoddard[1], Mary Beth Knight[1], Nikos K. Harakas[1], Joseph Feder[1], and Michael Klagsbrun[2]

[1]Monsanto Company, 800 N. Lindbergh Blvd., St. Louis, MO 63167; [2]Departments of Biological Chemistry and Surgery, Harvard Medical School and The Children's Hospital, Boston, Massachusetts 02115

Solid tumors are capable of directing the growth of new blood vessels presumably through the release of factors affecting vascular endothelial cell migration and mitosis (1,2). Human hepatoma cells (SK-HEP-1) produce a potent endothelial cell mitogen, hepatoma-derived growth factor (HDGF), which promotes both chemotaxis and growth of fetal bovine aortic endothelial (BAE) cells (3) _in vitro_, (Fig. 1) and thus, possesses two of the activities needed to promote angiogenesis. In addition, we present evidence suggesting that HDGF binds to a heparin-like proteoglycan on the endothelial cell surface (Fig. 2). The latter result may explain the general observation that endothelial cell mitogens have a high affinity for heparin, and other observations implicating heparin as a likely participant in angiogenesis.

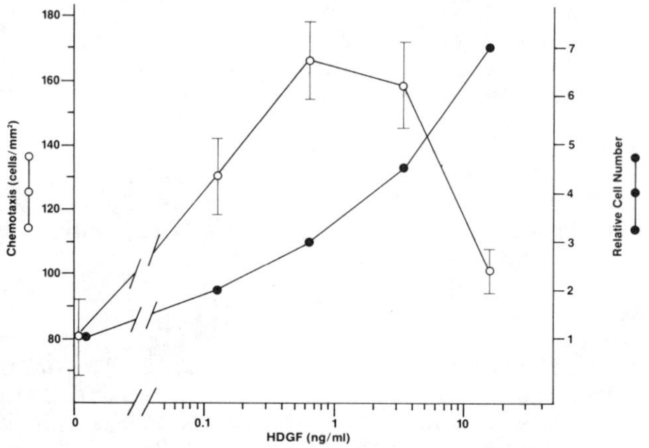

Fig.1. Stimulation of Endothelial Cell Chemotaxis or Growth by Hepatoma-Derived Growth Factor. Endothelial cell growth or chemotaxis were measured in the presence of different concentrations of HDGF which was purified as described (4). BAE cell growth assays were conducted by plating cells in 96-well plates (600 cells per well), and cell number determined after 6 days using a spectrophotometric assay for acid phosphatase (5). Boyden chamber chemotaxis assays were conducted using a 48-well apparatus (Neuroprobe). BAE cells and HDGF were placed on opposite sides of 5μm membranes (Nucleopore), and incubated for 4 hours at 37°C (6). After scraping cells from the top of the membrane, the cells which had migrated to the bottom surface were fixed, stained and counted.

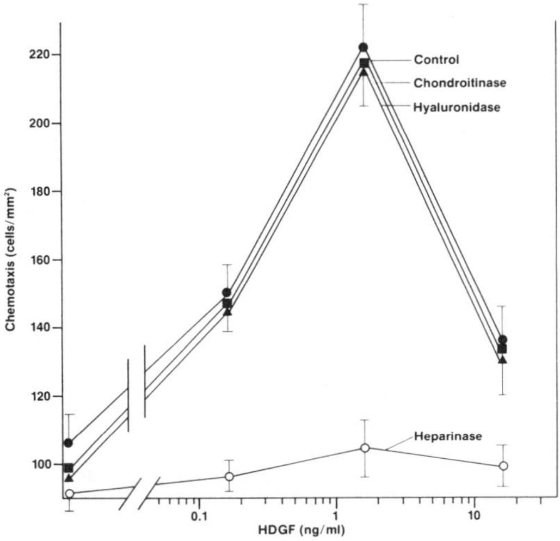

Fig. 2. Effect of Heparinase, Chondroitinase, or Hyaluronidase Treatments on Endothelial Cell Chemotaxis. BAE cell suspensions in 2 ml of serum free DMEM were incubated for 30 min. at 37°C with equal volumes of DMEM containing either heparinase (*Flavobacterium heparinum*, chondroitinase ABC (*Proteus vulgaris*), hyaluronidase (bovine testes), or PBS as control. The enzyme concentrations were adjusted to liberate 50-60 nanomoles per minute of product. After incubation, the cell suspensions were centrifuged and the supernatants containing the enzymes and reaction products were removed. The cells were resuspended in DMEM containing 10% calf serum and the chemotaxis assay performed as described in Fig. 1.

ACKNOWLEDGEMENTS: We thank Dr. Susan R. Doctrow (Harvard Medical School) for providing heparinase, and Dr. Jitka V. Olander (Monsanto) for providing endothelial cells.

REFERENCES

1. Folkman, J. (1985) Adv. Cancer Res. 43, 175-203.
2. Folkman, J. (1982) Annals N.Y. Acad. Sci. 401, 212-227; Ausprunk, D.H., and Folkman, J. (1977) Microvasc. Res. 14, 53-65.
3. Olander, J.V., Marasa, J., Kimes, R.C., Johnston, G., and Feder, J. (1982) In Vitro 18, 99-107.
4. Shing, Y., Folkman, J., Sullivan, R., Butterfield, C., Murray, J., and Klagsbrun, M. (1984) Science 223, 1296-1298.
5. Connolly, D.T., Knight, M.B., Harakas, N.K., Wittwer, A.J., and Feder, J. (1985) Anal. Biochem., in press.
6. Boyden, S. (1962) J. Exp. Med. 115, 453-466; Falk, W., Goodwin, R., and Leonard, E. (1980) J. Immun. Meth. 33, 239-247; Harvath, L., Falk, W., and Leonard E. (1980) J. Immun. Meth. 37, 39-45.

PRECISE LOCALIZATION OF THE HU-ETS-2 GENE TO THE CRITICAL REGION OF CHROMOSOME 21 IN t8;21 AML AND DOWN SYNDROME

H.A. Drabkin[1,2], M. Van Keuren[1], I. Hart[1], P Duesberg[3], N. Sacchi[4], T.S. Papas[4], and D. Patterson[1,5,6]
[1]Eleanor Roosevelt Institute for Cancer Research, Denver CO; [2]Division of Medical Oncology, [5]Dept. of Med., [6]Dept. of Biochem. Biophys and Genet, University of Colorado Health Sciences Center, Denver CO 80262; [3]Dept. of Molecular Biology and Virus Laboratory, University of California, Berkeley; [4]Laboratory of Molecular Oncology, Fredericks Cancer Facility.

Human DNA sequences homologous to v-ets have been isolated and localized to chromosome 11q23-24 (1). Recently, it has been demonstrated that in contrast to the single avian c-ets locus, the human gene, as well as both murine and feline genes, are split (2,3). Human DNA sequences homologous to the 5' region of the avian v-ets gene are located on chromosome 11 (Hu-ets-1), while those sequences homologous to the 3' v-ets region are located on chromosome 21 (Hu-ets-2). Both loci are transcriptionally active. We have used somatic cell hybrids to precisely localize the Hu-ets-2 gene within region q22.3 of chromosome 21, which appears to be critical to the development of t(8;21) acute myelogenous leukemia and also to the development of Down Syndrome. We have previously reported the isolation and analysis of the 21q+ chromosome from the AML 8;21 translocation (4). We now report the isolation of the 8q- portion of this translocation and demonstrate the reciprocal nature of this translocation.

METHODS: The following are CHO-human hybrids: cell lines 72532X-6 and 2FUr1 contain the entire chromosome 21 and the long arm of 21, respectively, as their only detectable human material. R2-10 contains a ring 21 as the only identifiable human material isolated from the fibroblast cell line GM 6137. The breakpoints in this ring chromosome are 21q22.3 and 21p11.2 (5). 21-8Ab5-23a contains the 21q+ chromosome as the only human material from the AML 8;21 translocation. J1 contains chromosome 11 (kindly provided by Dr. Carol Jones) as the only human material. 8;21/GB-12 contains a normal chromosome 8 as the only human material isolated from t(8;21) AML cells. Hybrid 13b1S8 contains the 8q- chromosome isolated from t(8;21) AML cells in the absence of a normal 8, 21 or 21q+ chromosome. t(8;21) AML cells were kindly provided by Drs. Jose Trujillo and Ann Cork. In agreement with our previous studies (4), hybrid 13b1S8 was found to contain human glutathione reductase activity (8p21), human c-mos DNA sequences (8q22), but did not contain human c-myc DNA sequences (8q24.1), nor human chromosome 21 superoxide dismutase (SOD-1) activity (21q22.1). Hybridization was to a nick translated v-ets specific probe (6) under moderately stringent conditions.

RESULTS: Digestion of total human DNA with EcoR1, produces four prominent fragments of 6.9, 3.6, 2.0, and 1.1 Kb. The 3.6 Kb EcoR1 fragment represents Hu-ets-2 DNA sequences, and is absent in the J1 hybrid containing human chromosome 11. In contrast, the remaining fragments are detected in the J1 hybrid. The Hu-ets-2 band is present in hybrids 72532X-6 and 2FUr1 which contain chromosome 21 and the long arm of No. 21, respectively. Hu-ets-2 sequences are also present in R2-10, which contains a ring 21, but absent in 21-8Ab5-23a which contains only the human 21q+ chromosome from the AML 8;21 translocation. Both the ring chromosome and the 21q+ chromosome have breakpoints in 21q22.3. We have examined a large number of chromosome 21 specific DNA sequences and have demonstrated that the 21q22.3 breakpoint in the ring chromosome is distal to the 21q22.3 breakpoint in the 8;21 translocation (Van Keuren et al., submitted). The DNA sequence pPW231C is located at the q22.3 breakpoint in the ring chromosome (7), and is germline in the 21q+ chromosome. Therefore, the Hu-ets-2 gene is proximal to the DNA sequence pPW231C. This localizes the Hu-ets-2 gene to the small overlap region of chromosome 21q22.3 between the ring and the t(8;21) breakpoints. Cytogenetically, the 8;21 translocation is felt to be reciprocal. The absence of Hu-ets-2 DNA sequences in the 21q+ chromosome and the presence of these sequences in the 8q- chromosome confirms the reciprocal nature of this translocation.

CONCLUSION: Using somatic cell hybrids, we have precisely localized Hu-ets-2 to region q22.3 of chromosome 21. At the molecular level, Hu-ets-2 is proximal to the DNA sequence pPW231C which is located in region q22.3. Translocation of 21q material to chromosome 8 is the constant feature in variant 3-way 8;21 translocations, an observation which led to speculation that an oncogene might be present on chromosome 21. The precise localization of the Hu-ets-2 to a subregion of band 21q22.3 near to the breakpoint observed in AML reinforces its possible involvement in this disease. Subregional assignment of Hu-ets-2 to this region of chromosome 21 is of additional importance because it is this region which is thought to be pathogenetic for Down Syndrome, the most frequent identifiable genetic cause of mental retardation which is associated with a large number of developmental abnormalities, including a markedly increased risk for the development of acute leukemia.

REFERENCES: (1) de Taisne, C., Gegonne, A. and Stehelin, D. (1984) Nature 310:581-583; (2) Watson, D.K., Smith, M.J., Kozak, C., Reeves, R., Gearhart, J., Nunn, M.F., Nash, W1, Fowle, J.R. III, Duesberg, P., Papas, T.S. and O'Brien, S.J. (1985) Proc. Natl. Acad. Sci USA, in press; (3) Watson, D.K., McWilliams-Smith, M.J., Nunn, M.F., Duesberg, P.H., O'Brien, S.J., and Papas, T.S. (1985) Proc. Natl. Acad. Sci USA, in press; (4) Drabkin, H.A., Diaz, M., Bradley, C.M., Le Beau, M.M., Rowley, J.D. and Patterson, D. (1985) Proc. Natl. Acad. Sci USA 82:464-468; (5) Stetten, G., Sroka, B., Corson, V.L., and Boehm, C.D. (1984) Hum. Genet. 68:310-313; (6) Nunn, M., Weiher, H., Bullock, P. and Duesberg, P. (1984) Virology 139:330-339; (7) Kittur, S., Antonarakis, S.E., Groner, Y., Phillips, J.A., Meyers, D. and Kazazian, H.H. (1985) Am. J. Hum. Genet. 36(suppl 4):1425.

Genomic Instability Associated with Tumor Progression in Hamster Brain Tumors. Duigou, G.[+], Fetherston, J.[+], Walsh, J.W.[*], and Zimmer, S.G.[+]. Department of Medical Microbiology and Immunology[+] and Department of Surgery[*], University of Kentucky Medical Center, Lexington, KY 40536-0084

Introduction

Primary intracranial tumors are a relatively common form of neoplasia, resulting in 10-15,000 operations in the U.S. each year (1). Over 40% of these tumors are of glial origin and most are highly invasive (2). This quality of invasiveness, which is poorly understood, makes surgical removal extremely difficult. In an attempt to elucidate the molecular mechanisms governing invasiveness in these tumors, we developed an experimental system using SV40-transformed hamster glial cells derived from the cerebral cortex (3). These cells were tumorigenic when injected intracranially into newborn hamsters. Using both in vivo selection of tumor forming cells and in vitro cloning procedures a panel of cell lines which were either tumorigenic non-invasive or tumorigenic invasive were developed. Interestingly, the original tumor forming cells exhibited increased invasiveness upon multiple in vivo passage. In order to monitor changes in the tumor cell population or the integrated viral DNA which might account for this phenotype we analyzed the SV40 DNA containing fragment patterns in each of our cell lines.

Materials and Methods

Changes in the SV40-viral DNA integration patterns were monitored by Southern blot hybridization (4) using ^{32}P-labeled SV40 DNA or SV40 DNA fragments (1-5 X 10^8 cpm/ug) as probes.

Results and Discussion

The pattern of SV40 DNA containing fragments which were generated by cleavage with EcoRI, BamHI, or BglI, changed as the cells were passed in vivo from Cx4T1 (first passage) to Cx4T3 (third passage). In general, the cloned cell lines derived from the non-invasive Cx4T1 (clones 1-3) and from the highly invasive Cx4T3 (clones 4-6) reflected, to some degree, the integration patterns observed in the tumor cell line of origin. Therefore, the non-invasive clones were similar to each other and to Cx4T1, but were quite distinct from the invasive clones (and vice versa). An XbaI digest (an enzyme which does not cut within the SV40 sequences) revealed the presence of a major band in the 25 Kb region in all cell lines, with a variable minor fragment pattern which differed for each cell line observed. These data suggested that the cell lines could have arisen either by selecting for pre-existing cell populations or by a more dynamic process of cellular rearrangement and selection.

While the question of origin could not be settled in an unequivocal manner, some characteristics of the more invasive cell lines could be investigated. We chose to analyze the stability of the integrated genome to determine if the progeny cells of the cloned invasive cell lines were homogeneous with respect to their SV40 DNA integration pattern. Subclones of the invasive cloned cell lines were derived by cloning in soft agar and the SV40 DNA-integration patterns in each of these cell lines was analyzed and compared with the cloned cell lines of origin. Indeed, BglI digests of subclones of the Cx4T3 derived invasive clones revealed a marked variation in the DNA integration patterns among the cell lines. Alterations of the EcoRI or BamHI patterns were more subtle, but could be detected.

Since the cloned invasive cell lines showed evidence for genomic instability and the fragment patterns changed as a function of *in vivo* passage, this would be due to changes in the flanking cellular sequences, within the viral genomic sequences, or various combinations of the two. We analyzed the Hind III integration patterns which allowed us to examine specific regions of the SV40 genome. We probed for early and late region SV40 sequences by using BglI-BamHI digested SV40 DNA to generate early and late region specific probes. These studies showed clearly that the highly invasive cloned cell lines (Cx4T3 clones 4-6) were missing all or part of the late region specific Hind III fragments. These studies also indicate that the BglI digests would be more likely to demonstrate a more marked heterogeneity in the subclones derived from the invasive cell lines. The EcoRI and BamHI sites may be missing in these cell lines, effectively making these enzymes noncutters resulting in the generation of a greatly simplified integration fragment pattern compared to that obtained with BglI.

All of these results, taken together, indicate, but do not prove, that the more invasive cell lines probably arose as a result of a dynamic process of rearrangement and selection with the resultant generation of a markedly altered cellular (but not necessarily viral) transcriptional program. These transcriptional alterations leading to the induction or suppression of affected gene products are very likely causally related to the acquisition of the invasive phenotype. Our future studies will focus on the identification of these important changes.

References

1. Bignor, D. and Pegram, C.M. (1976) Adv. Neurol. 15:57-83.
2. Rubinstein, L.J. (1976) Adv. Neurol. 15:1-25.
3. Walsh, J.W., Zimmer, S.G., Oeltgen, J. and Markesbery, W. (1982) J. Neuropathol. Exp. Neurol. 41:588-605.
4. Southern, E.M. (1975) J. Mol. Biol. 98:502-517.

Mitogen-Regulated Protein, a member of the prolactin/growth hormone family is regulated like prolactin at the transcriptional and post-translational levels.

R. T. Hamilton, M. Nilsen-Hamilton, V. R. Fienup, and M-H. Jeng.
Departments of Zoology and Biochemistry and Biophysics, Iowa State University, Ames, IA 50011

Mitogen Regulated Protein (MRP) is a secreted protein produced by Swiss 3T3 cells in response to growth factors. MRP is heterogeneously glycosylated with a median M_r of 34,000. The nonglycosylated form of MRP has an M_r of 21,000 [1].

For a series of growth regulators, we have found that the ability to induce MRP is correlated with their ability to stimulate DNA synthesis. Fibroblast growth factor (FGF), epidermal growth factor and platelet-derived growth factor all stimulate both MRP synthesis and DNA synthesis in Swiss 3T3 cells. Tumor promotors also induce MRP. Teleocidin, TPA (12-O-tetradecanoyl phorbol 13-acetate), mezerein and other strong, intermediate and incomplete tumor promotors stimulate the production of MRP to levels comparable to those induced by growth factors. Inactive phorbol esters do not induce MRP. Insulin and beta-TGF also do not stimulate MRP or DNA synthesis in these cells.

The amount of both intracellular and secreted MRP is increased in response to a proliferative signal such as FGF or TPA (Fig. 1). The amount of MRP mRNA is also increased by growth factors in 3T3 cells in parallel with the increase in newly synthesized protein. The increases in MRP protein and mRNA levels are inhibited by alpha-amanatin and actinomycin D. Thus it appears that growth factors and tumor promotors induce MRP by stimulating transcription.

As well as being regulated at transcription by agents that stimulate proliferation, we have found that the levels of MRP are regulated post-translationally by a mechanism that involves degradation of newly synthesized MRP by lysosomal proteases. Our results suggest that a proportion of newly synthesized MRP is degraded without being secreted by a mechanism that may include crinophagy. Crinophagy is a process that occurs when secretory vesicles fuse with lysosomes. The evidence for crinophagy as a means of modulating the secreted level of MRP includes the following. The amount of secreted MRP is increased 2- to 4-fold by lysosomotropic agents and the ionophores, monensin and nigericin. Leupeptin, a thiol protease inhibitor, increases the intracellular level of MRP up to 5-fold over the control [Fig. 1]. All of these agents inhibit proteolysis in the lysosomes. MRP does not seem to be a lysosomal protein as approximately 80% of the MRP synthesized in a six minute pulse is secreted. Once MRP is secreted its level is not altered by either growth factors, lysosomotropic agents, or ionophores.

Prolactin levels are also regulated by growth factors and crinophagy. Because of the similarity in their regulation we suspected a relationship between MRP and prolactin. This was confirmed when we found that MRP is probably the same protein as proliferin, the recently discovered new member of the prolactin/ growth hormone gene family. We have shown that MRP and proliferin are the same in two ways: First, antibodies raised against MRP specifically immunoprecipitate proliferin. Second, a cDNA clone to one MRP which includes the last third of the MRP mRNA sequence is identical to the proliferin sequence [2].

Thus we have shown that MRP and proliferin are in all probability the same protein and that therefore MRP is a member of the prolactin/growth hormone family. As well as being structurally related to prolactin the expression of MRP is regulated similarly to prolactin both at transcriptional and post-translational levels. Growth factors and tumor promotors increase the levels of mRNA coding for prolactin and MRP. At the post-translational level MRP and prolactin levels are modulated by crinophagy.

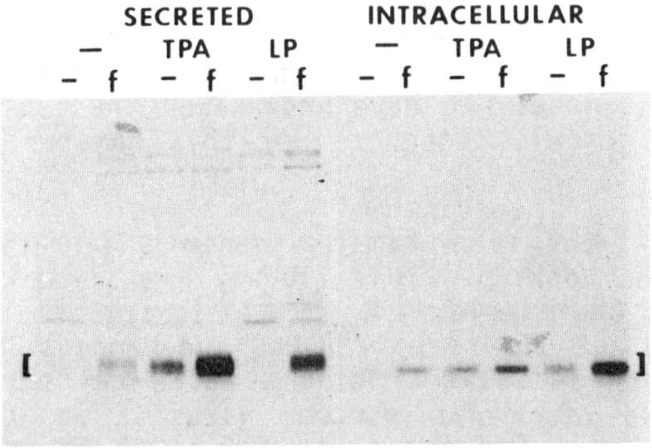

Figure 1. The effect of FGF, TPA, and Leupeptin on the level of MRP. Swiss 3T3 cells were incubated for 16 h with or without 100 ng/ml FGF, 10 ng/ml TPA and 200 ug/ml leupeptin. The cells were labeled for four hours with [^{35}S]methionine and then the medium and the cell layer was collected. The NP-40-soluble fraction of the cells was immunoprecipitated with anti-MRP antiserum. The immunoprecipitated intracellular fractions and samples of the medium were resolved by SDS polyacrylamide gel electrophoresis on gels consisting of a gradient of 7.5 to 15% acrylamide. The radiolabeled proteins were detected by fluorography. The position of MRP is indicated by the brackets. -, control; TPA, TPA; LP, Leupeptin; f, FGF

Acknowledgment: This work was funded by grant CDC-242 from the American Cancer Society

1. Nilsen-Hamilton, M., Shapiro, J. M., Massoglia, S. L., and Hamilton, R. T. (1980) Cell 20, 19-28
2. Nilsen-Hamilton, M. Hamilton, R. T., Allen W. R., and Massoglia, S. L. (1981) Biochem Biophys Res Commun 101, 411-417
3. Parfett, C. L. J., Hamilton, R. T., Howell, B. W., Edwards, D. R., Nilsen-Hamilton, M and Denhardt, D. T. (1985) Mol Cell Biol 5, 3289-3292

ISOLATION OF A SYRIAN HAMSTER PLATELET-DERIVED GROWTH FACTOR cDNA AND GENOMIC SEQUENCES WHOSE EXPRESSION IS REGULATED BY STEROIDS.

S.E. Harris+, J. Hall+, M. Harris+, R. Monk+, J.S. Norris*, and R.G. Smith°

+W. Alton Jones Cell Science Center, Lake Placid, NY, 12946, *Univ. of Arkansas Medical Center, Little Rock AK, °Bayler College of Medicine, Houston, TX.

The hamster ductus deferens tumor cell line, DDT_1-MF-2 is an excellent model system to study androgen stimulated growth of these cells on collagen gels and also how glucocorticoids inhibit their growth (1). Part of the mechanism of this steroid modulation of growth appears to involve the PDGF or c-sis gene in these DDT_1-MF-2 cells. Glucocorticoids added to the media of a 30-40% confluent culture results in the cells flattening out, growth arrest and a large decrease in two PDGF-like mRNAs (4.3 kb and 2.2 kb mRNA on Northern blots). PDGF added back to the media will result in a resumption of growth while the endogenous PDGF mRNA level remains suppressed (2). Androgen added to the media will induce PDGF mRNA under these conditions but is insufficient to induce growth. To further investigate this system, at the molecular level, we have undertaken the isolation of the PDGF-like cDNAs and genomic sequences for this hamster c-sis gene.

MATERIALS AND METHODS. A Syrian hamster genomic library was obtained from J.R. Wu at John Hopkins. This library has 12-18 kb Eco R1 fragments cloned into Charon 4A. A cDNA library to total poly(A)-RNA was prepared in λgt 11. From 250,000 independent recombinants, three cDNA clones were isolated using a twice gel purified probe from the v-sis region of simian sarcoma virus. Two of the clones contained a 4.3 kb insert and one contained a 2.2 kb insert. These fragments were subcloned into pUC13 and the inserts isolated. Using the 4.3 kb and 2.2 kb as probe, the genomic library was screened (3×10^6 plaques) and 25 signals have been purified and are presently being characterized. The 4.3 kb and 2.2 kb cDNA have been sequenced using synthetic primers and rapid deletion cloning in M13 with the dideoxy method using quasi-end labeling of M13 and pUC13 subcloned fragments.

RESULTS. On Northern blots, both the 2.2 kb and 4.3 kb mRNA homologous to v-sis are both down regulated by addition of glucocorticoids to a rapidly growing culture of DDT_1-MF2 cells. The cloned 4.3 kb and 2.2 kb cDNAs of PDGF thus appear to be full length representatives of those two mRNA seen in the Northern blots. By sequencing and restriction mapping, the 2.2 kb and 4.3 have identical 5'-ends. The entire coding region of PDGF is within the 2.2 kb mRNA. There is approximately 1.1 kb of 5'-non-coding region in both 4.3 and 2.2 kb forms. Within the 5'-non-coding region there are extensive areas that have homology to various sarcoma virus DNA sequences. The best homology was to the reverse transcriptase region in simian sarcoma virus. The 3'-non-coding 2.3 kb region of the 4.3 kb form has an extensive stem-loop structure with approximately a 600 bp stem with a 400-500 bp loop as seen by heteroduplex mapping.

When the 4.3 kb cDNA PDGF is used as a probe in a Southern blot, a smear on top of some specific unique bands is noted. The 2.2 kb when used as a probe in a Southern blot gives several unique, single copy bands with several restriction enzymes. When the genomic library was screened with the 4.3 kb cDNA, several hundred signals were observed indicating some repetitive structure within the 3'-non-coding region of the PDGF mRNA from hamster. The library was then rescreened with the 2.2 kb PDGF mRNA and 25 signals have been purified and are presently being characterized.

DISCUSSION. The significance of the extensive double-stranded region in the hamster PDGF mRNA is unknown but we may speculate that it may play some role in mRNA stability, interferon induction and/or inducer of ds RNA-dependent protein kinases. Further sequence information on that region may help in understanding the role of this 3'-non-coding region in this one form of PDGF mRNA. Finding regions in the 5'-non-coding region homologous to specific regions of simian sarcoma virus not related to the v-sis region was rather surprising. We speculate that possibly the extensive 5'-non-coding region of hamster PDGF gene(s) may play some important role in PDGF gene function and from the viral homology may in fact code for another small peptide. Isolation of the PDGF gene in our collection of 25 genomic clones and identification of the 5'-flanking region and transcription unit of this PDGF gene may help in understanding the role this gene plays in steroid modulated growth responses.

REFERENCES

(1) Syms, A.J., Norris, J.S. and Smith, R.G. (1983) In Vitro, 19, 929-936.

(2) Norris, J.S., Cornett, L.E., Hardin, J.W., Kohler, P.O., MacLeod, S.L., Srivastava, A., Syms, A.J. and Smith, R.G. (1984) Biochem. Biophys. Res. Commun. 122, 124-128.

CLONING AND SEQUENCE OF MONKEY MITOCHONDRIAL DNA ORIGIN OF REPLICATION

E. Karawya and R.G. Martin
Laboratory of Molecular Biology, NIADDK, National Institutes of Health, Bethesda, MD 20892

The mammalian mitochondrial genome, a closed circular duplex molecule, is replicated from a region on the L strand near an 18 bp consensus sequence. Replication of the majority of DNA molecules is terminated by an unknown mechanism after the synthesis of a short fragment which is referred to as 7S-DNA. These D looped molecules predominate when mitochondrial DNA is isolated. Significant differences have been found between the 5' ends of the 7S-DNA of rat and human mitochondria. Furthermore, the region just upstream of the 5' end is evolutionarily highly divergent. We therefore felt it to be of interest to determine the flanking sequences surrounding the origin of replication of monkey mitochondrial DNA.

Monkey mitochondrial DNA was purified from CV-1 cells according to the method of Bogenhagen and Clayton (1). Due to the difficulties of cloning a large fragment of mitochondrial DNA (our experience and (2)), two strategies were followed to clone the intact origin and the flanking sequences. In one case, the mitochondrial DNA was doubly digested with Bgl II and Hind III. The 1.2 Kb fragment was ligated to Bam H1 and Hind III sites of PΔ9 (a derivative of PBR322). E. coli strain, DH 1, was transformed with the recombinant plasmid according to the method of Hanahan (3). In the other case, the mitochondrial DNA was digested with Hind II. A 2.8-3.0 Kb Hind II fragment, containing the origin of replication, was ligated into the EcoR5 site of PΔ9. Screening for clones containing the origin of replication was made using a labeled probe (4). Several positive clones were identified in both cases. Subcloning of one plasmid containing a 2.8 Kb insert was carried out for sequencing. After restriction mapping, the sequencing was performed with both Maxam and Gilbert (5) and Sanger (6) methods. The complete sequence will be presented.

Acknowledgements

We thank Dr. Robert Craigie and Ms. Michiyo Mizuuchi for the helpful discussion and comments during this work.

References

(1) Bogenhagen, D. and Clayton, D.A. (1974) J. Biol. Chem. 249, 7991-7995.
(2) Drouin, J. (1980) J. Mol. Biol. 140, 15-34.
(3) Hanahan, D. (1983) J. Mol. Biol. 166, 557-580.
(4) Zannis-Hadjopoulos, M., Kaufmann, G., Wang, S., Lechner, R.L., Karawya, E., Hesse, J. and Martin, R.G. (1985) J. Mol. Biol. 5, 1621-1629.

(5) Maxam, A.M. and Gilbert, W. (1980) Methods in Enzymology 65, 499-580.
(6) Sanger, F., Nicklen, S. and Coulson, A.R. (1977) Proc. Natl. Acad. Sci. USA 74, 5463-5467.

HYDROCORTISONE PROMOTES THE NEODIFFERENTIATION OF KIRSTEN MURINE SARCOMA VIRUS TRANSFORMED HUMAN SKIN FIBROBLASTS TO ADIPOSE CELLS: RELEVANCE TO ONCOGENIC MECHANISMS

L. Kopelovich, R.F. Rich, and A.L. Wallace
Dept. Cancer Genetics and Cancer Prevention, Medical Research, VA Medical Center, Bay Pines, FL 33504.

Recent evidence supports the view that cellular oncogenes are involved in the malignant transformation of human cells. For example, a significant proportion of human tumor cells contain activated ras genes. However, little is known about how either the transforming or the normal ras gene regulates the expression of tissue-specific differentiation genes (1,2). Here we present evidence that transformation of human adult skin fibroblasts (SF) by the Kirsten murine sarcoma virus (KiMSV) is associated with their neodifferentiation into preadipose cells, and that hydrocortisone (HC) promotes the transformation/neodifferentiation of such preadipocytes into mature adipose cells.

Transformation of the human SF with KiMSV was assayed by focus formation as described (3). Thereafter, the cell cultures were fed twice weekly using tissue culture medium with or without HC. Scoring of adipocyte-containing foci (ACF) and total transformed foci was done through (a) direct visualization of live cultures under the light microscope (40X) and (b) specific staining with 0.2% Oil-Red-O and giemsa (3,4).

The results show that transformation of human SF by KiMSV is associated with their neodifferentiation into preadipose cells (Fig. 1A). HC or dexamethasone promote the transformation/neodifferentiation of such preadipocytes into mature fat cells (Fig. 1B).

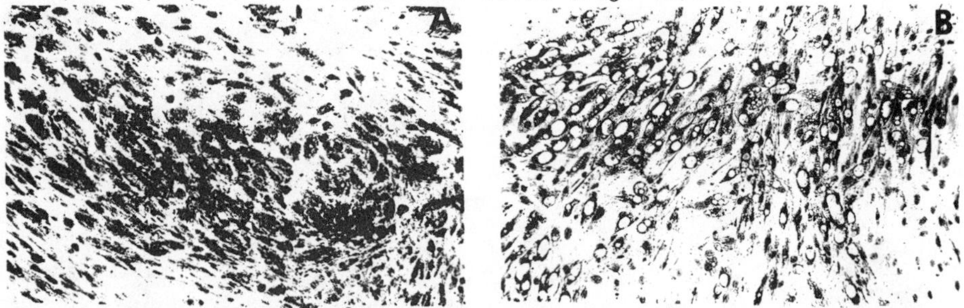

Fig. 1. TRANSFORMATION/NEODIFFERENTIATION OF HUMAN SF BY KiMSV AND HC A. Without HC. B. With HC. Magnification 25X. Shown are giemsa stained plates only.

The effects of HC on the expression of ACF and on total number of transformed foci present in KiMSV-treated SF cultures was optimal at a concentration of about 500 ng/ml, or 1.25×10^{-6}M (Fig. 2). In contrast, equimolar concentrations of estrogenic, androgenic, or progestational steroids were completely inactive. In addition, substitution of HC with azacytidine, insulin, or growth hormone in all possible permutations, including virus (Fig. 3), did not cause adipocyte conversion of these human SF. Although increasing serum concentrations

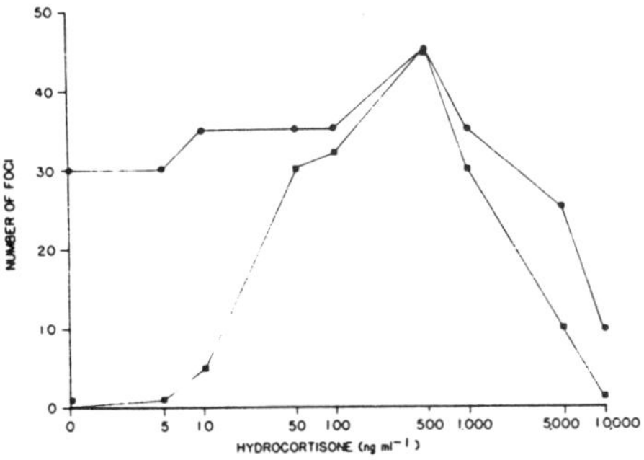

FIG. 2. EFFECT OF HC CONCENTRATION ON THE EXPRESSION OF TOTAL VIRUS INDUCED FOCI AND ACF. Cultures were treated as described in methods. HC was added after virus inoculation and foci were scored 14 days later. (■) ACF.

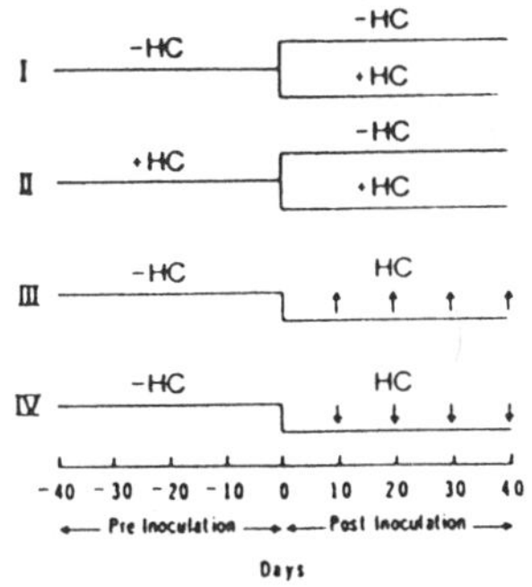

FIG. 3. KINETIC ANALYSES OF HC EFFECTS ON VIRUS-TREATED CELL CULTURES (SCHEME). Cells were infected with KiMSV on day zero. HC was present at time intervals either before, or after virus inoculation, or both as shown.

(2-15%) effected a proportionate increase in the total number of transformed foci, it had no effect on the expression of ACF in the presence of HC. Kinetic analyses (Fig. 3) demonstrated that cell cultures which were "primed" with HC for up to 30 days prior to virus inoculation showed the greatest yield of ACF post inoculation with KiMSV in the presence of HC. Furthermore, the continued presence of HC post inoculation was necessary for maximal adipocytic conversion in virus treated cultures.

It is likely that an activated ras oncogene and HC can effect transformation/neodifferentiation of cells in a variety of human tissues de novo. For example, a high incidence of steroid-induced lipomas has been observed in dogs systemically treated for a variety of inflammatory skin conditions. In humans, corticosteroid-induced episternal fatty tumors and various lipomatoses have also been reportes (5,6). In principal, however, the occurrence of activated ras oncogenes in "non tumor cells", or reversal of a cancer cell phenotype through mechanisms similar to those effected by KiMSV and HC should also be possible. Supported by NCI grants CA-31597 and CA-39081.

REFERENCES

(1) Weinberg, R.A. (1985) Science 230, 770-776.
(2) Kopelovich, L. (1985) In: Biomarkers, Genetics and Cancer (Guirgis, A., Lynch, H., eds.) in press. Van Nostrand Reinhold Press, New York.
(3) Pfeffer, L., and Kopelovich, L. (1979) Cell 313-320.
(4) Green, H., and Kehinde (1976) Cell 7, 105-113.
(5) Lucens, G.E., Bennett, W.M., Pierre, R.V. (1966) The New England J. Med. 275, 834-835.
(6) Pennisi, A.K., Meisler, W.J., and Dina, T.S. (1985) J. Computer Assis. Tomography 9, 595-598.

EXPRESSION OF CELLULAR PROTO-ONCOGENES AFTER IL 2 TREATMENT OF IL 2 INDEPENDENT T CELLS

E. J. KOVACS, H. A. YOUNG, F. W. RUSCETTI, W. L. FARRAR AND M. C. BIRCHENALL-SPARKS
Laboratory of Molecular Immunoregulation, Biological Response Modifiers Program, DCT, NCI, NIH, FCRF, Frederick, MD

Numerous reports have described the induction of cellular proto-oncogene (c-onc) expression as an early event in the reentry of a quiescent cell into the cell cycle following treatment of a cell with its appropriate growth factor. In contrast, a limited number of reports suggest that the expression of certain c-onc is independent of the cell cycle. It is the intent of these studies to distinguish between the expression of c-fos and c-myc as early events in the cell cycle from ones which are merely the result of the interaction of a receptor and its ligand. In the present study we compared the induction of two cellular proto-oncogenes in two related murine T cell lines, the IL 2 dependent T cell line (CT6) and a cell line derived from CT6 (BFS) which was selected by independence of IL 2 for growth, in response to treatment with IL 2.

Induction of interferon-gamma expression. Since it had previously been demonstrated that both cell lines constitutively express high affinity IL 2 receptor on the cell surface (1) and that BFS cells, like the parent line, CT6, secrete interferon-gamma (IFN-γ) in response to treatment with IL 2 in the absence of proliferation (2), we monitored IFN-γ DNA production as an indication of responsiveness to IL 2 in BFS cells. As shown in Figure 1, IFN-γ mRNA is clearly induced after 24 hour exposure of CT6 and BFS to recombinant IL 2 (100 units/ ml).

Figure 1. Induction of IFN-gamma mRNA production following treatment with IL 2.

1-10 μg; 2-5 μg. Hybridization with ^{32}P-labelled murine IFN-γ cDNA.

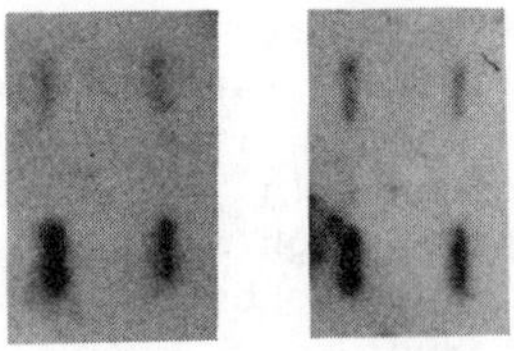

Cellular response to IL 2. We determined culture conditions under which CT6 and BFS cells reached quiescence and examined the response of quiescent cells to treatment with IL 2. After 24 hours of incubation in the absence of growth factors cells were incubated in the presence of IL 2 for varying periods of time and pulsed with ^{3}H-thymidine or ^{3}H-uridine for 1 hour. As shown in Table 1, both thymidine and uridine incorporation were markedly elevated in the CT6 cells following 48 hours of treatment with IL 2. In contrast, treatment of BFS cells with IL 2 did not influence isotope incorporation.

Table 1. Response of cells to IL 2 treatment

Cell Line	CPM/well			
	^{3}H-Thymidine		^{3}H-Uridine	
	+0	+IL 2	+0	+IL 2
CT6	4409	29142	378	21892
BFS	6039	5484	839	1043

Expression of c-onc. Evidence from cytoplasmic slot blot analysis (Figures 2 and 3) and nuclear run off transcription (data not shown) indicates that both CT6 and BFS cell lines enhanced their expression of c-fos and c-myc in response to incubation with IL 2. Low levels of c-fos are expressed by both cell lines prior to stimulation with IL 2. After 2 hours of treatment with IL 2 the level of c-fos mRNA was increased and returned to control levels after 6 hours. Similar kinetics were observed for the expression of c-myc in IL 2 treated cells.

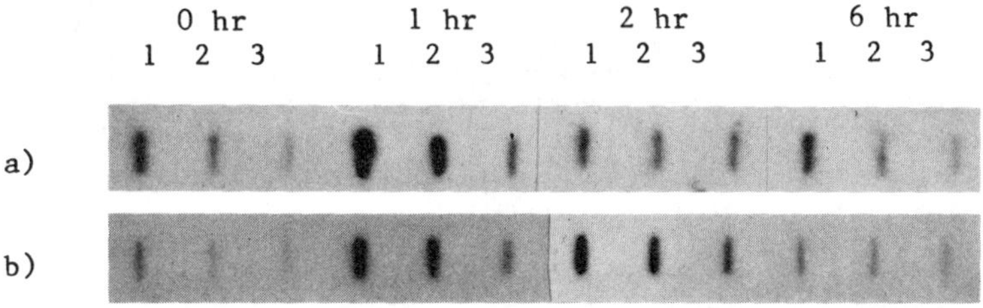

Figure 2. Slot blot analysis of CT6 cells treated with IL 2.

1-10 µg; 2-5 µg; 3-2.5 µg RNA. Filter a) was hybridized with ^{32}P-labelled c-fos cDNA and b) with c-myc.

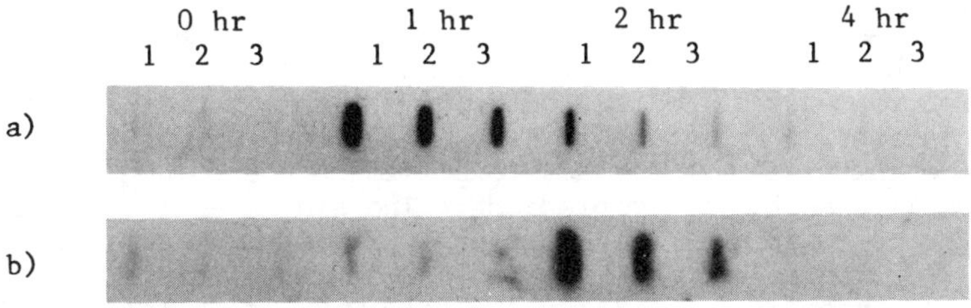

Figure 3. Slot blot analysis of BFS cells treated with IL 2.

1-10 µg; 2-5 µg; 3-2.5 µg RNA. Filter a) was hybridized with ^{32}P-labelled c-fos cDNA and b) with c-myc.

Since c-fos and c-myc are induced in both the IL 2 independent and IL 2 independent cell lines following treatment with IL 2, we conclude that the expression of c-onc in these cells is not associated with the entry of quiescent cells into the cell cycle. The data suggest, that the induction of c-onc expression may be regulated by the interaction of a receptor and its ligand.

REFERENCES

1) Farrar, W. L., F. W. Ruscetti, and H. A. Young (1985) J. Immunol. 135:1551.
2) Benjamin, W. R., P. S. Steeg, and J. J. Farrar (1982) Proc. Natl. Acad. Sci. 79:5379.

PURIFICATION OF TUMOR INHIBITORY FACTORS FROM COLON CARCINOMA CELLS

A.E. Levine, C.A. Crandall, L.C. Yeoman, and M.G. Brattain
Bristol-Baylor Laboratory, Department of Pharmacology, Baylor College of Medicine, Houston, TX 77030 U.S.A.

Several polypeptides have been described which inhibit the growth of transformed cells in vitro. One class of factors referred to as tumor inhibitory factors (TIF) are heat and acid stable polypeptides which have been partially purified from rat ascites fluid (1), human tumor cell conditioned medium (2,3), and a human colon carcinoma cell line designated MOSER (4). We have shown that the partially purified MOSER cell TIF (M_r 7000) inhibited the anchorage independent growth of well differentiated, but not poorly differentiated colon carcinoma cells (4). Addition of this TIF to responsive cells under anchorage dependent conditions resulted in fewer cells per colony and altered morphology characterized by a flattening of the cells and a larger surface area. These effects of TIF were reversible (4). In this report, we have further purified and characterized this M_r 7000 TIF and identified a second TIF of higher molecular weight (M_r 15,000).

Purification of Mr 7000 TIF. MOSER cells (grown in spinner culture) were extracted with acid/ethanol as previously described (4). The crude extract was applied to a Bio-Gel P-30 column and two major peaks (M_r 7000 and 15,000) which inhibit the anchorage independent growth of MOSER cells obtained. The M_r 7000 TIF was further purified using three reverse phase HPLC steps (Table 1). The Bio-Gel pool was applied to a C_8-silica column in 0.1% trifluoroacetic acid (TFA) and eluted with a linear 20-40% acetonitrile gradient. The single TIF activity peak (eluting at 32% acetonitrile) was pooled, reapplied to the column and eluted with a shallow acetonitrile gradient. The single activity peak eluting at 29% acetonitrile was further purified using a third HPLC step utilizing an isopropanol gradient in TFA. This TIF activity (21% isopropanol) was purified 400-fold with an overall yield of 1.5%.

Table 1. Purification of TIF from MOSER Cells

	Protein(mg)	Activity Units	U/mg	Fold purification	% recovery
Crude extract	383	812	4.2	1.0	100
Bio-Gel P-30					
M_r 15,000 Pool	110.3	216	2.0	0.45	27
M_r 7,000 Pool	94.6	179	1.9	0.45	22(100)
HPLC-acetonitrile	2.3	80	34.7	8.3	10(45)
HPLC-acetonitrile#2	0.3	40	133	31.7	5(22)
HPLC-isopropanol	0.007	12.5	1785	425	1.5(7)

Biological Effects of Mr 7000 TIF. As previously described (4),

TIF treatment of responsive colon carcinoma cell lines resulted in significant alterations in colony morphology. The effect of the Mr 7000 TIF on thymidine incorporation by the well differentiated CBS colon carcinoma cell line was examined (Table 2). The incorporation of ^{3}H-thymidine was reduced approximately 50% in the presence of TIF. If TIF was removed from the cells for 7 days before addition of ^{3}H-thymidine, the incorporation of ^{3}H-thymidine was similar to that of control untreated cells indicating that the effects of TIF were reversible.

Table 2. Effect of TIF on Anchorage-Dependent Growth

	^{3}H-Thymidine incorporation (cpm)
Control	47,655
+TIF	26,519
+TIF, remove TIF at 7d	41,969

CBS cells (1000/well) were grown in 9.6 sq cm tissue culture plates (4) and treated with partially purified TIF (0.9ug/ml) for 14 days or for 7 days in the reversal experiment. Cells were pulsed with ^{3}H-thymidine for 24 hrs and the incorporation of radioactivity into acid insoluble material determined.

Purification of Mr 15,000 TIF. The high molecular weight TIF peak from Bio-Gel P-30 was further purified by chromatography on CM-cellulose using ammonium acetate, pH 5.6. All of the TIF activity bound to the column and was eluted between 0.5 and 1M ammonium acetate. When applied to a C_8-silica reverse phase HPLC using TFA and a linear acetonitrile gradient the M_r 15,000 TIF eluted at 35% acetonitrile. This indicated that the two TIF's were chromatographically distinct molecules based on their elution properties from Bio-Gel and reverse phase HPLC. MOSER cells also produce transforming growth factors (4) and the balance between stimulatory and inhibitory factors may be important to the control of cell growth.

REFERENCES

(1) Levine, A.E., Hamilton, D.A., Yeoman, L.C., Busch, H., and Brattain, M.G. (1984) Biochem. Biophys. Res. Commun. 119, 76-82.
(2) Iwata, K.W., Fryling, C.M., Knott, W.B., and Todaro, G.J. (1985) Cancer Res. 45, 2689-2694.
(3) Fryling, C.M., Iwata, K.W., Johnson, P.A., Knott, W.B., and Todaro, G.J. (1985) Cancer Res. 45, 2695-2699.
(4) Levine, A.E., McRae, L.J., Hamilton, D.A., Brattain, D.E., Yeoman, L.C., and Brattain, M.G. (1985) Cancer Res. 45, 2248-2254.

EXPRESSION OF c-myc, JB, AND JE GENE SEQUENCES IS DIFFERENTIALLY REGULATED IN BALB-3T3, NIH-3T3 AND 3T3-ras CELLS. David H. Lynch and Kathy Kelly. Dept. of Ob/Gyn, Univ. of Utah Med. Ctr., Salt Lake City, UT 84132, and the Immunology Branch, NIH, Bethesda, MD 20205.

Introduction Control of cellular growth in fibroblasts by growth factors in the G1 phase of the cell cycle is exerted at two distinguishable control points. Platelet-derived growth factor (PDGF) acts at the initial competence phase of G1 while EGF and the somatomedins are required for progression of cells through a later stage of the G1 phase (1,2). BALB/c-3T3 (clone A-31) cells grown in the absence of PDGF become growth arrested in G0/G1. Treatment of these cells with PDGF results in the transcription of a group of gene sequences (of which c-myc is one; 3) that are not expressed merely as a consequence of cell growth, but instead appear to be "early genes" directly regulated by PDGF. Several of these "early" gene sequences from PDGF treated A-31 cells have been isolated and two of the genes used in this study (JB and JE) characterized (4,5). Although the functions of the products of neither of these genes is known, JB contains a domain with sequence homology to the 3rd exon of the murine c-fos gene (5).

Viral oncogenes and somatically altered cellular proto-oncogenes act as dominant growth transforming agents (6,7). A specific mutation in the c-ras proto-oncogene is responsible for converting this gene into a ras oncogene which induces cellular transformation (8). Microinjection of NIH-3T3 cells with the ras gene product causes transformation and initiates DNA synthesis (9). Further, microinjection of NIH-3T3 cells with monoclonal antibodies to the ras protein prevents them from entering S phase (10). Since the ras protein appears to be required for the initiation of S phase in NIH-3T3 cells, the relationship between the ras oncogene and the expres-sion of three "early" genes (c-myc, JB and JE) was examined.

Results Replicate cultures of BALB/c 3T3 (clone A-31) cells were incubated overnight in medium containing 5% platelet-poor plasma (PPP) to induce quiescence. One of the A-31 cell cultures was then changed to medium containing 15% newborn calf serum (NCS; which contains PDGF) and total RNA was extracted from both cultures 2 hours later. These procedures were simultaneously performed on cultures of NIH-3T3 and ras-transfected NIH-3T3 (3T3-ras) cells. Propidium iodide staining of the A-31 and NIH-3T3 cells grown in PPP confirmed that they were growth arrested. Northern blots of RNA from these cells were prepared and hybridized with ^{32}P-labeled c-myc, pBC-JB or pBC-JE probes. Relative levels of gene expression were estimated by integration of peaks obtained by densitometric scanning of the autoradiograms (Table 1).

Table 1

Probe	Cell culture Conditions	Cell Line Tested A-31	NIH-3T3	3T3-ras
c-myc	PPP	-0.05	0.32	3.48
	NCS	2.09	2.43	3.34
pBC-JB	PPP	-0.05	6.89	-0.02
	NCS	2.69	2.88	0.12
pBC-JE	PPP	0.02	5.32	5.28
	NCS	5.66	2.39	2.43

A-31 cells cultured overnight in PPP showed no detectable levels of c-myc RNA, while A-31 cells that had been transferred into NCS containing medium showed high levels of c-myc RNA. Extremely low levels of c-myc RNA were found in the NIH-3T3 cells cultured overnight in PPP, and were substantially increased in NIH-3T3 cells which were transferred into medium with NCS prior to harvest. High levels of c-myc expression were detected in the RNAs isolated from the 3T3-ras cells, regardless of whether the culture medium contained PPP or NCS. Hence transformation with the ras oncogene is sufficient to deregulate (either directly or indirectly) the expression of c-myc in NIH-3T3 cells.

To determine whether the ras oncogene deregulated other PDGF-inducible gene sequences these Northern blots were stripped and rehybridized with ^{32}P-labeled pBC-JB. Although the expression of the JB sequence is regulated by PDGF in A-31 cells, its expression in NIH-3T3 cells does not appear to require PDGF. Nor did expression of JB and c-myc appear to be coordinate since NIH-3T3 cells grown in PPP contained extremely low levels of c-myc sequences, but high levels of JB sequences. Surprisingly, no JB sequences were detected in the 3T3-ras cells, regardless of the culture medium used. However, it is possible that JB sequences may have been expressed at less than detectable levels in the 3T3-ras cells.

A duplicate Northern blot of these RNA preparations was hybridized with ^{32}P-labeled pBC-JE. Similar to the situation observed with JB sequences, PDGF was required for the expression of JE sequences in A-31 cells, but not in NIH-3T3 cells. However, JE sequences were found in 3T3-ras cells, regardless of whether these cells were cultured in PPP or NCS. Expression of JE sequences did not appear to be coordinate with the expression of c-myc since high levels of JE were detected in RNA from NIH-3T3 cells cultured in PPP. Nor did expression of JE appear linked to the expression of JB since JE sequences were detected in 3T3-ras cells cultured in either PPP or NCS, and yet no JB sequences were detected in these RNAs.

The data presented indicate that although JB and JE expression is regulated by PDGF in A-31 cells, they are not under PDGF control and appear to be constitively expressed in NIH-3T3 cells. It should be noted that A-31 and NIH-3T3 cells were independently derived and are of different genetic origins and NIH-3T3 cells may be slightly more transformed than A-31 cells. However, the results obtained indicate that expression of JB and JE sequences is not sufficient to induce competence since NIH-3T3 cells became quiescent when cultured in PPP. Induction of competence in both A-31 and NIH-3T3 cells by PDGF correlated best with the expression of c-myc sequences. Finally, the expression of JB sequences was inhibited by the ras oncogene, and may indicate that expression of JB sequences is not required for cell-cycle progression. Whether this is due to a trivial cause (such as insertion of the ras oncogene into the JB coding sequence), or interaction of ras gene products with JB is not known, and under study.

1. Stiles CD et al. Proc Nat Acad Sci, USA 76:1279, 1979.
2. Leof EB et al. Exp Cell Res 141:107, 1982.
3. Kelly K et al. Curr Top Microbiol Immunol 113:117, 1984.
4. Cochran BH, Reffel AC, Stiles CD. Cell 33:939, 1983.
5. Cochran BH et al. Science 226:1080, 1984.
6. Cooper GM. Science 217:801, 1982
7. Bishop JM. Ann Rev Biochem 52:301, 1983.
8. Tabin CJ et al. Nature 300:143, 1982.
9. Stacey DW, Kung H-F. Nature 310:508, 1984.
10. Mulcahy LS, Smith MR, Stacey DW. Nature 313:241,1985.

EFFECT OF INSULIN ON THE GROWTH AND C-MYC ONCOGENE EXPRESSION OF HUMAN HEPATOMA CELLS PLC/PRF/5

Y. Motoo, M. Mahmoudi, K. Osther, and A.P. Bollon
Wadley Institutes of Molecular Medicine, 9000 Harry Hines Blvd., Dallas, Texas 75235

INTRODUCTION

Insulin has 2 major effects: a metabolic effect and a growth promoting effect. The rat hepatoma cell line H35 is known to be highly sensitive to insulin (1). On the other hand, c-myc oncogene is considered to play an important role in carcinogenesis and cell growth (2). In this study, we report the effect of insulin on the growth and c-myc expression of a human hepatoma cell line PLC/PRF/5.

MATERIALS AND METHODS

Assay for growth promoting activity. Promotion of cell growth was assayed as previously described by Massagué et al. (3). Briefly, cells were cultured as monolayers in serum free medium for at least 48 hrs. Then insulin was added to the culture medium. At indicated times, ^{3}H-thymidine incorporation was determined.

Assay of oncogene expression. Dot blots were performed using the Quick-Blot Kit (Schleicher & Schuell). Briefly, cells were treated with proteinase K and NaI, then dotted onto nitrocellulose paper. The immobilized mRNA from the cells was hybridized with a nick-translated human c-myc probe. The human c-myc probe obtained from American Type Culture Collection is a 9.0 Kb EcoRI-HindIII fragment from human c-myc clone in bacteriophage; subcloned into pBR322.

RESULTS

In a time course study, 10^{-8} M insulin enhanced the c-myc expression in the hepatoma cells with a peak 9 hrs after the addition of insulin (Fig. 1A). The DNA synthesis was also promoted by insulin with a peak at 30 hrs (Fig. 2A). A dose response study revealed that the maximal effect was obtained with 10^{-8} M insulin both in the c-myc expression and the DNA synthesis (Fig. 1B, 2B).

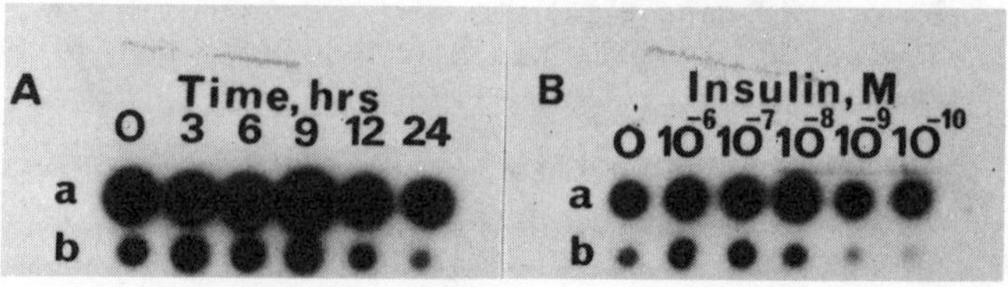

Fig. 1 Dot blot analysis of c-myc mRNA from the hepatoma cells.

A. Time course study after the addition of 10^{-8} M insulin. B. Dose response study 9 hrs after the addition of insulin. a. 1:1, b. 1:10 dilution of the original samples.

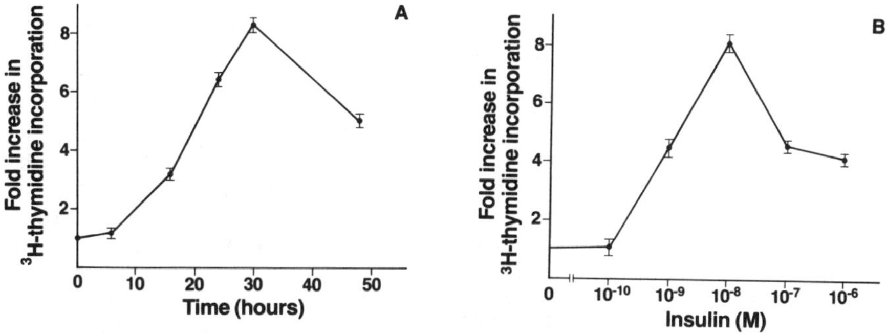

Fig. 2. ^{3}H-thymidine incorporation into DNA of the hepatoma cells. A. Time course study after the addition of 10^{-8} M insulin. B. Dose response study 30 hrs after the addition of insulin.

DISCUSSION

Insulin promoted the growth of the human hepatoma cells and enhanced the c-myc expression. The expression of c-myc has been reported to be induced 40-fold after 3 hrs in fibroblasts treated with platelet-derived growth factor, PDGF (4). Our results show that the maximal enhancement of c-myc expression by insulin occurs later than that by PDGF. Furthermore the enhancement by insulin is not so pronounced as in the experiment with PDGF. These differences might be due to a deregulation of c-myc expression in malignant cells or due to the differences in growth-promoting mechanisms of the growth factors.

REFERENCES

(1) Koontz, J.W., and Iwahashi, M. (1981) Science 211, 947-949.
(2) Armelin, H.A., Armelin, M.C.S., Kelly, K., Stewart, T., Leder, P., Cochran, B.H. and Stiles, C.D. (1984) Nature 310, 655-660.
(3) Massagué, J., Blinderman, L.A., and Czech, M.P. (1982) J. Biol. Chem. 257, 14958-13963.
(4) Kelly, K., Cochran, B.H., Stiles, C.D., and Leder, P. (1983) Cell 35, 603-610.

PURIFICATION AND PARTIAL CHARACTERIZATION OF PROSTATE-DERIVED GROWTH FACTOR

H. NANRI, S. MAEHAMA, D. LI, AND T. F. DEUEL

Department of Medicine, Jewish Hospital at Washington University Medical Center, 216 S. Kingshighway, St. Louis, MO 63110

A number of growth promoting polypeptides have been found in extracts of animal tissues and in conditioned media from cultures of transformed cells. The isolation and characterization of these growth factors are important to understand the mechanisms of cell growth regulation. A close relationship between growth factors and products of oncogenes suggested the importance of elucidating the structure and function of growth factors as they may relate to mechanisms of transformation. We report the purification and partial characterization of a novel growth factor isolated from rat prostate.

PURIFICATION. A growth promoting polypeptide was purified 16,400-fold from acid extracts of rat prostate using ion-exchange, reverse-phase, and gel filtration chromatography (Table 1). A single protein peak with growth promoting activity was obtained on a reverse-phase C_{18} HPLC. This active peak was also eluted as a single peak on a TSK gel filtration HPLC and migrated as a single silver-stained band on SDS-PAGE.

PURIFICATION OF PrGF FROM RAT PROSTATES (Table 1)

Purification Step	Volume (ml)	Protein (mg)	Total Activity (dpm)	Yield (%)	Purification (- fold)
Crude Extraction	2700	6.99×10^{4}	2.32×10^{10}	100	1
SP-Sephadex	6800	2.06×10^{3}	8.54×10^{9}	37	12.5
DEAE-Sephadex	6150	3.08×10^{2}	8.89×10^{9}	38	87
Ammonium Sulfate Precipitation	50	2.55×10^{2}	6.45×10^{9}	28	93
Sephadex G-75	256	1.89×10^{1}	7.21×10^{8}	3.1	115
DEAE-HPLC					
peak II	24	2.74×10^{-1}	4.04×10^{8}	1.7	4442
(peak I)	(20)	(–)	(1.58×10^{8})	(0.7)	(–)
(peak III)	(16)	(–)	(1.57×10^{8})	(0.7)	(–)
C_{18}-HPLC	10	N/D[a]	3.16×10^{8}	1.4	N/D
TSK-2000	14	4.48×10^{-2} [b]	2.44×10^{8}	1.1	16385

[a]N/D = not determined
[b]protein was quantitated by amino acid analysis

CHARACTERIZATION. The molecular weight of prostate-derived growth factor (PrGF) determined by SDS-PAGE is 25 kDa for non-reduced PrGF and 6-8 kDa for reduced one. The isoelectric point of PrGF is 5.0. The radiolabeling by use of sodium metaperiodate-Na[^{3}H]BH_4 and the appearance of an unidentified peak on amino acid analysis consistent with an amino sugar suggested that PrGF is a glycoprotein. The mitogenic activity of the purified PrGF has a linear dose-response with maximum activity at about 10 ng/ml. PrGF is heat and acid stable, inactivated by a treatment of protease or β-mercaptoethanol, and has no transforming activity. The initially characterized properties of PrGF indicate that PrGF is a previously undescribed growth factor.

PROPERTIES OF PrGF (Table 11)

Molecular weight	non-reduced	25,000
	reduced	6,000-8,000
Isoelectric point		pH 5.0
Carbohydrate		+
Concentration of maximum activity		10 ng/ml
Heat stability		+
Acid stability		+
Inactivation by protease		+
reduction		+
Transforming activity		-

A CHANGE IN CALCITONIN GENE RNA PROCESSING DURING GROWTH OF HUMAN MEDULLARY THYROID CARCINOMA CELLS IN CULTURE.

B.D. Nelkin, K.Y. Chen, A. de Bustros, and S.B. Baylin.
Johns Hopkins Oncology Center, Baltimore, Maryland 21205

The calcitonin gene has been found, in both rat[1] and man[2-4], to generate a single transcript which, by alternative RNA processing, produces two distinct mRNAs. The mRNA encoding calcitonin (CT) is composed of sequences from exons 1,2,3 and 4, while the mRNA encoding calcitonin gene related peptide is composed of sequences from exons 1,2,3,5 and 6. The processing pathway is tissue specific; mainly CT mRNA is produced in the thyroid C-cells, and mainly CGRP mRNA is produced in cells of the central nervous system[5].

We have been studying CT gene expression in the human medullary thyroid carcinoma cell line TT. This cell line produces mRNA for both CT and CGRP. We have previously shown that, during growth in culture, this cell line exhibits substantial changes in CT peptide production[6]. Here, we show that, while overall CT gene transcription fluctuates only slightly, the ratio of CT to CGRP mRNA during growth in culture varies dramatically, suggesting changes in the posttranscriptional RNA processing pathway.

Cells were plated at $5x10^4$ cm^{-2} in RPMI 1640 with 16% FBS. Cytoplasmic RNA was isolated and CT gene mRNAs were assayed by Northern blot hybridization using cloned cDNAs specific for exons 2 and 3 ("common" region, to measure total CT gene transcripts), exon 4 (CT specific), or exons 5 and 6 (CGRP specific). β-actin cDNA was used as a control. A summary of densitometric tracings of the resultant autoradiograms is in the Table. The level of total cytoplasmic CT gene mRNA (common region probe) remains fairly constant early in culture, then rises nearly two-fold as cells reach confluence (day 9). Consistent with our earlier data for CT peptide[6], CT specific mRNA decreases somewhat between days 2 and 5, then rises in parallel with the increase in total CT gene transcript accumulation measured by the common region probe. In contrast, CGRP specific mRNA begins to increase dramatically from days 2-5 after plating when CT specific mRNA levels are lowest. Subsequently, from days 6-9, CGRP specific mRNA increases further, in parallel with the rise in total CT gene transcripts. CGRP specific mRNA decreases sharply again after day 9, at which time CT specific mRNA levels do not fall. Thus, early in the growth period, the ratio of CGRP to CT mRNA is relatively low, but then rises, establishing a new, higher ratio which is then maintained through day 9, but drops sharply by day 11.

RELATIVE LEVELS OF HYBRIDIZATION*

DAY	COMMON	CT	CGRP	RELATIVE CGRP/CT RATIO
0	1.00	1.00	1.0	1.00
2	.90	1.40	.8	.57
4	.80	.88	1.7	1.93
5	.85	.77	3.5	4.55
6	.92	1.17	5.8	4.96
7	1.27	1.62	7.6	4.69
9	1.58	1.85	10.0	5.41
11	1.39	2.08	3.4	1.63

*normalized to day 0 (day cells were plated)

Since both CT and CGRP mRNAs derive from a single pre-mRNA transcript, variation in the ratio of CT to CGRP mRNA must be mediated at a posttranscriptional level: i.e., mRNA splicing, transport, or stability. We are currently examining these possibilities.

For any mechanism involved, cellular cofactors must change during growth in culture in order to differentially process CT and CGRP mRNA. The dynamic changes we observe in this cell line should provide an outstanding opportunity to develop in vitro systems to study the RNA processing cofactors involved.

REFERENCES

(1) Amara, S.G., Jonas, V., Rosenfeld, M.G., Ong, E.S., and Evans, R.M. (1982) Nature 298, 240-244.
(2) Nelkin, B.D., Rosenfeld, K.I., de Bustros, A., Leong, S.S., Roos, B.A., and Baylin, S.B. (1984) Biochem. Biophys. Res. Commun. 123, 648-655.
(3) Steenbergh, P.H., Hoppener, J.W.M., Zandberg, J., van de Ven, W.J.M., Jansz, H.S., and Lips, C.J.M. (1984) J. Clin. Endocrinol. Metab. 59, 358-360.
(4) Edbrooke, M.R., Parker, D., McVey, J.H., Riley, J.H., Sorenson, G.D., Pettengill, O.S., and Craig, R.K. (1985) EMBO J. 4, 715-724.
(5) Rosenfeld, M.G., Mermod, J.-J., Amara, S.G., Swanson, L.W., Sawchenko, P.E., Rivier, J., Vale, W.W., and Evans, R.M. (1983) Nature 304, 129-135.
(6) Berger, C.L., de Bustros, A., Roos, B.A., Leong, S.S., Mendelsohn, G., Gesell, M.S., and Baylin, S.B. (1984) J. Clin. Endocrinol. Metab. 59, 338-343.

LEVELS OF FOS, ETS-2 AND MYB RNAs CORRELATE WITH TUMORIGENICITY OF HeLa/HUMAN FIBROBLAST HYBRIDS

B. M. O'Hara*, H. P. Klinger** and D. G. Blair*
*Laboratory of Molecular Oncology, National Cancer Institute, Frederick, MD 21701-1013, and **Department of Genetics, Albert Einstein College of Medicine of Yeshiva University, Bronx, NY 10461

The tumorigenicity in nude mice of HeLa cells is suppressed when hybrids are formed with normal human fibroblasts. Derivatives of the non-tumorigenic hybrids which have lost a small number of chromosomes are often found to be tumorigenic. These observations suggest that a chromosome(s) donated by the normal parent suppresses the tumorigenicity of HeLa cells and that its loss from a hybrid allows reexpression of tumorigenicity (1). We have examined a panel of tumorigenic and non-tumorigenic hybrids to determine if the mechanism of tumorigenicity control might be reflected in the levels of oncogene RNAs. Of 23 oncogenes examined, 7 were not detected in polyadenylated RNA. A further 13 oncogene-specific RNAs were detected but showed no correlation with the tumorigenic phenotype of the hybrids. Table 1A shows the levels for a subset of this group expressed as a percentage of actin RNA, the level of which was found to be relatively invariant throughout the cell types. Table 1B shows a similar analysis for the <u>ets</u>-2, <u>fos</u> and <u>myb</u> RNAs.

Table 1: RNA Expression of Oncogenes in Tumorigenic and Non-Tumorigenic HeLa/Human Fibroblast Cell Hybrids

RNA (size in kb)	Non-Tumorigenic Hybrids						Tumorigenic Segregants		HeLa
	A	B	C	D	E	F	G	H	I	J
A.										
abl (7.0)	5	39	39	6	37			38	40	8
abl (6.0)	25	130	108	12	67			83	88	36
H-ras-1 (1.3)	77	148	48	18	87	38	73	69	46	74
P53 (2.4)	62	62	60	75	157	87	81	73	81	69
HPV-18 (4.2)	73	62	105	56	76	113	5	47	96	89
HPV-18 (1.5)	70	95	70	13	70	240	24	80	100	46
β2M (1.3)	61	65	174	72	48	200	225	73	150	88
B.										
ets (4.8)	17	69	31	78	23	76	233	243	386	219
ets (3.3)	80	102	83	152	71	359	581	461	413	439
ets (2.8)	26	47	21	36	15	113	302	118	81	184
myb (4.1)	28	63	35	36	202	19	1	1	1	1
fos (2.4)	3	10	3	2	10	717	791	26	78	28
myc (2.4)	39	43	52	34	30	85	63	25	30	30

RNA was prepared and analyzed by Northern blot analysis using probes specific for the indicated genes. In each case the blots were also analyzed with an actin probe. The exposed films were scanned and the expression of each oncogene was calculated relative to the level of actin RNA detected in each lane. Cells analyzed were: A, Col1; B, Col3; C, 2μCol1; D, 2μCol1Col1; E, 3K; F, Col1Col1; G, 146; H, Col2; I, A70; J, D98 (HeLa) cells. F-K are all tumorigenic in nude mice, while A-E do not form tumors or show a much reduced tumorigenicity.

Ets-2 (located on chromosome 21 and homologous to a portion of the *E26* retrovirus oncogene (2)) and *fos* RNAs were found to be higher in the tumorigenic hybrids. *Myb* RNA was not detected in either parent, was evident in the non-tumorigenic hybrids and was much reduced in the tumorigenic hybrids. While these correlations do not necessarily identify mechanisms controlling suppression of tumorigenicity, they appear to be significant because (a) they closely reflect the tumorigenic phenotype in the absence of comparable variations for the other oncogenes mentioned and for several other genes, (b) the correlations extend to log phase and confluent cells, and (c) they are not affected by murine sarcoma virus-mediated transformation and thus are not a necessary consequence of transformation. These data therefore suggest a role for cellular oncogenes in the control of tumorigenicity and they also suggest coordinate regulation of the *fos*, *ets*-2 and *myb* oncogenes.

1. Klinger, H. P. *Cytogenet. Cell Genet*. 27:254-266, 1980.

2. Watson, D. *et al*. *Proc. Natl. Acad. Sci. USA* 82:7294-7298, 1985.

MAMMARY TUMOR VIRUS RNA EXPRESSION IN SPLENIC B LYMPHOCYTES FROM MMTV-NEGATIVE BALB/C MICE.

Robert J. Pauley and Diana M. Lopez. Department of Microbiology and Immunology, University of Miami School of Medicine, Miami, FL 33101

The Balb/c strain, as well as all inbred mouse strains, contain multiple copies of germinally-transmitted mouse mammary tumor virus (MMTV) proviral DNA. Balb/c MMTV proviral DNA has been characterized by restriction endonuclease mapping and molecular hybridization with either a MMTV complementary DNA (cDNA) (1) or cloned probes of specific regions of the MMTV genome (2) and has been found to consist of two genome size MMTV proviruses distinguished from each other by their integration sites within different regions of cellular DNA. In addition, the Balb/c strain contains a subgenomic, or defective MMTV provirus shown to contain the LTR region and at least a portion of the env gene region but lacking most of the gag-pol sequences (3).

We have previously observed the expression of an antigen capable of reacting with antisera raised against purified MMTV and with monoclonal antibodies directed to gp52, the major structural protein of MMTV (4). Approximately 25% of the nylon adherent, SIg+ lymphocytes obtained from spleens of Balb/c mice express such antigen(s) on their surfaces, even though this strain does not harbor an exogenous MMTV and whole viral particles cannot be detected in its tissues. This antigen is absent from normal or neoplastic Balb/c mammary cells, as well as from liver and lymphoid cells of thymic derivation.

The organization of MMTV DNA sequences was examined in tissues and cells that lack or contain the MMTV antigen. It was found that identical size MMTV DNA-containing restriction fragments were observed in liver, mammary gland, carcinogen-induced mammary tumor, thymus and splenic nylon nonadherent cells which do not express the MMTV antigens, or in Balb/c spleen and splenic nylon adherent cells that have the MMTV antigen. Mammary tumors from Balb/c mice infected with the milk-transmitted MMTV contained additional copies of MMTV proviral DNA. Therefore, there was no detectable amplification of the MMTV DNA copy number, alteration in the cellular sites of interaction, or alteration of the Balb/c MMTV proviral DNA organization in tissues or cells that contain or lack the MMTV antigen.

To determine whether the expression of the MMTV antigen on Balb/c spleen cells, which was absent from both normal or neoplastic Balb/c mammary cells and from thymic cells, was due to the regulation of MMTV RNA transcription. Balb/c liver, thymus, multiparous retired breeder mammary gland, and the D1-DMBA-3 carcinogen-induced mammary tumor were examined. All contained MMTV RNA at (0.0001%) or below the limits of detection, that demonstrated a very limited extent of hybridization to the MMTV cDNA probe even at high equivalent Rot values. In contrast, virgin female Balb/c spleen contained a significant amount of MMTV RNA, however, this was about 100-fold lower than the level of MMTV RNA observed in a Balb/cfC3H mammary tumor that contained additional copies of the milk-transmitted MMTV DNA.

In order to elucidate whether MMTV RNA expression is restricted to a specific subpopulation of Balb/c spleen lymphocytes, total cellular RNA from various sources was isolated and bound to a nitrocellular filter for hybridization with radiolabeled MMTV DNA cloned probes. As seen in Figure 1, the splenic T lymphocyte enriched subpopulations

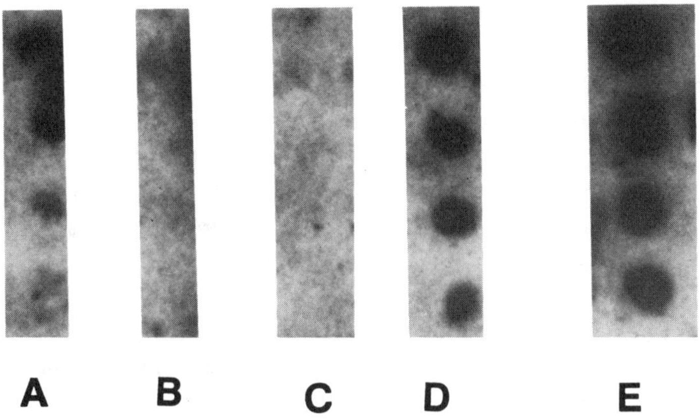

Figure 1: Dot blot hybridization patterns of mRNA from: (A) Balb/c multiparous lactating mammary gland; (B) virgin Balb/c liver; (c) nylon nonadherent, T cell enriched, spleen cells from virgin Balb/c; (D) nylon adherent, B-cell enriched spleen cells from virgin Balb/c; (E) and Balb/cfC3H mammary tumor RNA.

lacked detectable MMTV RNA. The splenic B lymphocyte subpopulations, on the other hand, contained MMTV RNA, although at a level of less than one-tenth the Balb/cfC3H mammary tumor. Therefore, the level of MMTV RNA expression in Balb/c tissues and splenic cell subpopulations correlates positively with the presence of MMTV antigen(s) in the same tissues and splenic cell subpopulations. In combination, with the restriction mapping data, these observations indicate that the germinally-transmitted MMTV provirus(es) are preferentially expressed in Balb/c splenic B lymphocytes.

REFERENCES

(1) Cohen, J.C., Majors, J.E. and Varmus, H.E. (1979) J. Virol. 32, 483-490.
(2) Pauley, R.J., Parks, W.P. and Popko, B.J. (1984) Virus Res. 1, 381-400.
(3) Popko, B.J. and Pauley, R.J. (1984) J. Virol. 52, 328-335.
(4) Lopez, D.M., Charyulu, V. and Paul, R.D. (1985) J. Immunol. 134, 603-607.

TSP-180 EXPRESSION AND METASTATIC CAPACITY ON LEWIS LUNG CARCINOMA VARIANTS

Sacchi A.*,Falcioni A.*,Kennel S.J.§,Heldin K.** and Caputo A.*
* "Regina Elena" Cancer Institute,V.le Regina Elena 291,00161 Rome, Italy,§ Oak Ridge National Laboratory,37831 Tennessee,U.S.A.,**Box 575,University of Uppsala,S-72523,Sweden.

The metastases are the most dramatic event of malignancy in human cancer. Recent studies have indicated that metastases may differ from primary tumor cell population in a number of parameters. In the attempt to correlate metastatic potential with specific properties of the tumor cells, homogeneous subpopulations which are endowed with low to high metastatic potential have been isolated from single tumor. Since interactions of tumor cells with their environment,and possibly immune-cells, are mediated by cell surface constituents, these structures are possibly involved in the metastatic process. In particular, changes in antigen expression have been correlated with metastatic potential of tumor cells.Expression of a tumor associated antigen, recognized by a MoAb to lung carcinoma cells, has been studied in Lewis lung carcinoma (3LL) tumor lines endowed with different metastatic potential. These lines have been show to be stable for metastatic phenotype along the *in vivo* passaging. MoAb 135-13C recognizes a protein (TSP-180) that appears on cell surface of several murine lung carcinoma (1) but is not detected on normal cells in culture.

<u>Tumor Lines</u>: *in vivo* M1087 and BM21548 lines(1) and the parental line (original) of 3LL were passaged in C57Bl/6 mice. Each mouse was injected in the leg muscle with $2.5x10^5$/0.1ml of viable tumor cells. CCL is a melanoma tumor maintained in DBA/2 mice by injection of$1x10^6$ viable cells.Line 1 is a murine type II alveolar carcinoma that arose spontaneously in a Balb/c.We used an *in vitro* cell line developed from line 1 tumor which is highly malignat and metastatic (3). <u>Monoclonal Antibodies:</u>the generation and the characterization of MoAb135-13C and of the policlonal antibody anti-P-tyr have been previously described (1,4).Proteins were radiolabelled with ^{125}I using the Chloramine T method. Control MoAb 225.28S to a human high molecular weight melanoma associated antigen,was constructed as described (5). Antibody binding and cell protein analysis were performed as described (1).

Table 1 summarizes the metastatic capacity of the tumor lines as

Table I summarizes the metastatic capacity of the tumor lines as compared with the ability to bind the MoAb 135-213C.

TABLE I

Tumor lines	ng of ^{125}I MoAb135-13C	Metastases n° ± S.E.
CCL	0.5	0
Line 1	65	>150
3LL p.	30	35 ± 4
BM21548	3	15 ± 3
M1087	50	106 ± 6

The amounts (ng) of bound MoAb corresponds to the values attained at the plateau level of the binding curves, when $2x10^5$ viable tumor cells are assayed with 3 μg of purified protein. The order of binding of MoAb135-13C to the different tumor cells is: line 1>M1087> 3LL parent>BM21548>CCL. Background binding is demonstrated by cells derived from melanoma tumor CCL. Lysates from primary tumor cells suspensions of M1087 line labelled with ^{35}S methionine were immunoprecipitated by MoAb 135-13C and 225.28S as control. Autoradiograms of SDS-PAGE gels demonstrated that MoAb 135-13C specifically precipitates three components (m.w.135,150,180kd). The fact that a 180 kd protein can be detected in the lysate of the most metastatic line of 3LL (M1087)is in good agreement with previous results (1). Immunoprecipitates from M1087 lysates labelled with ^{32}P,also, show in presence of the MoAb135-13C a band migrating at 180kd which is not evident for MoAb 225.28S. Figure 1 shows that antiP-tyr precipitates from the same lysates a unique band at 180kd (lane 3) which disappears in presence of an excess of cold phosphotyrosyne (lane 4-5) and corresponds to the same band precipitated by MoAb 135-13C (lane 1)(lane 2 MoAb225.28S).

In conclusion we demonstrate that, in these 3LL variants, metastatic phenotype and the surface protein/s detected by MoAb135-13C are correlated and that a band migrating at 180kd, immunoprecipitated by MoAb 135-13C, contains a residue of phosphotyrosine. The possible role of TSP-180 protein as receptor of growth factor is discussed.

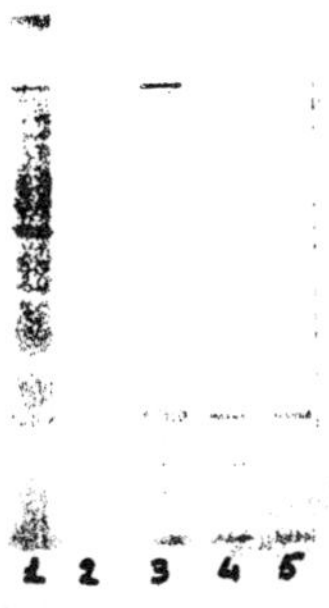

Fig. 1

REFERENCES:

1) Kennel S.J. et al.(1981) Cancer Res.40:2153-2159.
2) Starace G. et al.(1982) Europ.J.Cancer 18: 973-978.
3) Yuhas J.M. et al.(1974) Cancer Res. 34:722-728
4) Ek B.and Heldin C.H.(1982) J.Biol.Chem. 259:
5) Imai K. et al.(1982) In: Peeters (ed),Protides and biological fluids,Pergamon Press,893-897.

ETS GENES IN HUMAN ACUTE LEUKEMIAS

N. Sacchi, D. K. Watson and T. S. Papas
Laboratory of Molecular Oncology, NCI, Frederick, MD 21701

We have previously established that the ets sequence of the transforming avian erythroblastosis virus, E26, has homologs in chicken, mouse, cat and man. The ets related sequence of human DNA, located on chromosome 11 (ets-1) and chromosome 21 (ets-2), are discontiguous except for a small overlap region encoding for 14 amino acids, of which 12 are conserved between these two loci (1). Further, ets-1 and ets-2 behave as separate unique loci in the mouse and cat as well as man; these ets domains are situated within syntenic gene groups known to be conserved among the three diverse mammalian species (2). Both human ets-1 and ets-2 genes are transcriptionally active; the human ets-1 locus encoding a single mRNA of 6.8 kb, while the ets-2 encodes mRNAs of 4.7, 3.2 and 2.7 kb (1). We have also determined, by in situ hybridization, that human ets-2 is located in the 21q22.1-22.3 region (2); while human ets-1 maps to the 11q23-24 region (3).

We have demonstrated that both Hu-ets-1 and Hu-ets-2 genes translocate from their normal position as a consequence of translocations involving the 11q23 and 21q22 breakpoints. This conclusion is based on analysis of two panels of somatic cell hybrids retaining, in a chinese hamster cell background, either the normal or the recombinant chromosomes deriving from the (4;11) and (8;21) translocation (4).

We determined if the translocations of human ets-1 and ets-2 affected the transcription patterns of these genes. This could only be performed on a limited number of patients which were cytogenetically characterized. In addition fresh bone marrow blasts specimens are used to preserve the integrity of the RNA. We have, therefore, been able to assay for the expression of mRNA in fresh leukemic samples. Total RNA was isolated from leukemic cells and compared to normal human lymphocyte RNA in Northern blot experiments. In one AUL t(4;11) leukemia we observed only low levels of Hu-ets-1 mRNA; similar results were also obtained using RNA from the RS4;11 cell line. The expression of Hu-ets-2 gene in the t(8;21) AML-M2 leukemias is much lower than the control lymphocytes. In addition, we did not observe all the human ets-2 mRNA species present in normal control lymphocytes (Fig. 1), and known to be present in several other tissues and cell lines of human origin (1). The 4.7 kb and 3.2 kb mRNA species are notably absent in one patient sample, and the 4.7 kb species is absent in the other. It is possible that the altered expression pattern of ets-1 and ets-2 genes is a consequence of the translocations observed.

Our data makes our investigations into the involvement of this proto-oncogene most promising and support the use of the Hu-ets probes to study the pathogenesis of the above mentioned, suspect, leukemic malignancies.

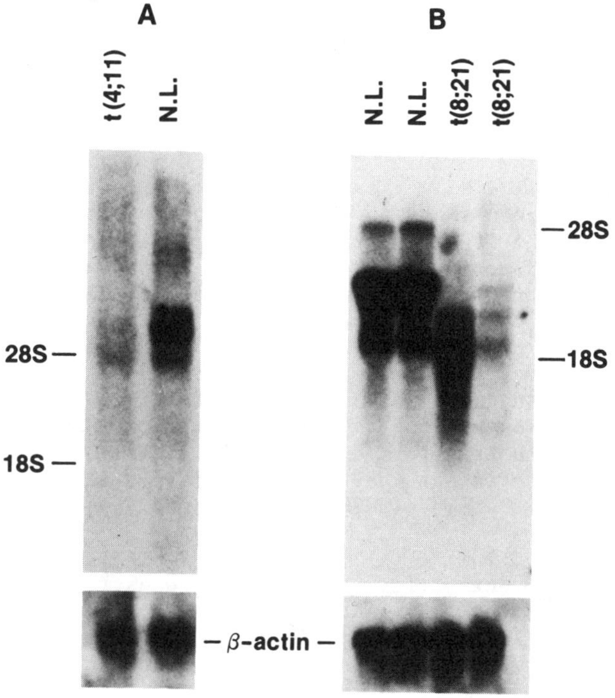

Figure 1. Northern blot analysis of total RNA extracted from: A) blasts cells derived from a t(4;11) AUL patient and normal lymphocytes (N. L.), and B) blasts cells derived from two t(8;21) AML-M2 patients and normal lymphocytes using (A) the ets-1 (RD6K) probe and (B) the ets-2 (H33) probe. The same blots (bottom) have been rehybridized with a β-actin cDNA probe to compare the amount of RNA in these samples.

REFERENCES

1. Watson, D. K., McWilliams-Smith, M. J., Nunn, M. F., Duesberg, P. H., O'Brien, S. J. and Papas, T. S. (1985) Proc. Natl. Acad. Sci. U.S.A. 82, 7294-7298.
2. Watson, D. K., McWilliams-Smith, M. K., Kozak, C., Reeves, R., Gearhart, J., Nuun, M. F., Nash, W., Fowle III, J. R., Duesberg, P. H., Papas, T. S., and O'Brien, S. J. (1985) Proc. Natl. Acad. Sci. U.S.A., in press.
3. de Taisne, C., Gegonne, A. and Stehelin, D., Bernheim, A. and Berger, R. (1984) Nature 310, 581.
4. Sacchi, N., Watson, D. K., Geurts van Kessel, A. H. M., Hagemeijer, A., Kersey, J., Drabkin, H. D., Patterson, D., and Papas, T. S. (1985) Science, in press.

ENHANCED CASEINKINASE II ACTIVITY DURING MOUSE EMBRYOGENESIS

H.R.Schneider, G.H.Reichert, and O.-G.Issinger
Institut für Humangenetik, Universität des Saarlandes
D-6650 Homburg-3, Fed.Rep.Germany

INTRODUCTION

Caseinkinase II (CKII) is a cyclic-nucleotide independent protein kinase that has been shown to phosphorylate translational factor eIF-3 *in vitro* and *in vivo*(1,2). The enzyme can utilize ATP and GTP as a phosphoryl donor and is specifically inhibited by heparin(3). Established and transformed human tumor cell lines show an enhanced CKII activity which is about 5 times higher than in fibroblasts and primary human tumor cell cultures derived from tumor biopsy material (4). Since this activity increase was independent from the type of tumor cells investigated we concluded that it was a specific effect which might probably be due to higher proliferation kinetics common to established and transformed tumor cell lines.
Here, we present evidence that CKII activity is also increased during embryogenesis of the mouse(NMRE), i.e. in normally developing tissue.

RESULTS AND DISCUSSION

I. Protein kinase activities in mouse embryo extracts during different developmental stages. Whole mouse embryos(gestation day 8,10,12,16,18 at birth and 6 days after birth were analysed for protein kinase activity(CKII,cAMP and cGMP-dependent kinase). It is shown(Fig. 1A) that CKII activity changes significantly during fetal development reaching a peak activity at the 12th gestation day. When ATP is replaced by GTP a similar CKII activity profile is obtained,albeit at lower rates(results not shown).Addition of heparin leads to a strong reduction of CKII activity(Fig.1A). At day 12 the CKII activity is about 300% above the average activity found at other times of fetal development but it is still not so high as in ascites tumor cells.

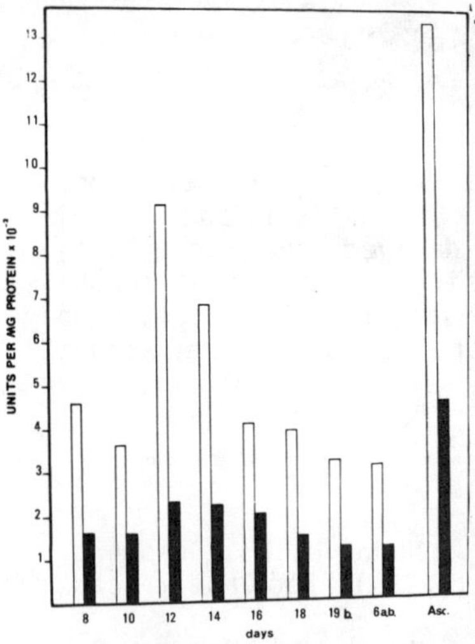

Fig.1A CKII activity at various developmental stages during mouse embryogenesis. Open bars, no inhibitor,solid bars in the presence of heparin(1 µg/ml). b.at birth; a.b. after birth; asc. ascites

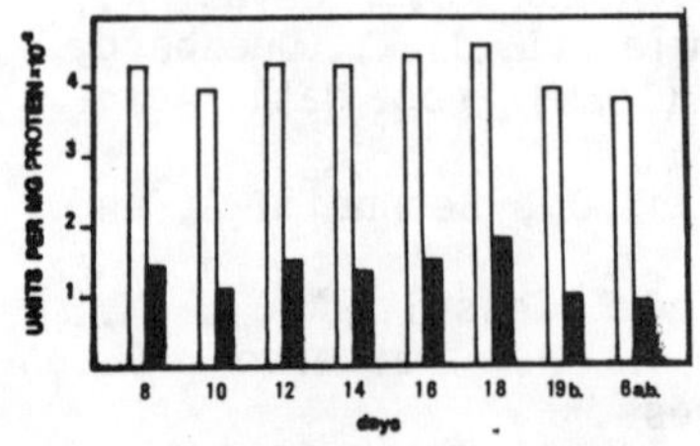

Fig.1B cAMP-dependent protein kinase activity.Open bars no inhibitor,solid bars in the presence of heat stable inhibitor(200 µg/ml).

All other kinases tested(Fig.1B) showed a basal level of enzyme activity with only minor alterations(data for cGMP-dependent kinase not shown). The latter result is in agreement with observations made in established and transformed tumor cells.

II. Autophosphorylation of a 110kDa protein. When mouse embryo extracts were incubated in the presence of ATP^{32} or GTP^{32}, a major phosphoprotein(mol.mass 110 kDa) was observed. Phosphorylation of this pp110 in mouse embryo extracts was inhibited by heparin. Together with the observation that CKII activity was highest in day 12 embryos it is tempting to speculate that the observed phosphoprotein might be identical with eIF-3 pp110. In order to establish identity of the 2 phosphoproteins(from purified eIF-3 and from mouse extracts) 2D tryptic peptide maps will be presented.

	pp110	
Enzmye source	- heparin	+ heparin
ASCITES	100	18
10 d	6	<1
12 d	31	<1
19.b.	<1	-

Table I. Comparison of the amount of pp110 in mouse embryo and ascites cell extracts.
A phosphoprotein of mol.mass 110 kDa (pp110) which might be identical to a corresponding polypeptide from eIF-3 was found in autophosphorylated extracts from ascites cells and mouse embryos. The radioactivity was compared with each other using the ascites protein as a reference(100%). The increase in phosphorylation in the autophosphorylated extracts was 6% and 31% in 10 day and 12 day old embryos, respectively. It declines till birth to less than 1%. In the presence of heparin(1 μg/ml) the phosphorylation of pp110 was strongly reduced.

ACKNOWLEDGEMENTS
This work was supported by DFG grant Is 19/9-1. H.Schneider is a fellow from the Konrad-Adenauer-Stiftung.

REFERENCES

(1) Issinger,O.-G., Benne,R., Hershey,J.W.B., and Traut,R.R.(1976) J.biol.Chem. 251, 6471-6474
(2) Schuck,J., Reichert,G., and Issinger,O.-G.(1979) Biochem.J. 194, 1007-1009
(3) Feige,J.J., Pirollet,F., Cochet,C., and Chambaz,E.M.(1980) FEBS Lett. 121, 139-142
(4) Prowald,K., Fischer,H., and Issinger,O.-G.(1984) FEBS Lett. 176, 479-483

IN VITRO ANALYSIS OF PORCINE MAMMARY-DERIVED GROWTH FACTORS

F. A. Simmen, K. Cera, and D. C. Mahan
Dept. of Animal Science and Laboratories of Molecular and Developmental Biology, OARDC, The Ohio State University, Wooster, OH 44691

Murine and human milks are known to contain appreciable quantities of epidermal growth factor (EGF), a potent mitogen for a wide variety of animal cells in vitro. Mammary-derived EGF is implicated in mammary gland development (1) and may be involved in growth and development of the small intestine. With this in mind, we have recently begun an analysis of mitogenic activities in porcine mammary secretions. The pig was chosen since large amounts of early milk (colostrum) can be obtained (in contrast to mouse and human systems). Also, pig intestinal physiology is markedly similar to human, thus providing a useful model system for studying effects of mammary-derived growth factors on neonatal intestine. Here we present preliminary characterization of the mitogenicity of these mammary secretions and its temporal expression during lactation.

RESULTS AND DISCUSSION. Sow colostrum, collected within 12 hr postpartum, was defatted (2) and filter-sterilized. This material when combined with DMEM medium at 5% (v/v) supported proliferation of neonatal pig kidney fibroblasts and murine AKR-2B cells to saturation densities in vitro. This suggested the presence of one or more polypeptide growth factors in the early mammary secretions. Further tests of this were carried out by monitoring stimulation of DNA synthesis in confluent, density-arrested cell cultures (Table I) and in growing cells (Fig. 1). Porcine colostrum stimulated DNA synthesis in AKR-2B cells, Balb/c 3T3s and MDCK canine kidney epithelial cells when tested at confluence (Table I). The degree of stimulation was dose-dependent and varied for each cell type (Fig. 1).

Table I. Cell-type specific mitogenic responses to porcine colostrum[1]

Cells	TCA precipitable cpm[2] Basal	+ pig colostrum (5% v/v)
Mouse embryo-derived AKR-2B cells	41,961	744,640
Murine Balb/c 3T3	3,863	463,582
MDCK canine kidney epithelial cells	17,253	67,885

[1] Mitogenicity was tested by supplementation of colostrum to density-arrested, quiescent monolayer cultures after 48 hrs in 2% serum (3). After 20 hrs, ^{3}H-thymidine was added and the cells incubated for 4 additional hrs. Thymidine uptake was determined as described (3).
[2] Mean of triplicate determinations.

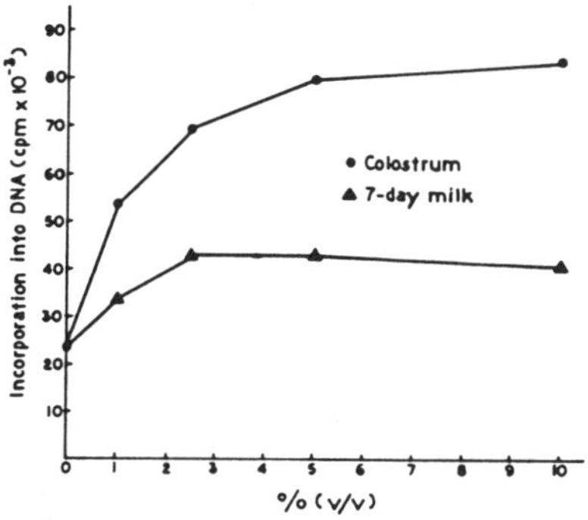

Fig. 1. Stimulation of DNA synthesis in porcine kidney fibroblasts by porcine mammary secretions. Fibroblasts (3rd passage) obtained from neonatal pig kidney were incubated (during logarithmic growth) in the presence of DMEM medium containing various concentrations of milk or colostrum. DNA synthesis was monitored by uptake of ^{3}H-thymidine over a 12-h period. Media formulations were filter (0.2 μm) sterilized.

Total mitogenic activity in porcine colostrum (day 0) and milk (day 7) was compared using growing porcine fibroblasts (Fig. 1). Colostrum was more mitogenic than the milk at all concentrations tested, suggesting temporal regulation of expression of these activities during lactation.

Table II. Antibodies to mouse EGF do not inhibit mitogenicity of porcine mammary secretions for AKR-2B cells[1]

Additions	TCA precipitable cpm ± S.D.[2]
PBS	47,131 ± 3,349
Colostrum (2.5%)	585,953 ± 34,396
Colostrum + anti-mEGF IgG	558,776 ± 33,497
Colostrum + Control Ab	516,455 ± 37,594
mEGF	318,222 ± 32,243
anti-mEGF IgG	54,656 ± 8,731
EGF + anti-mEGF IgG	38,245 ± 3,563
EGF + Control Ab	276,814 ± 41,541
d 21 porcine milk	134,525 ± 28,146
d 21 milk + anti-mEGF IgG	123,455 ± 24,547

1 Mitogenicity was determined as for Table I.
2 Mean and standard deviation of triplicate determinations.

Porcine mammary secretions were examined for growth factors antigenically related to murine EGF by use of rabbit polyclonal IgG raised to purified mouse EGF (Table II). Addition of 160 μg of anti-EGF IgG failed to significantly inhibit the mitogenic activity of colostrum and day 21 milk below that of control antibody. We conclude that the porcine mitogens are structurally distinct from mEGF although it remains to be determined whether they represent porcine EGF or EGF-like molecules.

REFERENCES

(1) Okamoto, S. and Oka, T. (1984) Proc. Natl. Acad. Sci. U.S.A. 81, 6059-6063.
(2) Klagsbrun, M. (1978) Proc. Natl. Acad. Sci. U.S.A. 75, 5057-5061.
(3) Carpenter, G. and Cohen, S. (1976) J. Cell Phys. 88,227-237.

EXPRESSION OF A CYTOSKELETON-ASSOCIATED PROTO-ONCOGENE PRODUCT IN ACTIVATED MACROPHAGES

M. M. Soong, H. Duy, E. S. Didier, S. Fan, and W. A. F. Tompkins
Department of Pathobiology, University of Illinois, Urbana, IL 61801

Fan (1) recently identified 2 major phosphoproteins with molecular weights of 60 and 58 Kd in the actin-rich fractions of murine peritoneal macrophages (MP) and 2 MP cell lines. The level of phosphorylation in these 2 proteins correlated with the activation states of MP and the level of cytotoxicity. Preliminary studies in collaboration with Christie King (University of Illinois, Chicago) indicated that the MP pp60 was phosphorylated, at least in part, at the tyrosine residue. This observation, plus the similarity in M. Wt. of MP pp60 to $pp60^{src}$ led us to investigate if the two proteins were related. B6MP102, a C57BL/6 bone marrow-derived MP cell line which displays MP properties, was used for the molecular characterization of MP pp60. Monoclonal antibody to $pp60^{c\text{-}src}$ of rodent and human cultured cells (2) was used to immunoprecipitate [^{32}P]-labeled B6MP102 cells. As shown in Fig 1, anti-$pp60^{src}$ precipitated a major phosphoprotein (Fig 1A, Lane 2) from RIPA-extracted MP which moved a little slower than $pp60^{v\text{-}src}$ (Fig 1A, Lane 1). Partial peptide mapping of immunoprecipitated MP pp60 and $pp60^{src}$ showed that V-8 protease cleaved $pp60^{v\text{-}src}$ into a 34 Kd amino-terminal fragment and a 26 Kd carboxy-terminal fragment (Fig 2C), while MP pp60 was cleaved into 34 Kd and 28 Kd fragments (Fig 2B). The V-8 protease maps of $pp60^{c\text{-}src}$ from mammalian cells have also been shown to contain a longer carboxy terminal fragment than the avian v-src (3). An immune-complex kinase reaction using α-casein as an exogenous substrate showed that α-casein was phosphorylated by both $pp60^{src}$ and MP pp60. The above results suggest that MP pp60 is related to $pp60^{src}$.

To determine if this src-related MP pp60 was associated with cytoskeletal structures, B6MP102 was extracted with 1% TX-100 as described (1). The detergent-insoluble fraction was resuspended in kinase-assay buffer (20 mM Tris, pH 7.2, 10 mM Mn^{2+}) and incubated with 20 uCi [γ-^{32}P]-ATP at 28 C for 10 min, followed by SDS-PAGE analysis. As shown in Fig 1B, Lane 3, the major protein phosphorylated in the TX-insoluble fraction was a 53 Kd protein. In addition, a minor 60 Kd phosphoprotein, the amount of which varied from experiment to experiment, was present. Sodium vanadate, a potent tyrosine phosphatase inhibitor which has been shown to stimulate $pp60^{src}$ phosphorylation (4), greatly stimulated the phosphorylation of the 53 Kd protein (Fig 1B, Lane 2). Furthermore, preincubation of TX-insoluble fraction with 10 mM N-tosyl-L- lysyl chloromethyl ketone (TLCK), an inhibitor of $pp60^{src}$ and the EGF receptor-associated tyrosine-specific kinase activities, greatly reduced the phosphorylation of pp53. Treatment of the gel with 1N NaOH at 50 C for 1.5 hr, which removed most of phosphoserine and to a lesser extent phosphothreonine, did not reduce the amount of pp53 (Fig 1C). The immune-complex kinase assay also showed that the 53 Kd protein in the TX-insoluble fraction phosphorylated an exogenous substrate, α-casein, and that the activity was inhibited by TLCK. Proteolytic breakdown of pp^{src} to 45-52 Kd polypeptide by cellular proteases has been documented (5), and depended on the cell extraction method and the handling time before the samples were analyzed. Immunoprecipitation of RSV-transformed cells extracted with hypotonic buffer at neutral pH with Triton X-100 showed only a 52 Kd polypeptide (6). A 53 Kd c-src related phosphoprotein has also been reported as the major phosphoprotein in fish brain which has extremely high protease activity (7). MP contain high levels of protease activity, and the extraction buffer we employed favored the proteolytic cleavage despite the presence of various protease inhibitors.

To check the possibility that pp53 was a degradation product of pp60, the *in vitro* phosphorylated TX-insoluble fraction was dissolved in RIPA buffer and immunoprecipitated with Ab to c-src followed by SDS-PAGE analysis. A 53 Kd phosphoprotein and, after longer exposure, a 60 Kd phosphoprotein, were detected. The V-8 peptide map of the 53 Kd protein showed 30 Kd and 28 Kd fragments (Fig 2A). The 30 Kd protein probably represented the proteolytic cleavage product of the 34 Kd amino-terminal fragment of MP pp60.

These data show a correlation between phosphorylation of a cytoskeleton-associated proto-oncogene product pp60/53 and expression of MP cytotoxicity. This suggests that triggering of certain proto-oncogenes may be involved in MP responses to activation signals and that these gene products may exert their influence through phosphorylation of cytoskeleton proteins. In support of this, we have demonstrated that addition of 1-50 $_{u}$M Na_3VO_4 to the MP cytotoxicity assay augments tumoricidal activity by as much as 10-fold and TLCK significantly inhibits this response.

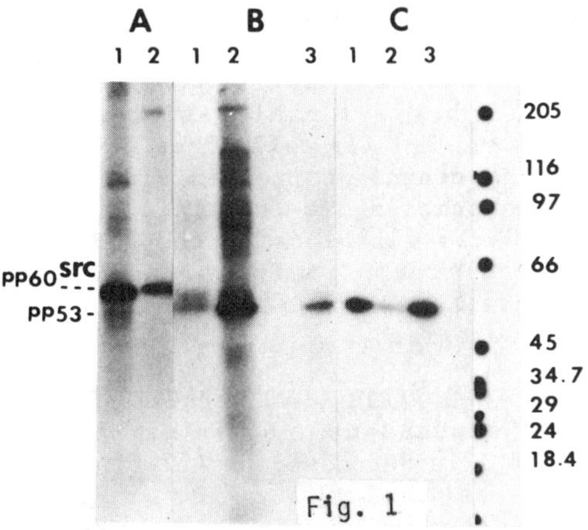

Fig. 1

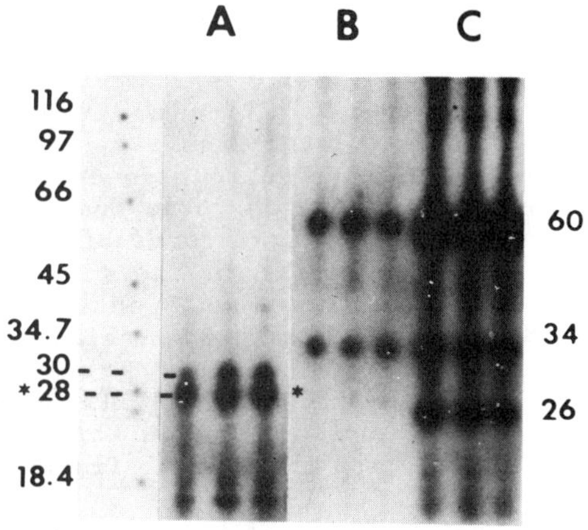

Fig. 2

References

1. Fan, S., 1985. Ph.D. Thesis, University of Illinois.
2. Parsons, S. J. *et al.*, 1984. J. Virol. 51:272-282.
3. Oppermann, H. *et al.*, 1979. Proc. Nat'l. Acad. Sci. 76:1804-1808.
4. Resh, M. D. and R. L. Erikson, 1985. Mol. Cell. Biology 5:916-922.
5. Goldberg, A.R. *et al.* Cold Spring Harbor Symp. Quant. Biol. 44:991-1005.
6. Erikson, R. L. *et al.*, 1980. Cold Spring Harbor Symp. Quant. Biol. 44:907-917.
7. Barnekow, A. *et al.*, 1982. Cancer Research 42:2429-3433.

8. Supported by U.S PHS NCI Training Grant No. CA24930.

SEPARATION OF PROTEIN KINASE ACTIVITIES FROM MDCK AND DB^{r}3

Joseph A. Syracuse, and Mary L. Taub
SUNYAB, Dept. Biochemistry, Buffalo, N.Y. 14214

DB^{r}3 is a variant of the cell line MDCK (isolated by its resistance to 1 mM dibutyryl cAMP and 4 mM theophylline) which has lost the ability to respond to prostaglandin E_1 (PGE_1) by increased expression of differentiated transport functions resulting in the formation of hemicysts or domes in confluent monolayer cultures grown in serum free hormonally defined medium (1). The loss of this response to PGE_1 does not affect the growth stimulatory response of DB^{r}3 to PGE_1 in subconfluent cultures (1). The effects of PGE_1 on both transport and growth are mimicked by the addition of 1 mM dibutyryl cyclic AMP to the culture medium (1), indicating that the PGE_1 effects are mediated through cAMP dependent protein kinase activity. This conclusion is supported by the data which shows that the rate of phosphorylation of calf thymus histone by cAMP dependent protein kinase from DB^{r}3 is 50% of the rate observed in 4 additional DB^{r}3 type variants (1) further strengthening the conclusion that PGE_1 regulates these functions through a cAMP dependent protein kinase. In addition, dibutyryl cAMP resistant variants isolated from S49 (3), CHO (4) and Y-1 (5) cell lines have all been observed to have decreased cAMP dependent protein kinase activity. Towards these ends, we are attempting to correlate the loss of one or more forms of kinase activity with loss of the PGE_1 induced increase in the differentiated transport functions by separating the cAMP dependent protein kinase activities of both MDCK and DB^{r}3 using DEAE-cellulose chromatography.

PROTEIN KINASE ACTIVITY OF SOLUBLE AND PARTICULATE FRACTIONS. The data in Table I show that the cAMP depdendent protein kinase activity from the soluble fraction of DB^{r}3 is decreased by 45% from that of MDCK. The cAMP dependent protein kinase activity of the particulate fraction of DB^r is not significantly decreased from that of MDCK. Chromatography on DEAE-cellulose revealed that all of the kinase activity from this fraction elutes at a salt concentration of 0.1 M NaCl (data not shown).

TABLE I. Protein Kinase Activity of MDCK and DB^{r}3

	Rate of Phophorlyation of Histone (p mole ^{32}P/min/mg protein) -cAMP	+cAMP	Protein Kinase: Activity Ratio $\frac{\text{rate (-cAMP)}}{\text{rate (+cAMP)}}$	cAMP dependent Protein Kinase Activity
Soluble Fraction				
MDCK	76.9±4.5	194.6±12.1	.40	117.7±14.6
DB^{r}3	67.3±11.8	132.2±24.4	.51	64.9±34.2
Particulate Fraction				
MDCK	192.8±52.2	384.5±7.6	.50	191.6±44.6
DB^{r}3	196.4±15.4	332±9.8	.59	135.9±25.1

The soluble fraction was prepared as described in (1) and the particulate fraction prepared in 0.15% Triton X-100 as described in (2). The protein kinase activity of both fractions was determined by phosphorylation of calf thymus histone II A in the presence and absence of 2 mM cAMP as described (1). The cAMP dependent protein kinase activity was determined by subtracting the rate of protein phosphorylation in the absence of cAMP from the rate in the presence of cAMP.

PROTEIN KINASE ACTIVITY OF THE SOLUBLE FRACTION FROM MDCK AND DB^{r}3. When the soluble fraction is applied to a

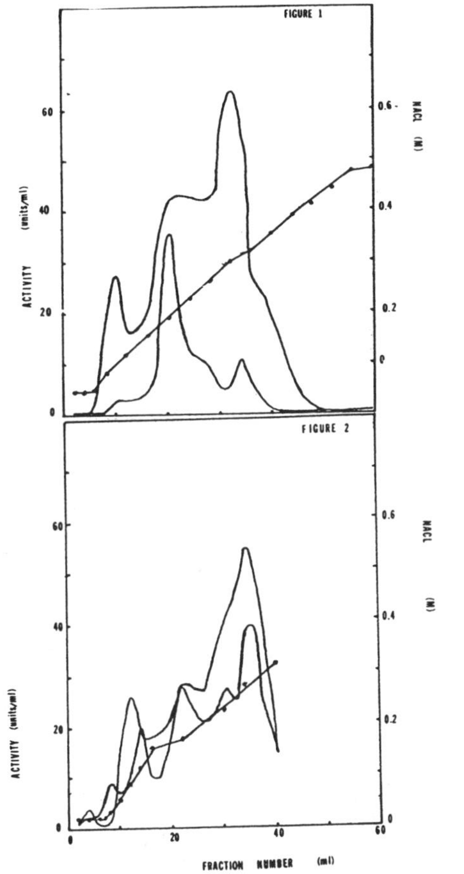

The soluble fraction from MDCK and DB^r3 was prepared, and the fractions assayed for kinase activity as described in (1). Units is pmoles ^{32}P/min.

DEAE-celulose column (0.9x6 cm) and eluted with a gradient of 0 to 0.5 M NaCl the profile of the protein kinase activity presented in Figure 1 is obtained. There are 2 distinct peaks of cAMP dependent protein kinase activity which elute at concentrations of 0.1 and 0.3 M NaCl and a large shoulder of cAMP dependent protein kinase activity which eluted at 0.2 M. When the soluble fraction of DB^r3 is subjected to the same chromatographic conditions (Figure 2), there are again two distinct peaks of cAMP dependent protein kinase activity at 0.1 and 0.3 M. The shoulder of cAMP dependent activity at 0.2 M NaCl appears to be eliminated. In addition, the total area under the cAMP dependent peaks which elute at 0.1 and 0.3 M, is unchanged. Further, there is apparently an increase in the activity of the cAMP independent peaks which elute at 0.1 and 0.3 M NaCl while there is no change in the cAMP independent activity at 0.2 M. These data indicate that the loss of PGE_1 regulation of differentiated transport functions in DB^r3 may be due to a generalized loss of the cAMP dependent protein kinase activity or, may even be due to a shift in kinase activity from cAMP dependent to cAMP independent types.

REFERENCES

1. Devis, P.E., Hiller Grohol, S., and Taub, M. (1985) J. Cell. Physiol. 125, 23-35.
2. Rubin, C.S., Rangel-Aldas, R., Sarkar, D., Erlichman, J. and Fleischer, N. (1975) J. Biol. Chem. 254, 3797-3805.
3. Lemaire, I., and Coffino, P. (1977) J. Cell. Physiol. 92, 437-446.
4. Gottesman, M.M., LeCam, A., Bukowski, M., and Pastan, I. (1980) Somat. Cell Genet. 6, 45-61.
5. Gutmann, N.S., Rae, P.A. and Schimmer, B.P.. (1978) J. Cell. Physiol. 97, 451-460.

Type β Transforming Growth Factors, Epidermal Growth Factor and Tumor Promotors Selectively Induce Secreted Proteins in Mink Lung Epithelial Cells

Frederic W. Thalacker, Lisa J. Crabill, Scott J. Miller and Marit Nilsen-Hamilton, Department of Biochemistry and Biophysics, Iowa State University, Ames, IA

Transforming growth factor type β and 12-O-tetradecanoyl phorbol acetate (TPA) specifically increase the secreted levels of a 48 KDa protein in two epithelial cell lines - African green monkey kidney (BSC-1) cells and Mink lung epithelial (CCL 64) cells. This protein, called "Inhibitor Inducible Protein" (IIP48) was first identified in BSC-1 cells when it was shown to be induced by the BSC-1 derived growth inhibitor [1]. It has since been shown that the BSC-1 growth inhibitor secreted by African green monkey kidney epithelial (BSC-1) cells [2] is a TGF-β [3].

(I) IIP48. The rate of production of secreted IIP48 in response to GI/TGF-β, human platelet TGF-β, and TPA was measured using [^{35}S]methionine-labeling followed by SDS polyacrylamide gel electrophoresis and fluorography. Quantitative analysis of the results of these experiments showed that GI/TGF-β induced IIP48 in CCL 64 by 2 to greater than 800-fold over the control levels. The increase in IIP48 was rapid, occurring within 2 h of addition, and the rate of production of IIP48 reached a maximum within 4 to 6 h of adding GI/TGF-β. The time course of production of IIP48 by CCL 64 cells in response to GI/TGF-β was similar to the time course of induction of IIP48 originally reported for BSC-1 cells [1]. The increase in IIP48 did not occur if inhibitors of RNA synthesis were present. The inhibitors decreased basal levels and GI/TGF-β-stimulated levels of IIP48. These results suggest that the mRNA coding for IIP48 turns over rapidly.

Epidermal growth factor (EGF) also induces CCL 64 cells to produce IIP48, but less effectively than does GI/TGF-β. Together, EGF and GI/TGF-β act synergistically to produce IIP48 (Fig. 1). Greatest induction of IIP48 in GI/TGF-β-treated CCL 64 cells is achieved with as little as 0.5 ng/ml EGF. As well as EGF, TPA induces CCL 64 cells to produce IIP48, but TPA does not act synergistically with GI/TGF-β. TPA stimulates the production of IIP48 to the same extent as a combination of EGF and GI.

Because TPA also stimulates the synthesis of urokinase, we explored the possibility that IIP48 might be urokinase. Antibody against human urokinase did not immunoprecipitate IIP48. Also IIP48 did not adsorb to benzamidine-Sepharose, an affinity column that has been used to purify urokinase. A number of serine proteases specifically bind to benzamidine-sepharose. These data also suggest that IIP48 is not one of these serine proteases.

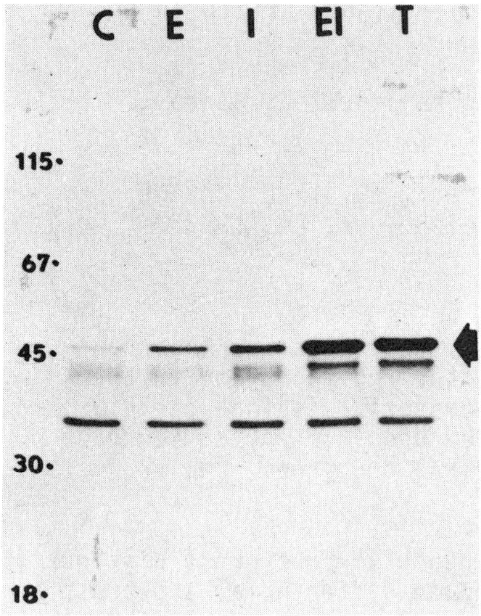

Fig. 1. Effect of EGF, GI/TGF-β, EGF and GI/TGF-β combined, and TPA on the induction of IIP48. CCL64 cells (near term mink lung epithelial cells) were incubated with or without EGF or GI/TGF-β for 2.5 h, then labeled for 4 h with [^{35}]methionine. The cell density was 1.9 x 10^5 cells/cm^2. Shown is a fluorogram of an SDS polyacrylamide gel. IIP48 is indicated by the arrow. In this experiment, there was a 2.1-fold increase over the control in IIP48 after treatment with EGF, a 4.5-fold increase in IIP48 after treatment with GI/TGF-β, a 19.2-fold increase with EGF and GI/TGF-β, and a 16.5-fold increase with TPA. The molecular weight standards used on the gel were (from top to bottom): β-galactosidase, BSA, Ovalbumin, carbonic anhydrase, and myoglobin. C: control, E: 5 ng/ml EGF, I: 1 unit/ml GI/TGF-β, EI: EGF with GI/TGF-β, and T: 10 ng/ml TPA.

(II) OTHER PROTEINS INDUCED BY GI/TGF-β AND TPA. As well as inducing IIP48, GI/TGF-β also stimulates the production of a 73 KDa protein (IIP73) by CCL 64 cells. The time course of induction of IIP73 was much slower than that for IIP48, with the maximum rate of production of IIP73 occurring about 20 h after the addition of GI/TGF-β. Neither EGF nor TPA induce IIP73 nor do they act synergistically with GI/TGF-β to induce IIP73. TPA does not induce IIP73 but does induce the synthesis of a 67 KDa that we have called "Promotor Inducible Protein" (PIP67).

(III) CONCLUSIONS. EGF, TPA and GI/TGF-β each alter the expression of certain genes that code for secreted proteins. The set of proteins induced by each agent is different. GI/TGF-β induces IIP48 and IIP73 whereas EGF only induces IIP48. TPA induces a larger set of secreted proteins that includes the proteins induced by EGF and GI/TGF-β but also includes some proteins induced by neither growth factor. EGF and TGF-βs regulate the expression of genes coding for secreted proteins by separate but interacting pathways.

REFERENCES

(1) Nilsen-Hamilton, M., and Holley, R.W. (1983) Proc. Natl. Acad. Sci. USA 80, 5636-5640
(2) Holley, R.W., Bohlen, P., Fava, R., Baldwin, J.H., Kleeman, G., and Armour, R. (1980) Proc. Natl. Acad. Sci. USA 77, 5989-5992
(3) Tucker, R.F., Shipley, G.D., Moses, H.L., and Holley, R.W. (1984) Science 226, 705-707

ACKNOWLEDGEMENT - This work was funded by NIH grant GM 33528.

A NEW MEMBER OF THE TYROSINE KINASE GENE FAMILY EXPRESSED IN A HUMAN T-CELL LEUKEMIA

J.M. Trevillyan, Y. Lin, S-J. Chen, C.A. Phillips, C. Canna, T.J. Linna.

Central Research and Development Department, E. I. du Pont de Nemours and Co., 500 S. Ridgeway Ave., Glenolden, PA 19086

Introduction

Protein tyrosine kinase (PTK) activity appears to be important in the signal transduction of growth factor receptors and in the regulation of cell proliferation. At least six distinct cellular genes for PTKs have been identified based upon nucleotide sequence homology with molecularly cloned retroviral oncogenes, the products of which express PTK activity (1).

Human B and T lymphocytes have been reported to express distinct membrane associated PTK activities based on differential substrate specificities (2,3). The relationship between the human lymphocyte PTKs and those encoded by known PTK oncogene-protooncogene sequences is unknown. We report below the molecular cloning of a PTK from the human T-cell leukemia, JURKAT. The JURKAT PTK is homologous to, but distinct from previously identified retroviral PTKs. Preliminary data suggest that the expression of the JURKAT PTK is restricted to lymphocytes of the T-lineage.

Results and Discussion

A JURKAT cDNA library was constructed in lambda phage using standard molecular biology techniques(4). An oligonucleotide probe based upon a highly conserved PTK autophosphorylation sequence, Glu-Asp-Asn-Glu-Ty-Thr, was used to screen the JURKAT cDNA library. A 0.86 Kbp partial cDNA designated λptk-JURKAT, was isolated and the nucleotide sequence determined (Fig. 1). The λptk-JURKAT clone

```
    10                    30                    50
AlaLeuSerCysLysIleAlaAspPheGlyLeuAlaArgLeuIleGluAspAsnGluTyr
GCCCTGAGCTGCAAGATTGCAGACTTTGGCCTAGCACGCCTCATTGAGGACAACGAGTAC

    70                    90                   110
ThrAlaArgGluGlyAlaLysPheProIleLysTrpThrAlaProGluAlaIleAsnTyr
ACAGCCAGGGAGGGGGCCAAGTTTCCCATTAAGTGGACAGCGCCAGAAGCCATTAACTAC

   130                   150                   170
GlyThrPheThrIleLysSerAspValTrpSerPheGlyIleLeuLeuThrGluIleVal
GGGACATTCACCATCAAGTCAGATGTGTGGTCTTTTGGGATCCTGCTGACGGAAATTGTC

   190                   210                   230
ThrHisGlyArgIleProTyrProGlyMetThrAsnProGluValIleGlnAsnLeuGlu
ACCCACGGCCGCATCCCTTACCCAGGGATGACCAACCCGGAGGTGATTCAGAACCTGGAG

   250                   270                   290
ArgGlyTyrArgMetValArgProAspAsnCysProGluGluLeuTyrGlnLeuMetArg
CGAGGCTACCGCATGGTGCGCCCTGACAACTGTCCAGAGGAGCTGTACCAACTCATGAGG

   310                   330                   350
LeuCysTrpLysGluArgProGluAspArgProThrPheAspTyrLeuArgSerValLeu
CTGTGCTGGAAGGAGCGCCCAGAGGACCGGCCCACCTTTGACTACCTGCGCAGTGTGCTG

   370                   390                   410
GluAspPhePheThrAlaThrGluGlyGlnTyrGlnProGlnPro
GAGGACTTCTTCACGGCCACAGAGGGCCAGTACCAGCCTCAGCCTTGAGAGGCCTTGAGA

   430                   450                   470
GGCCCTGGGGTTCTCCCCCTTTCTCTCCAGCCTGACTTGGGGAGATGGAGTTCTTGTGCC

   490                   510                   530
ATAGTCACATGGCCTATGCACATATGGACTCTGCACATGAATCCCACCCACATGTGACAC

   550                   570                   590
ATATGCACCTTGTGTCTGTACACGTGTCCTGTAGTTGCGTGGACTCTGCACATGTCTTGT

   610                   630                   650
GCATGTGTAGCCTGTGCATGTATGTCTTGGACACTGTACAAGGTACCCCTTTCTGGCTCT

   670                   690                   710
CCCATTTCCTGAGACCACAGAGAGAGGGGAGAAGCCTGGGATTGACAGAAGCTTCTGCCC

   730                   750                   770
ACCTACTTTTCTTTCCTCAGATCATCCAGAAGTTCCTCAAGGGCCAGGACTTTATCTAAT

   790                   810                   830
ACCTCTGTGTGCTCCTCCTTGGTGCCTGGCCTGGCACACATCAGGAGTTCAATAAATGTC

   850
TGTTGATGACTGCCG
```

Fig. 1. Nucleotide and derived a.a. sequence of λptk-JURKAT cDNA. Oligonucleotide probe, stop codon, and polyadenylation sequences are underlined.

shared 70% nucleotide sequence homology with exon 10, 11 and 12 of the human c-src protooncogene (5). Alignment of the nucleotide sequence to correspond to the hexapeptide autophosphorylation sequence (above), resulted in an open reading frame coding 135 amino acids with a 447 nucleotide 3' untranslated region containing the polyadenylation signal AATAAA (Fig. 1). The derived amino acid sequence from the λptk-JURKAT clone shared extensive homology with, but was distinct from the carboxy terminal amino acid sequence of PTKs encoded by the v-src, v-yes and v-fgr oncogenes as well as the human c-src protooncogene(Fig. 2). Less homology was found between the PTKs encoded by the v-abl, v-fps, v-fes, and v-ros oncogenes. Analysis of human genomic DNA, using the λptk-JURKAT probe, revealed the JURKAT PTK gene to be present in single copy number and was distinct from the human c-src protooncogene. The λptk-JURKAT probe hybridized with an approximately 2 Kb RNA transcript from both JURKAT cells and the human T-cell lymphoma MOLT-4, but failed to hybridize with poly A+ RNA from either human B cell lymphomas, RAJI and IM-9 or the human erythroid-myeloid leukemia, K562. Our data, taken together, establishes the expression of a unique PTK gene in a human T-cell leukemia. The expression of this human protein tyrosine kinase may be restricted to lymphocytes of the T lineage.

Fig. 2 Homology between the JURKAT PTK and PTKs encoded by c-src, v-src, v-yes and v-fgr. Highly conserved sequences are boxed.

Human c-ptk JURKAT	L	S	CK	I	ADFGLARLIEDNEY	TA	R	E	GAKFPIKWTAPEA	INY	G	T
Human c-src	L	V	CK	V	ADFGLARLIEDNEY	TA	R	Q	GAKFPIKWTAPEA	ALY	G	R
v-src	L	V	CK	V	ADFGLARLIEDNEY	TA	R	Q	GAKFPIKWTAPEA	ALY	G	R
v-yes	L	V	CK	I	ADFGLARLIEDNEY	TA	R	Q	GAKFPIKWTAPEA	ALY	G	R
v-fgr	L	V	CK	I	ADFGLARLIEDNEY	NP	R	Q	GAKFPIKWTAPEA	ALF	G	R

FTIKSDVWSFGILLTE	IVTH	GR	I	PYPGM	T	N	P	EV	IQNL	E	R
FTIKSDVWSFGILLTE	LTTK	GR	V	PYPGM	V	N	R	EV	LDQV	E	R
FTIKSDVWSFGILLTE	LTTK	GR	V	PYPGM	V	N	R	EV	LDQV	E	R
FTIKSDVWSFGILLTE	LVTK	GR	V	PYPGM	V	N	R	EV	LEQV	E	R
FTIKSDVWSFGILLTE	LISK	GR	V	PYPGM	N	N	R	EV	LEQV	E	H

GY	R	M	VR	P	DN	CP	EE	L	YQL	M	RLC	W	KER	P	ED	RPTF	D	Y
GY	R	M	PC	P	PE	CP	ES	L	HDL	M	CQC	W	RKE	P	EE	RPTF	E	Y
GY	R	M	PC	P	PE	CP	ES	L	HDL	M	CQC	W	RKD	P	EE	RPTF	K	Y
GY	R	M	PC	P	QG	CP	ES	L	HGL	M	KLC	W	KKD	P	DE	RPTF	E	Y
GY	H	M	PC	P	PG	CP	AS	L	YEA	M	EQT	W	RLD	P	EE	RPTF	E	Y

LRSV	L	EDFFTATEGQYQPQP
LQAF	L	EDYFTSTEPQYQPGENL
LQAQ	L	LPACVLEVAE
IQSF	L	EDYFTAAEPSGY
LQSF	L	EDYFNGPQQN

References

(1) Hunter T. and Cooper J.A. (1985) Ann. Rev. Biochem. 54:897-930.
(2) Trevillyan, J.M., Nordstrom, A. and Linna, T.J. (1985) Biochem. Biophys. Acta 845:1-9.
(3) Harrison, M.L., Low, P.S. and Geahlen, R.L. (1984) J. Biol. Chem. 259:9348-9350.
(4) Maniatis, T., Fritsch, E.F., and Sambrook J. (1982) in Molecular Cloning (a Laboratory Manual). Cold Spring Harbor Laboratory, Cold Spring Harbor, NY.
(5) Anderson, S.K., Gibbs C.P., Tanaka, A., Kung, H. and Fujita, D.J. (1985) Mol. and Cell. Biol. 5:1122-1129.

THE CELLULAR MYC ONCOGENE OF RAINBOW TROUT

R. J. Van Beneden*†, D. K. Watson†, T. T. Chen‡, T. S. Papas†

†Laboratory of Molecular Oncology, NCI, Frederick, MD 21701;

Cellular sequences homologous to the MC29 v-*myc* gene have been identified by Southern blot analysis in a wide variety of species, but confirmed by sequence analysis only in chicken (1), mouse (2), human (3), and most recently in trout (*Salmo gairdneri*) (4). A genomic library was prepared from rainbow trout testes DNA and clones identified by hybridization to v-*myc* under relaxed conditions. A single clone which contained sequences homologous to both chicken exon II and exon III was subjected to sequence analysis. The trout *myc* gene contains an exon II which is smaller than that of other vertebrates; exon III is larger. Here we present a comparison of the predicted *myc* gene products (Fig. 1). Overall, the third exon is the most highly conserved, showing 69% homology between trout and chicken and 66% homology between trout and human. Although the overall homology is less within exon II (60% between trout and chicken; 58% between trout and human), several specific regions are highly homologous. These regions include the *myc* boxes A and B which are the sequences of highest conservation between c-*myc*, N-*myc* and L-*myc*. These regions show greater than 89% deduced amino acid homology among trout, chicken, and human.

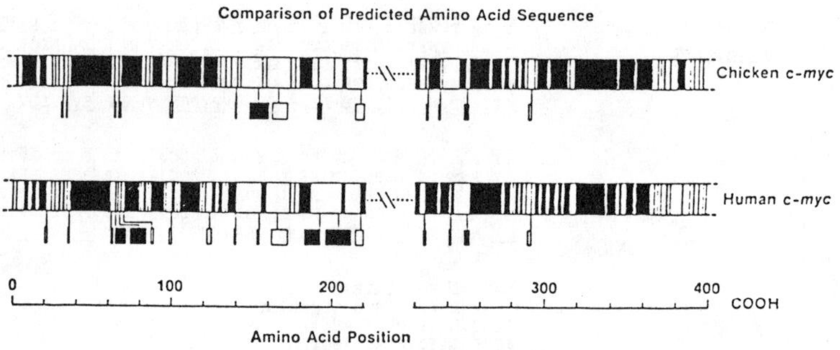

Figure 1. Comparison of the predicted amino acid sequence of rainbow trout c-*myc* to those of chicken and human c-*myc*. Left, exon II; right, exon III. Solid regions of the bars indicate conserved sequences; open regions indicate variable regions. The solid and open boxes below the bars indicate insertions and deletions, respectively.

*Guest Researcher of Chesapeake Bay Institute, Johns Hopkins University, Shadyside, MD 20764; ‡Presently at the Department of Biology, McMaster University, Hamilton, Ontario, Canada L8S 4K1

Restriction Polymorphism of myc in Fish Tumors. DNA isolated from normal and tumor tissues of northern pike was used to prepare Southern blots (Fig. 2). Different restriction patterns are apparent between Eco RI digests of DNA derived from normal kidney and lymphosarcoma tissues. These findings are consistent with a rearrangement and/or translocation of the myc gene trout which may have occurred in the northern pike lymphosarcoma cells.

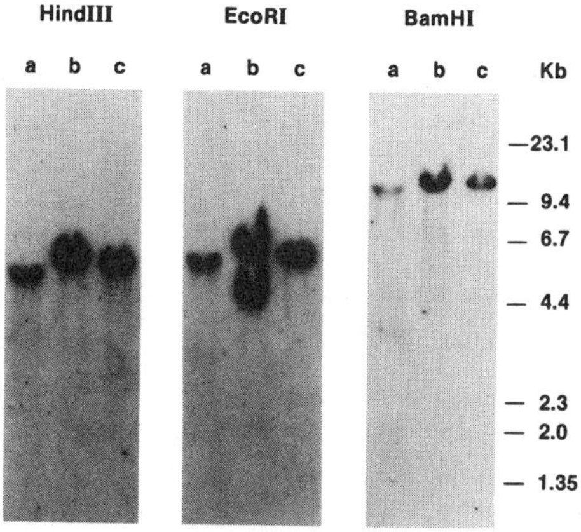

Figure 2. Southern blot of DNA from tumor and normal tissue of northern pike: a) lymphosarcoma, spontaneously arising in a laboratory-reared fish; b) lymphosarcoma, spontaneous tumor from a feral fish; c) normal kidney. Samples (20 µg) were digested with either Bam HI, Eco RI, or Hind III as indicated and fragments resolved on a 0.8% agarose gel. Immobilized DNA was hybridized to a trout myc probe (containing exons II and III) under stringent conditions.

REFERENCES

1. Watson, D. K., Reddy, E. P., Duesberg, P. H. and Papas, T. S. (1983) Proc. Natl. Acad. Sci. U.S.A. 80, 2146-2150.
2. Stanton, L. W., Fahrlander, P. D., Tesser, P. M. and Marcu, K. B (1984) Nature (London) 310, 423-425.
3. Watson, D. K., Psallidopoulos, M. C., Samuel, K. P., Dalla-Favera, R. and Papas, T. S. (1983) Proc. Natl. Acad. Sci. U.S.A. 80, 3642-3645.
4. Van Beneden, R. J., Watson, D. K., Chen, T. T., Lautenberger, J. A., and Papas, T. S. Proc. Natl. Acad. Sci. U.S.A., in press.

THE p135 TRANSFORMING PROTEIN OF E26 IS NOT CO-TERMINAL WITH THE CHICKEN PROTO-ETS GENE PRODUCT.

D. K. Watson, M. J. McWilliams-Smith, C. S. Flordellis*, and T. S. Papas
Laboratory of Molecular Oncology, NCI-FCRF, Frederick, MD 21701

E26 is a replication-defective avian retrovirus that induces erythroblastosis and myeloblastosis in chickens and transforms erythroblasts and myeloid cells in culture. The E26 provirus has been cloned and sequence analysis has identified two cell derived sequences (Figure 1), myb and ets, which are fused with gag in the p135 transforming protein (1). Comparison of the oncogenic properties of E26 and AMV suggests that the ets domain of E26 may be responsible for the erythroblastic tropism of this virus.

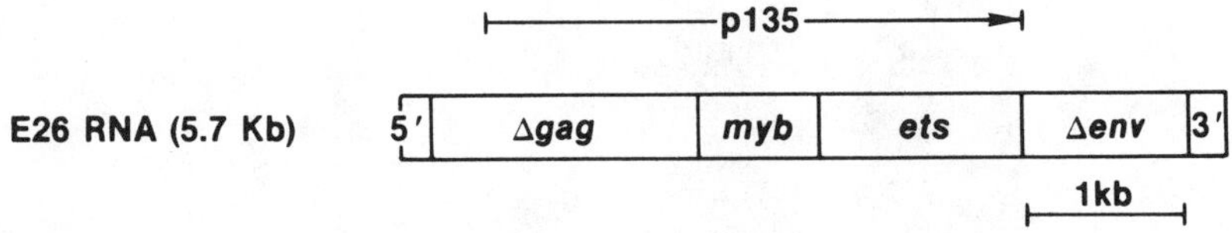

Figure 1. Genetic organization of the E26 transforming virus.

To eludicate the origin of E26 and to understand the function of the ets gene, we have initiated the characterization of the chicken proto-ets gene and the c-ets genes from mouse and man. We found that the ets sequence is present on two chromosomes in mouse, cat and man (2). Both human ets genes contain unique domains of v-ets homology and are transcriptionally active. The human ets-1 locus on chromosome 11 encodes a single mRNA of 6.8 kb; the second locus, ets-2 on chromosome 21, encodes three mRNAs of 4.7, 3.2, and 2.7 kb. At the predicted amino acid level, the human ets genes and v-ets gene are over 95% conserved (3). A number of leukemias show chromosomal abnormalities where the human ets genes reside (11q23;21q22), and we haved demonstrated that Hu-ets-1 and the Hu-ets-2 genes are transposed in leukemias with translocation t(4;11) or translocation t(8;21) (4).

We have determined the nucleotide sequence of the v-ets homologous exons of a genomic chicken clone. Whereas the mammalian ets genes are present on two chromosomes, the chicken ets gene is contiguous with the ets-1 and ets-2 sequences located on one chromosome (Figure 2). The chicken locus is primarily expressed in normal chicken cells as a major 7.5 kb mRNA transcript. Alignment of the 3' end of v-ets with the sequences of genomic chicken clone, λC51, identifies a region of complete homology followed

*Presently at Dana-Farber Cancer Institute, Boston, MA 021115

by a region of non-homology. In spite of this non-homology, the open reading frame (ORF) extends into this region of the chicken gene. It seems that this (ORF) extension continues within the last chicken exon, rather than be representative of an intron. The following criteria support this hypothesis: (i) absence of splice doner signal (ii) homology with Hu-ets-2 and (iii) presence of the sequence in human cDNA clones (3). The origin of the carboxy-terminus of p135 is unclear, but is not the same as that of the chicken gene. Because ets-1 and ets-2 sequence can be found either on different chromosomes (mammals) or as contiguous sequences (chicken), we conclude that the v-ets is likely to contain at least two dissociable functional domains. In conclusion, E26 may actually include a total of four domains (Δgag, myb, ets-1 and ets-2).

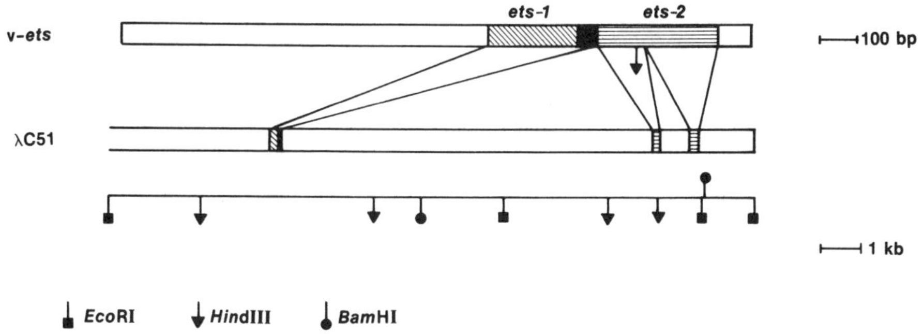

Figure 2. Ets-1 and ets-2 sequence are contiguous in chicken. Allignment of v-ets sequence with the ets homologous regions of chicken clone λC51.

REFERENCES

1. Nunn, M. F., Seeburg, P. H., Moscovici, C., and Duesberg, P. H. (1983) Nature 306, 391-395.
2. Watson, D. K., McWilliams-Smith, M. J., Kozak, C., Reeves, R., Gearhart, J., Nuun, M. F., Nash, W., Fowle III, J. R., Duesberg, P. H., Papas, T. S., and O'Brien, S. J. (1985) Proc. Natl. Acad. Sci. U.S.A., in press.
3. Watson, D. K., McWilliams-Smith, M. J., Nunn, M. F., Duesberg, P. H., O'Brien, S. J. and Papas, T. S. (1985) Proc. Natl. Acad. Sci. U.S.A. 82, 7294-7298.
4. Sacchi, N., Watson, D. K., Geurts van Kessel, A. H. M., Hagemeijer, A., Kersey, J., Drabkin, H. D., Patterson, D., and Papas, T. S. (1985) Science, in press.

ACUTE LYMPHOBLASTIC LEUKEMIA-ASSOCIATED ANTIGEN, GP24, AND ITS RELATIONSHIP TO PLATELET-DERIVED GROWTH FACTOR

N.L. Wood,* E. Westin,#+ and T. Mohanakumar,*+ Departments of Surgery,* Microbiology,+ and Medicine,# Medical College of Virginia, Richmond, VA 23298-0001

Leukemia-associated antigens (LAA) have been useful in phenotyping and subclassifying childhood leukemias, however, there has been little information regarding the function of these antigens. Several growth factors and their receptors have homology with oncogene products. Thus, it seems intriguing to consider the possibility that some of the LAA may have a functional role in growth and differentiation. In this report, we demonstrate an association between the 24 kd non-T, non-B acute lymphocytic leukemia (ALL) associated antigen, gp24, defined by monoclonal antibodies (MOAB) (1,2) and the platelet-derived growth factor, PDGF, which has sequence homology with the oncogene, sis (3).

PRESENCE OF LAA gp24, DEFINED BY MOAB IN PDGF PREPARATIONS. Three sources of PDGF [1) Collaborative Research, Lexington, MA; 2) Cellular Products Inc., Buffalo, NY; and 3) Seragen, Boston, MA] were tested for LAA gp24 using dot blot analysis with a specific MOAB followed by a secondary ^{125}I-labeled antibody. Figure 1 shows that all three contained LAA gp24. Commercial preparations of PDGF generally contain less than 10% PDGF leaving the possibility that anti-LAA gp24 detects some other molecule in the PDGF preparation.

Figure 1. Densitometer tracing of dot blot analysis of serial dilutions of three different preparations of PDGF and affinity purified LAA gp24 from REH cells using monoclonal antibody to LAA gp24. PDGF was blotted at 4, 2 and 1 unit/ml, respectively. LAA gp24 was applied at concentrations of 0.24, 0.12 and 0.06 μg/ml, respectively.

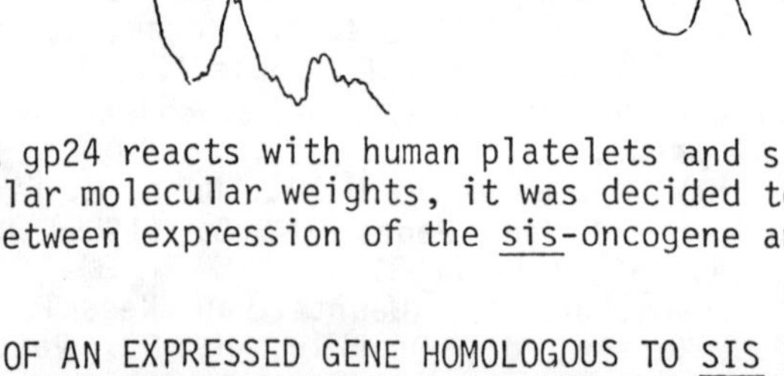

Since anti-LAA gp24 reacts with human platelets and since LAA gp24 and PDGF have similar molecular weights, it was decided to examine the relationship between expression of the sis-oncogene and LAA gp24 expression.

PRESENCE OF AN EXPRESSED GENE HOMOLOGOUS TO SIS IN REH CELLS. To further establish a relationship between LAA gp24 and PDGF, we examined DNA and RNA from REH cells by Southern and Northern blotting analysis for homologous sequences to a c-sis specific gene probe. Examination of the DNA revealed no gross amplifications or rearrangements of the c-sis gene. Preliminary data suggests that a sis specific mRNA is present in phorbol ester stimulated REH cells which also express increased amounts of surface LAA gp24, thus indicating expression of the c-sis/PDGF product in these cells.

PRESENCE OF LAA gp24 IN IMMUNOPRECIPITATES FROM SIS-TRANSFECTED 3T3 CELLS. To examine the similarity between LAA gp24 and PDGF, extracts of either REH, NIH-3T3 cells, or sis-transfected NIH-3T3 cells were labeled with ^{125}I and precipitated with anti-LAA gp24. As seen in figure 2, all three cell lines expressed LAA gp24. Additionally biosynthetic labeling with ^{35}S-methionine showed that both 3T3 and sis-3T3 synthesized an 18kd molecule precipitable with anti-LAA gp24 (Fig. 3).

Figure 2: Densitometer tracing of immunoprecipitation analysis of ^{125}I-labeled REH, 3T3 and sis-3T3 using anti-LAA gp24.

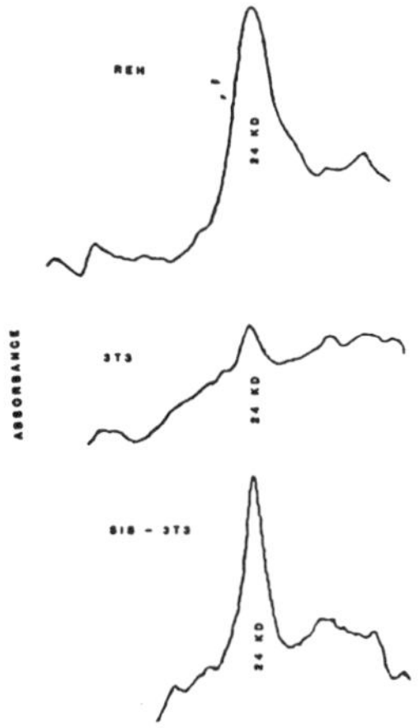

Figure 3: Densitometer tracing of immunoprecipitation analysis of ^{35}S-methionine labeled 3T3 or sis-3T3 using anti-LAA gp24.

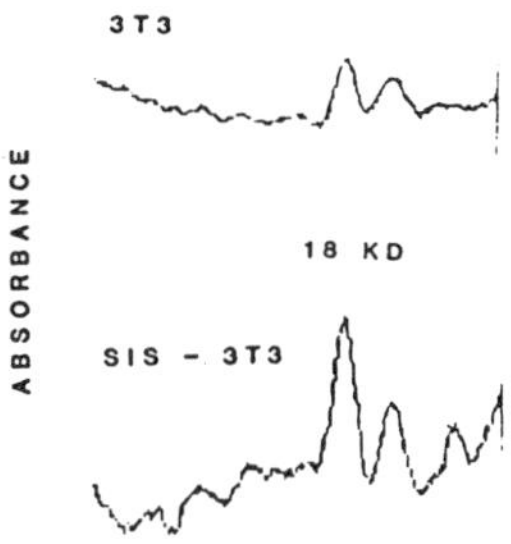

Our results demonstrate a close similarity between LAA gp24, defined by MOAB, and the growth factor, PDGF. Thus far, LAA have served as markers with little knowledge of their function. This study suggests that these molecules may have growth factor or growth factor receptor activity or may be the product of cellular oncogenes. The presence of RNA sequences sharing homology with sis in LAA gp24 positive cells, as well as the presence of gp24 in PDGF preparations suggests a relationship between these molecules. Since 3T3 express LAA gp24, it appears that this antigen may not be identical but closely related to PDGF. Studies are ongoing to establish this relationship.

REFERENCE

1. Kersey, J.H., et al. (1981) J. Exp. Med. 153, 726-731.
2. Jones, N.H., et al. (1981) Proc. Am. Assoc. Cancer Res. 22, 1210.
3. Waterfield, M.D., et al. (1983) Nature 304, 35-39.

Supported by NIH CA 27416 and ACS CH 270. TM is a recipient of ACS FRA 246.

Peptide and Protein Receptors

TRANSMEMBRANE SIGNALLING BY EGF: EVIDENCE FOR AN ALLOSTERIC-OLIGOMERIZATION MECHANISM

Y. Yarden* and J. Schlessinger**
*Department of Molecular Biology, Genentech, Inc., 460 Pt. San Bruno Blvd., South San Francisco, CA 94080 and **Department of Chemical Immunology, The Weizmann Institute of Science, Rehovot 76100, Israel

Epidermal growth factor (EGF) stimulates cell growth by binding to a 170 kilodalton membrane receptor. The latter is composed of a large extracellular EGF-binding domain connected to a cytoplasmic tyrosine kinase domain by a single membrane spanning region (1). Stimulation of the intrinsic phosphotransferase activity is probably the first cytoplasmic effect induced by EGF binding. Moreover, no other membranal component seems to be involved in this process. Thus, elucidation of the molecular mechanism which functionally couples ligand binding to kinase activation may explain how the hormonal signal is transmitted across the plasma membrane. We addressed this question by considering two potential mechanisms. According to the first, an intramolecular model, ligand binding induces a molecular change which is transmitted across the membrane spanning domain. On the contrary, we tentatively assumed that a monomeric receptor having a single transmembrane region lacks the rigidity required for this kind of mechanism. Therefore an alternative intermolecular model was suggested where EGF binding confers the essential molecular rigidity by an allosteric mechanism (2). This model, presented in Figure 1, assumes that EGF binding favors an oligomeric state of the receptor. Furthermore, it is suggested that the ligand-induced oligomerization is sufficient to stimulate the cytoplasmic kinase domain. Receptor aggregation, upon EGF binding, was previously demonstrated by electron microscopy (3) and on living cells (4), and it was further suggested to play a role in the cascade of events leading to the mitogenic signal (5).

(I) FUNCTIONAL EVIDENCE. To examine the necessity of an intermolecular step for kinase stimulation by EGF, we employed an *in vitro* system composed of detergent-solubilized receptor and contrasted the two types of mechanisms by the following approaches:

1. EGF-stimulated phosphorylation of the receptor depends on receptor concentration as if the reaction is bimolecular.
2. Cross-linking of receptors by bivalent antibodies or multivalent lectins stimulated the kinase function; therefore the possibility is raised that simple juxtaposition of receptors is sufficient to replace EGF binding.
3. Prevention of interactions among receptor molecules by immobilization on a solid support abolished their EGF stimulability capacity, indicating that receptor interaction, in addition to ligand binding, is crucial.
4. Aggregation of receptors by means of a bivalent antibody increased their affinity toward EGF.

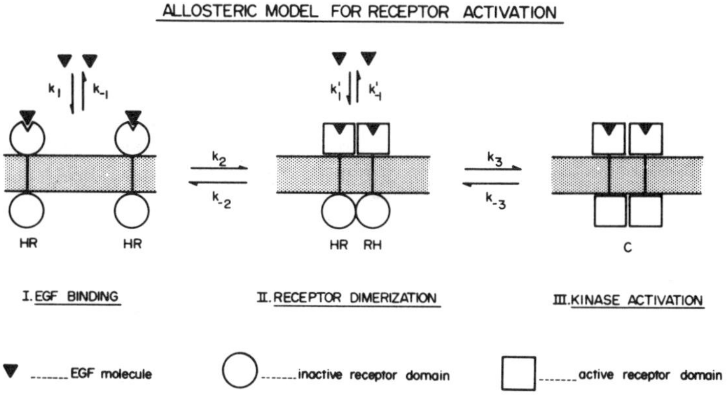

Fig. 1. EGF receptor is schematically depicted as a bilobular transmembranal structure. The model assumes that a ligand-dependent equilibrium exists between the receptor monomeric state and an oligomeric state (for simplicity represented here as a dimer). EGF binding shifts the equilibrium to the right by having higher affinity toward the aggregated receptor.

In conclusion, our functional approaches favor the intermolecular model. It was further indicated that a minimal receptor oligomerization, namely dimerization, is sufficient for signal transduction.

(II) STRUCTURAL EVIDENCE. The increased ligand-affinity of the aggregated receptor suggested that the oligomeric state is energetically stabilized by at least 1 kcal/mol, which may enable direct detection. To this end we subjected an affinity-purified receptor, internally radiolabeled, to a non-denaturing polyacrylamide gel electrophoresis. Autoradiography of the gel revealed that the receptor exists in two forms: a lower form, having high electrophoretic mobility, and a higher form. In the absence of EGF the lower form dominated, whereas upon EGF binding the higher form is induced. False migration of the EGF receptor under non-denaturing conditions prevented reliable molecular weight determination. Other investigators (6), using sucrose-density gradient centrifugation, established the existence of receptor dimers in addition to receptor monomers. The molecular shift observed in the non-denaturing gel seems to represent the oligomerization process predicted by the intermolecular model, based on the following observations:

1. EGF binding induces, in a dose-dependent manner, the conversion of the lower form into the higher form.
2. The ligand-induced molecular shift is rapid (complete within a few minutes) and moderately affected by temperature.

3. The appearance of the higher molecular form has a parabolic dependence on the concentration of EGF receptor, thus excluding the possibility that an intramolecular conformational change is responsible for the reduced electrophoretic effect.
4. The higher molecular state, once formed, is stable under neutral pH in non-ionic detergents. Both extreme pH and treatment with ionic detergents fully reversed the higher form into the lower form.

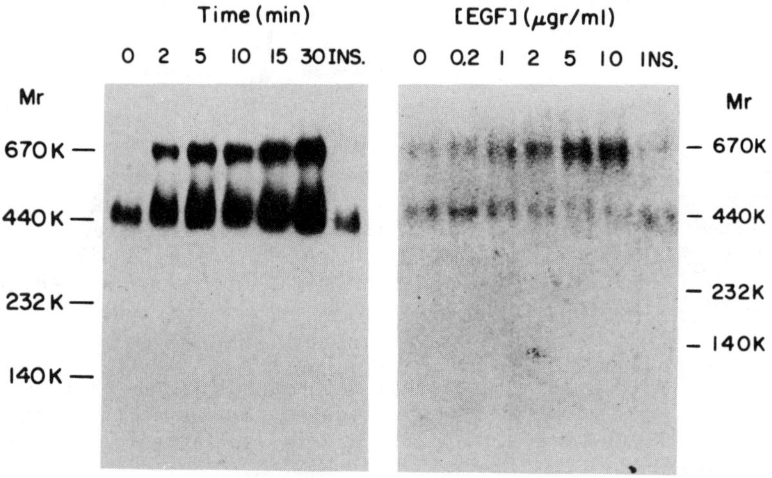

Fig. 2. Receptor functions in non-denatured polyacrylamide gel. Left panel: Affinity purified receptor (0.2 fmoles) was incubated at 0°C with saturating concentrations of EGF, insulin or buffer alone for the indicated periods of time. Self-phosphorylation was then initiated by adding [γ-^{32}P]-ATP and $MnCl_2$. The reaction was stopped after 90 seconds at 0°C by quenching with non-labeled ATP, and the samples were loaded on a non-denatured polyacrylamide gel (2-15 percent linear gradient of acrylamide; essentially Triton X-100 replaces sodium dodecyl sulfate). An autoradiogram of the dry gel is shown. Right panel: Affinity-purified receptor was preincubated at 22°C with the indicated concentrations of EGF or insulin (1.8 μM), and then subjected to gel electrophoresis under non-denaturing conditions. The gel was washed twice with a buffer containing Triton X-100 and albumin and then incubated with the same buffer containing 100 ng/ml of radiolabeled EGF. Binding was allowed for 1 hr at 22°C and followed by rapid washes. An autoradiogram of the dry gel is shown. The molecular weights indicated were obtained by using a commercial mixture of water-soluble proteins (Pharmacia).

5. The formation of the higher form seems to involve non-covalent interactions, as it is fully reversible upon dilution.

In conclusion, our structural approach may indicate the existence of an equilibrium between two receptor states: a monomer and an oligomer, possibly a dimer, and that EGF binding favors the oligomer.

(III) COMBINED STRUCTURAL AND FUNCTIONAL EVIDENCE. In order to correlate the functional and the structural approaches, we undertook a study of the functional properties of both receptor states. When an affinity-purified, fully active receptor is first self-phosphorylated and then subjected to gel electrophoresis (Fig. 2, left panel), two receptor forms are detected, the higher form being much less phosphorylated. Upon EGF binding the phosphorylation of both forms is greatly enhanced. Under certain conditions we could detect an earlier enhanced phosphorylation of the higher receptor form, followed by an elevated phosphorylation of the lower form. These experiments, though preliminary, may suggest the existence of a "collision-activation" mechanism. The relative affinities of both forms toward EGF were examined by binding of radiolabeled EGF to the receptor states preserved within the gel. As is evident in Figure 2 (right panel), short preincubation of the receptor with the hormone prior to the electrophoresis step results in enhanced labeling by EGF, mostly of the higher form. The more intense labeling observed after preincubation with EGF is consistent with the notion that the oligomeric state may have an increased ligand affinity.

In summary, the work described here raises the possibility that EGF binding is followed, at least in vitro, by a rapid receptor oligomerization step which may play a role in signal transduction across the plasma membrane. It may further suggest that the oligomerization function is intrinsic to the receptor molecule.

REFERENCES

(1) Ullrich, A., Coussens, L., Hayflick, J.S., Dull, T.J., Gray, A., Tam, A.W., Lee, J., Yarden, Y., Libermann, T.A., Schlessinger, J., Downward, J., Mayes, E.L.V., Whittle, N., Waterfield, M.D., and Seeburg, P.H. (1984) Nature 309, 418-425.
(2) Yarden, Y. and Schlessinger, J. (1985) Biochemistry (submitted).
(3) Haigler, H.T., McKanna, T.J., and Cohen, S. (1979) J. Cell. Biol. 83, 82-90.
(4) Zidovetzki, R., Yarden, Y., Schlessinger, J., and Jovin, T.M. (1981) Proc. Natl. Acad. Sci. 78, 6981-6985.
(5) Schreiber, A.B., Libermann, T.A., Lax, I., Yarden, Y., and Schlessinger, J. (1983) J. Biol. Chem. 258, 846-853.
(6) Biswas, R., Basu, M., Sen-Majumdar, A., and Das, M. (1985) Biochem. 24, 3795-3802.

PDGF RECEPTORS: STRUCTURAL AND FUNCTIONAL STUDIES

L.T. Williams[1], T.O. Daniel[1], J.A. Escobedo[1], V.A. Fried[2] and S.R. Coughlin[1]
[1]Cardiovascular Research Institute and Howard Hughes Medical Institute, U-426, University of California, San Francisco, 94143 and [2]Department of Biochemistry, St. Jude Children's Hospital, Memphis, Tennessee, 38101

PDGF AND RELATED PEPTIDES

PDGF is a potent mesenchymal cell mitogen. Although initially its proposed role was in vascular repair and atherogenesis (1), recent studies have suggested that it may be involved in cell transformation (2) and in development (3,4). The biologically active native molecule is a disulfide-linked dimer. At least one of the polypeptide chains is encoded by the c-sis gene (5,6). The PDGF protein or the c-sis message has been found in several normal tissues including platelets, endothelial cells (7), macrophages, placenta (3), kidney, lung, and brain. Recent studies in our lab have shown that the expression of c-sis mRNA can be regulated by activation of protein kinase C.

Certain human tumor cell lines express high levels of sis mRNA and release PDGF-like peptides (8,9,10). These findings are especially provocative in light of the discovery that the simian sarcoma virus, an acutely transforming retrovirus, carries in its genome the v-sis oncogene that is highly homologous to the c-sis coding sequence of PDGF (11,12). Cells transformed by the simian sarcoma virus produce peptides that bind and activate PDGF receptors and are functionally indistinguishable from PDGF. Simian sarcoma virus cell transformation appears to require the presence of PDGF receptors for expression of the transformed phenotype. Thus in these cases the v-sis encoded peptides act by an autocrine mechanism involving the continuous stimulation of the PDGF receptor system. Whether this stimulation involves intracellular receptor activation or extracellular activation has not been resolved.

PURIFICATION OF THE PDGF RECEPTOR USING ANTIPHOSPHOTYROSINE ANTIBODIES

The PDGF receptor is a 180 kDa plasma membrane glycoprotein (13-15) found in most fibroblast and smooth muscle cell lines and in some intact tissues. Some cells, including endothelial cells, are notably devoid of PDGF receptors, an observation that is important in view of the ability of the endothelium to produce PDGF-like peptides that probably act on adjacent receptor-bearing smooth muscle cells in blood vessels. The binding of PDGF to its receptor induces rapid tyrosine phosphorylation of the receptor (16). We have shown that antiphosphotyrosine antibodies recognize the tyrosine phosphorylated form of the receptor but not the unphosphorylated form (17). Using monoclonal and polyclonal antiphosphotyrosine antibodies we have shown that the major tyrosine phosphorylated protein recognized in PDGF stimulated cells is the PDGF receptor (18). Thus we have used immobilized antiphosphotyrosine antibodies as a method of purifying the PDGF receptor from mouse 3T3 cells. Purification of the receptor to homogeneity requires additional steps including lectin affinity chromatography and sizing by HPLC or SDS polyacrylamide gels. Using these procedures we have purified 400 ug of receptor to homogeneity. The purified receptor retains activity as a tyrosine kinase, binds ^{125}I-PDGF with the same affinity (K_D=0.1 nM) as the membrane-bound receptor, and has a 10,000-20,000 fold purification of specific binding activity.

STRUCTURAL AND BIOSYNTHETIC STUDIES OF THE PDGF RECEPTOR

We digested purified PDGF receptor by treatment with trypsin followed by separation of the peptides using reversed phase HPLC. The primary amino acid sequences of a number of these peptides have been determined by automated Edman degradation on a gas-phase sequenator. Three of the sequenced peptides are highly homologous to the predicted amino acid sequence of tyrosine kinase domains of the v-*fms*, v-*abl*, and v-*erb B* oncogene products respectively. Thus the PDGF receptor is predicted to be a tyrosine kinase on the basis of this sequence information.

We have used monoclonal antiphosphotyrosine antibodies to provide information about the rate of receptor appearance and disappearance from the surface activatable pool of receptors. Metabolically labeled receptors appear on the surface of Balb c/3T3 cells in an activatable form within 30-45 minutes of receptor synthesis. They are removed from that pool in the absence of ligand with an apparent half life of six to eight hours, a rate considerably faster than that described for EGF and insulin receptors in other fibroblast lines.

Biosynthetically labeled surface receptors bear sialic acid and both N-and O-linked oligosaccharides. The presence of sialic acid residues is not required for activation of receptors stimulated at 4°C. Surface activated receptors from murine fibroblasts undergo an apparent 35 kDa reduction in molecular weight with enzymatic removal of N-linked oligosaccharides. Trypsin treatment of activated receptors in intact cells protects the cytoplasmic domain of the receptor and yields a 100 kDa fragment that retains sialic acid and a small portion of the total N-linked sugar. Thus the receptor is highly glycosylated, turns over at a rapid rate, is homologous to the tyrosine kinase family of transforming proteins, and has a large cytoplasmic domain.

THE ROLE OF THE C-MYC GENE AND PROTEIN KINASE C IN PDGF RECEPTOR STIMULATION

The mechanism by which the PDGF receptor stimulates mitogenesis is unknown. Several groups of investigators have shown that the most rapid responses to PDGF include phosphoinositide turnover (19), activation of protein kinase C, and the induction of the expression of specific genes including the c-myc and c-fos proto-oncogenes (20,21). We have focused on the role of phosphoinositide turnover-protein kinase C pathway in mediating c-myc expression and cell proliferation (23). These studies have shown that both direct activators of kinase C (e.g. phorbol ester analogues) and hormones that activate kinase C via receptor-mediate phosphoinositide turnover (e.g. PDGF, bradykinin, or vasopressin) elicit a rapid increase in c-myc mRNA expression. Desensitization of the kinase C pathway by prolonged exposure to phorbol esters (24) abolishes the induction of c-myc by subsequent phorbol ester challenge and attenuates the c-myc induction by PDGF. The stimulation of c-myc expression is a common response to a diverse group of agents that elicit phosphoinositide turnover and activate protein kinase C.

Although the protein kinase C/c-myc pathway may be involved in cellular response to PDGF, there clearly are additional independent pathways important in PDGF-stimulated mitogenesis. Phorbol esters and bradykinin activate protein kinase C and stimulate c-myc expression to levels similar to those seen in response to PDGF, but elicit less than 1/10 of the mitogenic response as PDGF in Balb/c 3T3 cells. Densensitization of the protein kinase C pathway by phorbol esters causes a total loss of protein kinase C activity and an attenuation of the c-myc response, but has no effect on the mitogenic response to PDGF. Additional work will be necessary to determine whether these pathways involve tyrosine kinase activity, receptor internalization, or as yet unrecognized mechanisms.

REFERENCES

(1) Ross, R. and Glomset, J.A. (1976) New Engl. J. Med. 295, 420-427.
(2) Heldin, C-H. and Westermark, B. (1984) Cell 37, 9-20.
(3) Goustin, A.S., et al. (1985) Cell 41, 301-312.
(4) Slamon, D.J. and Cline, M.J. (1984) Proc. Natl. Acad. Sci. USA 81, 7141-7145.
(5) Chiu, I-M. (1984) Cell 37, 123-129.
(6) Josephs, S.F., et al. (1984) Science 223, 487-491.
(7) Barrett, T.B., et al. (1984) Proc. Natl. Acad. Sci. USA 81, 6772-6774.
(8) Betsholtz, C., Westermark, B., Ek, B. and Heldin, C-H. (1984) Cell 39, 447-457.
(9) Nister, M., Heldin, C-H., Wasteson, A. and Westermark, B. (1984) Proc. Natl. Acad. Sci. USA 81, 926-930.
(10) Pantazis, P., et al. (1985) Proc. Natl. Acad. Sci. USA 82, 2404-2408.
(11) Waterfield, M.D. (1983) Nature 304, 35-39.
(12) Doolittle, R.F. et al. (1983) Science 221, 275-277.
(13) Heldin, C-H., Wasteson, A. and Westermark, B. (1982) J. Biol. Chem. 257, 4216-4222.
(14) Glenn, K., Bowen-Pope, D.F., and Ross, R. (1982) J. Biol. Chem. 257, 5172-5176.

(15) Williams, L.T., et al. (1984) J. Biol. Chem. 259, 5287-5292.
(16) Nishimura, J., Huang, J.S., and Deuel, T.F. (1982) Proc. Natl. Acad. Sci. USA 79, 4303-4308.
(17) Frackelton, A.R., Jr., Tremble, P.M., and Williams, L.T. (1984) J. Biol. Chem. 259, 7909-7915.
(18) Daniel, T.O., et al.(1985) Proc. Natl. Acad. Sci. USA 82, 2684-2687.
(19) Habenicht, A. et al. (1981) J. Biol. Chem. 256, 12329-12335.
(20) Kelly, K. et al. (1983) Cell 35, 603-610.
(21) Greenberg, M.E. and Ziff, E.B. (1984) Nature 311, 433-438.
(22) Coughlin, S.R. et al. (1985) Cell 43, 243-251.
(23) Collins, M.K.L. and Rozengurt, E. (1984) J. Cellular Physiol. 118, 133-142.

ISOLATION, ORGANIZATION, AND EXPRESSION OF THE TRANSFERRIN RECEPTOR AND THYMIDINE KINASE GENES.

F. H. Ruddle

Department of Biology, Yale University, Kline Biology Tower, P. O. Box 6666, New Haven, CT 06511

The acquisition of iron by cells is mediated through transferrin receptors (TR) which bind and internalize iron-carrying transferrin. Iron is required by cells for hemoglobin synthesis, respiratory enzyme activity, and the function of several other iron-dependent enzymes. Therefore, some level of cell surface membrane expression of the transferrin receptor is found on nearly all cells. However, the level of TR expression is greatly elevated on rapidly proliferating normal cells and transformed on tumor cells. Functional TR appears to be essential for cells to complete the S phase of the cell cycle.

We have isolated the human gene for TR (1) and defined a 365 base pair fragment that contains a promoter element. Sequencing of this fragment reveals the typical TATA box sequence and a unique GC rich sequence just upstream. This GC rich site was found to have strong homology to a region at a similar position of the human dihydrofolate reductase (DHFR) gene. Like TR, DHFR provides an important S phase function and is found at elevated levels in proliferating cells. This suggests that the homologous region in the promoters of the two genes may provide a regulatory function which allows these genes and other genes in this class to be expressed at higher levels in growth stimulated cells. Such a sequence might be expected to interact with specific regulatory proteins which stimulate or inhibit transcription from this promoter site. To investigate this possibility, we have tried to identify proteins that interact with the promoter region of the transferrin receptor gene. We have developed a procedure in which electrophoretically separated proteins are transferred to nitrocellulose and then incubated with labelled DNA. Using this procedure, we have identified several high molecular weight proteins which bind with high affinity and specificity to the 365 base pair fragment which contains the TR gene promoter. When quiescent 3T3 cells are induced to grow by increasing serum concentrations, there is a rapid increase in the level of these proteins. This increase reaches a maximum approximately three hours after stimulation and is followed by a dramatic decrease in the level of these binding proteins. The increase in level of these DNA binding proteins precedes an increase in cytoplasmic TR mRNA by several hours.

These results have led us to the hypothesis that a class of genes that code for products that are necessary for S phase share common regulatory sequences. These sequences interact with specific proteins which modulate expression of these genes. Regulation of these DNA binding proteins thus may be a critical process in control of cell proliferation.

REFERENCES

(1) Kühn, L. C., A. McClelland and F. H. Ruddle. (1984) Cell 37: 95-103.

STRUCTURE-FUNCTION RELATIONSHIPS IN THE HUMAN LOW DENSITY LIPOPROTEIN RECEPTOR

D.W. Russell, R.W. Bishop, C.G. Davis, M.A.Lehrman, and T. Yamamoto
Department of Molecular Genetics, University of Texas Health Science Center at Dallas, 5323 Harry Hines Blvd., Dallas, TX 75235

Receptor-mediated endocytosis is a process by which mammalian cells internalize nutrients, viruses, toxins, and hormones (1). The process is initiated when receptors on the cell surface bind macromolecules and move through the membrane into clathrin-coated pits. Within minutes the coated pits invaginate into the cell and pinch off to form coated vesicles. After removal of their clathrin coats by an ATP-driven uncoating enzyme, the vesicles fuse with one another to form endosomes whose internal milieu is rapidly acidified by an ATP-driven proton pump. This reduction in pH usually brings about a dissociation event between the ligand and its receptor. Following dissociation, the ligand is frequently sorted to the lysosome and degraded, while the receptor is recycled to the cell surface where it participates in additional endocytic events.

Since its discovery more than thirteen years ago (2), the low density lipoprotein (LDL) receptor has served as a paradigm for receptor-mediated endocytosis. Its characterization at the cellular, biochemical, and genetic levels has revealed many details in this important process. Recently, we have gained new insights into the LDL receptor through the application of the powerful techniques of molecular biology. Biochemical tools developed with the purified LDL receptor protein have allowed the isolation of cDNA clones corresponding to the bovine and human receptor mRNAs (3,4). DNA sequence analysis of these cDNAs revealed that the mature receptor protein is composed of at least five discrete domains: an amino-terminal ligand binding domain, a domain homologous to the epidermal growth factor (EGF) precursor, a carbohydrate-rich domain, a transmembrane segment, and at the COOH terminus, a cytoplasmic domain of fifty amino acids. When introduced into cultured cells by transfection, a cDNA encoding these domains expressed functional LDL receptors (4).

The predicted domain structure of the protein is reflected in the intron-exon organization of the LDL receptor gene (5). A strong correlation exists between the position of introns in the gene and subdomains in the ligand binding, EGF-homologous, and carbohydrate-rich regions of the encoded protein. Furthermore, homologies detected at the protein level between the LDL receptor and five other proteins are mirrored in the gene structure: homologous regions are encoded by discrete exons. These results suggest that the LDL receptor is a mosaic protein whose gene has been constructed through evolutionary time by exon shuffling (6).

To define roles these predicted protein domains play in receptor-mediated endocytosis of LDL, we have taken two experimental approaches. First, advantage has been taken of naturally-occurring mutations in the human LDL receptor gene that occur at a high frequency (1/500) and give rise to the genetic disease familial hypercholesterolemia (7). Mutations causing FH have been divided into several discrete classes at the biochemical level (1). They disrupt the synthesis of the protein, transport to the cell surface, LDL binding, and clustering in coated pits on the cell surface. Their analysis at the DNA level has revealed the roles three domains in the protein play in the receptor- mediated endocytosis of LDL. Deletions in the gene which remove the transmembrane domain encode proteins that are secreted into the media (8). Thus, this domain functions to anchor the LDL receptor in the plasma membrane. Mutations that truncate (9) or change (10) sequences in the cytoplasmic domain encode proteins that do not cluster in coated pits. Thus, this domain contains signals which sort the LDL receptor to coated pits, entry into which is an absolute prerequisite for the internalization of bound ligand.

An animal model of familial hypercholesterolemia, the WHHL rabbit (11), has a mutation in a third domain of the LDL receptor. Previous biochemical studies revealed that the WHHL mutation encodes an LDL receptor that is slowed in transport to the cell surface (12). Molecular analysis of cDNA clones derived from normal and WHHL rabbit LDL receptor mRNAs revealed a four amino acid deletion in the ligand binding domain (13). This domain of the protein is composed of a single 40 amino acid unit that is tandemly repeated seven times (5). Each of these repeats contains six highly conserved cysteine residues that probably form three intra-repeat disulfide bonds. A likely explanation for the slowed transport kinetics in this mutant is that the four amino acid deletion impairs normal disulfide bond formation which in turn disrupts folding of the protein. Transport of the unfolded protein to the cell surface may be slowed to prevent an autoimmune response. In addition, these studies revealed that sequences in the various domains of the LDL receptor are highly conserved between the human and rabbit species. The domains in order of decreasing % homology are: cytoplasmic (86%), EGF precursor homology (84%), ligand binding (75%), transmembrane (68%), and clustered O-linked sugar (40%).

A second approach to elucidating the functional roles of predicted protein domains has involved the construction of mutations in the LDL receptor cDNA <u>in vitro</u> followed by transfection analysis in receptor-defective hamster fibroblasts (14). A 48 amino acid region of the protein has been deleted to which clustered Ser- and Thr-linked carbohydrate chains are attached during posttranslational processing (14). The LDL receptor encoded by the deletion-bearing cDNA bound and internalized LDL normally, recycled with normal kinetics, and exhibited a normal half-life. Thus, at the present time it is not known what role the clustered O-linked sugars play in the LDL receptor. Finally, site-specific mutagenesis and transfection analysis have been used to further map the coated pit targeting sequence in the cytoplasmic domain of the LDL receptor (15).

REFERENCES

1. Goldstein, J.L., Brown, M.S., Anderson, R.G.W., Russell, D.W., and Schneider, W.J. (1985) Annual Reviews of Cell Biology 1: 1-39.
2. Goldstein, J.L., and Brown, M.S. (1974) J. Biol. Chem. 249: 5153-5162.
3. Russell, D.W., Yamamoto, T., Schneider, W.J., Slaughter, C.J., Brown, M.S., and Goldstein, J.L. (1983) Proc. Natl. Acad. Sci. USA 80: 7501-7505.
4. Yamamoto, T., Davis, C.G., Brown, M.S., Casey, M.L., Goldstein, J.L., and Russell, D.W. (1984) Cell 39: 27-38.
5. Südhof, T.C., Goldstein, J.L., Brown, M.S., and Russell, D.W. (1985) Science 228: 815-822.
6. Gilbert, W. (1978) Nature 271: 501.
7. Goldstein, J.L., and Brown, M.S. (1983) In The Metabolic Basis of Inherited Disease, eds. J.B. Stanbury et al., pp. 672-712. New York, McGraw-Hill.
8. Lehrman, M.A., Schneider, W.J., Südhof, T.C., Brown, M.S., Goldstein, J.L., and Russell, D.W. (1985) Science 227: 140-146.
9. Lehrman, M.A., Goldstein, J.L., Brown, M.S., Russell, D.W., and Schneider, W.J. (1985) Cell 41: 735-743.
10. Lehrman, M.A., Davis, C.G., Russell, D.W., Goldstein, J.L., and Brown, M.S. (1985), manuscript in preparation.
11. Goldstein, J.L., Kita, T., and Brown, M.S. (1983) N. Engl. J. Med. 309: 288-296.
12. Schneider, W.J., Brown, M.S., and Goldstein, J.L. (1983) Mol. Biol. Med. 1: 353-367.
13. Yamamoto, T., Bishop, R.W., Goldstein, J.L., Brown, M.S., and Russell, D.W. (1985), manuscript in preparation.
14. Davis, C.G., Elhammer, A., Russell, D.W., Schneider, W.J., Kornfeld, S., Brown, M.S., and Goldstein, J.L. (1986) J. Biol. Chem., in press.
15. Davis, D.G., Anderson, R.G.W., Lehrman, M.A., Russell, D.W., Brown, M.S., and Goldstein, J.L. (1985), manuscript in preparation.

PURIFICATION OF THE HUMAN PDGF-RECEPTOR: A POLYPEPTIDE WITH INTRINSIC TYROSINE KINASE ACTIVITY

Subal Bishayee[1], Alonzo H. Ross[2], Richard B. Womer[1], and Charles D. Scher[1]
[1]The Children's Hospital of Philadelphia, The University of Pennsylvania, and [2]The Wistar Institute, Philadelphia, PA 19104

Introduction

The mitogenic action of platelet derived growth factor (PDGF) is mediated through a cell surface receptor which appears to have tyrosine kinase activity. To understand the role of ligand-receptor interaction in mitogenic signal transduction, we have purified and characterized the PDGF receptor from a human source.

Results

The human osteogenic sarcoma cell line, MG-63, which neither expresses c-sis mRNA nor secretes PDGF (1), was found to have nearly 23,000 PDGF-binding sites per cell with a Kd of about 10 pM. Other human cell lines tested had fewer number of PDGF-binding sites.

Plasma membranes from MG-63 cells were found to contain a 180,000 dalton protein which became phosphorylated on tyrosine in response to PDGF. Covalent affinity labeling with ^{125}I-PDGF revealed that the 180,000 dalton protein is the PDGF-receptor. Purification of this receptor was achieved by using anti-phosphotyrosine monoclonal antibody (2). The first step involved phosphorylation of MG-63 plasma membranes with ATP in the presence of PDGF. The tyrosine phosphorylated receptor was solubilized with NP-40 and passed through a column of a Sepharose containing covalently bound monoclonal anti-phosphotyrosine antibody. The bound receptors (and other minor tyrosine phosphorylated proteins) were eluted with phenyl phosphate. The receptor was further purified by wheat germ agglutinin-agarose chromatography and DEAE-cellulose chromatography, resulting in the removal of the minor contaminants. Receptor activity was monitored during purification using a newly developed ^{125}I-PDGF binding assay. The final purified preparation was at least 80% pure as judged by silver staining and by autoradiography after iodination with ^{125}I. PDGF-stimulatable tyrosine kinase activity of the purified preparation was demonstrated by autophosphorylation of the receptor protein and also by phosphorylation of exogeneous substrates. Incubation of the freshly purified receptor with gamma-^{32}P-ATP resulted in the incorporation of ^{32}P into the PDGF-receptor in a PDGF-dependent fashion. Half maximal phosphorylation was achieved at 0.5 nM PDGF. Tyrosine kinase specific substrates, angiotensin II and a src related synthetic tridecapeptide were also phosphorylated by the purified receptor in response to PDGF.

Discussion

One of the early consequences of interaction of PDGF with cells is phosphorylation of the PDGF-receptor on tyrosine residues (3). Two other well-characterized growth factor receptors - EGF - and insulin-receptors - are tyrosine kinases with autophosphorylating ability (4,5). By analogy, it has been suggested that PDGF-receptor is also a tyrosine kinase (6,7). Recently, Daniel et al (8) reported purification of the murine PDGF-receptor but were unable to demonstrate PDGF-stimulatable tyrosine kinase activity in the purified preparation. In contrast, the results reported in this communication demonstrate that the human PDGF-receptor can be purified to near homogeneity with full retention of its PDGF-stimulatable tyrosine kinase activity. These results are consistent with the idea that tyrosine kinase activity is intrinsic to the PDGF-receptor.

References

(1) Graves, D.T., Owen, A.J., Barth, R.K., Tempest, P., Winoto, A., Fors, L., and Hood, L.E. (1984) Science 226, 972-974.
(2) Frackelton, A.R., Ross, A.H., and Eisen, H.N. (1983) Mol. Cell. Biol. 3, 1343-1352.
(3) Frackelton, A.R., Tremble P.M., and Williams, L.T. (1984) J. Biol. Chem. 259, 7909-7915.
(4) Ushiro, H. and Cohen, S. (1980) J. Biol. Chem. 255, 8363-8365.
(5) Kasuga, M., Zick, Y., Blithe, D.L., Crettaz, M., and Kahn, C.R. (1982) Nature 298, 667-669.
(6) Nishimura, J., Huang, J.S., and Deuel, T.F. (1982) Proc. Natl. Acad. Sci. 79, 4303-4307.
(7) Pike, L.J., Bowen-Pope, D.F., Ross, R., and Krebs, E.G. (1985) J. Biol. Chem. 258, 9383-9390.
(8) Daniel, T.O., Tremble, P.M., Frackelton, A.R., Jr., and Williams, L.T. (1985) Proc. Natl. Acad. Sci. 82, 2684-2687.

IS COPPER ASSOCIATED WITH ANGIOTENSIN II NUCLEAR RECEPTORS?

S.E. Bryan, L. LeGros, J. Brown and R.N. Re. Department of Biological Sciences, University of New Orleans, New Orleans, LA 70148 and Alton Ochsner Medical Foundation, New Orleans, LA 70121

Previous experiments demonstrated high-affinity, specific angiotensin II (AII) acceptor sites in micrococcal nuclease-generated nuclear fragments following incubation with labeled AII in the presence or absence of unlabeled hormone (1). Nanometer concentrations of unlabeled AII produced detectable displacement of labeled AII binding, however there was no displaceable binding when digestions were terminated by the addition of EDTA. Other studies revealed elevated levels of copper and zinc in nuclease digested non-chelated soluble chromatin (2,3). Here we present further evidence for a possible link between copper and AII acceptor sites in chromatin.

In solubilized, dialyzed chromatin the metal ratio of μg copper /mg DNA in AII treated samples to untreated control is approximately 3:1. This elevation appears to be specific for copper since the zinc ratio is unchanged. Gel filtration metal profiles of the dialyzed samples shown in Fig. 1 are distinctive: Prominent copper peaks appear on the leading edge of the nucleosome peak (V/V_o 1.7) where di, tri nucleosomes elute (3). An accumulation of the metal is expected in this region because of the high content of internucleosomal linker DNA. A less prominent copper peak appears near or adjacent to linker DNA at V/V_o approx. 2.0. In the case of AII, this copper peak coincides with fragments containing specific AII receptors (V/V_o 2.2). Thus, copper appears to be localized in linker DNA fragments released in the initial stage of digestion and is therefore a likely component of active chromatin. The data further suggest that copper may be associated with AII receptor protein, or perhaps another DNA binding protein.

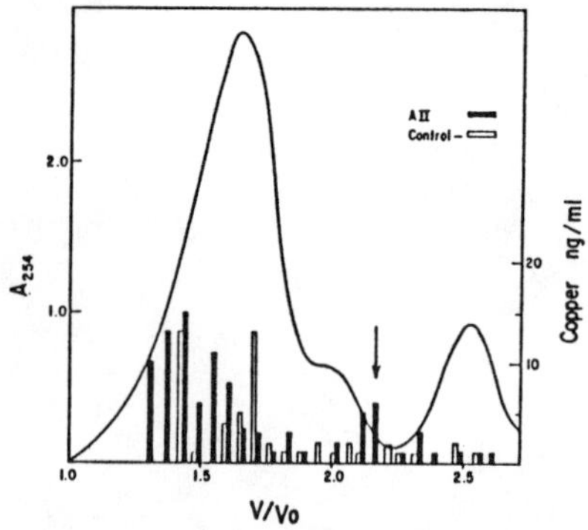

Fig. 1. A representative A-5 M metal profile for chromatin digested at 30° for 5 min, following incubation with 10^{-8} M AII or without AII and dialyzed 3 hr at 4° C. Copper analysis by flameless AA denotes V/V_o 2.2. See reference 3 for further details.

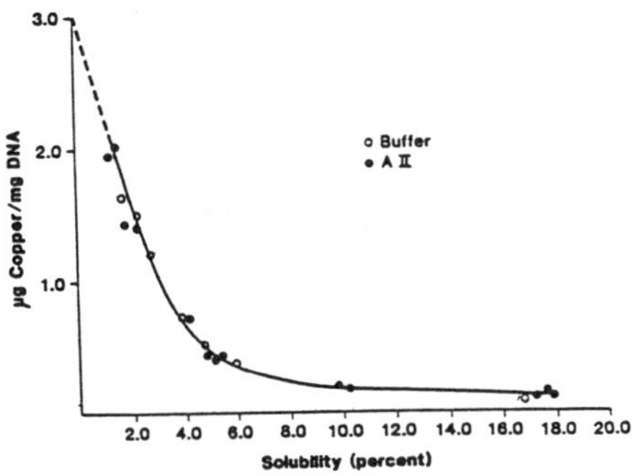

Fig. 2. The inverse relationship between copper (released into solubilized chromatin) and solubility following digestion. Nuclei (10-20 A_{260}/ml were incubated with either 10^{-8} M unlabeled AII or with $MgCl_2$ buffer at room temperature for 10 min prior to digestion (0.059 enzyme units/A_{260}) for various times (1.5 min-5 min) at 30° C.

Copper was essentially the same in non-dialyzed samples in either the presence or absence of AII (Fig. 2). Of special interest is the finding that samples with lowest solubilities (1-2%) contained the highest level of copper. Thus, in both AII treated and buffer control, the enzyme appeared to preferentially cleave a copper rich nucleoprotein region in chromatin. The data in Fig. 2 indicates that, following the initial digestion, no additional copper is released. When increasing amounts of nuclei were digested, there was an increased solubilization and an increased copper content. A plot of µgCu/mg DNA vs µL enzyme again shows an inverse relationship where the highest copper/DNA ratio corresponded to the least digested sample (data not shown). This could indicate a limited number of copper rich regions in chromatin.

Whether the metal is complexed to protein, to DNA, or exists in a protein-Cu-DNA ternary complex is not known. Experiments are in progress to further identify AII receptor protein and to determine specific location(s) for nuclear copper. Other laboratories have reported a chelation-sensitive metaphase scaffold that appears to be stabilized by copper and have proposed that a reorganization of this structure drives chromosome condensation (4). Therefore, it is possible that copper serves more than one function in chromatin.

REFERENCES

(1) Re, R.N., Vizard, D.L., Brown, J., LeGros, L. and Bryan, S.E. (1984) J & Hyper. 2 (Supple. 3) 271-273.

(2) Bryan, S.E., Vizard, D.L., Beary, D.A., LaBiche, R.A., Hardy, K.J. (1981) Nucleic Acid Res. 4, 5811-5823.

(3) Beary, D.A., Vizard, D.L., LaBiche, R.A., Hardy, K.J., and Bryan, S.E. (1982) Bioch. and Bioph. Res. Comm. 104, 491-499.

(4) Lewis, C.D. and Laemmli, V.K. (1982) Cell, 29-171-181.

EGF RECEPTOR EXPRESSION IN YOUNG AND SENESCENT WI-38 CELLS C.R. Carlin and B.B. Knowles
The Wistar Institute of Anatomy and Biology, 36th Street at Spruce, Philadelphia, PA, 19104

We have been using human fetal lung-derived WI-38 cells, which display a limited replicative lifespan in culture [1], as a model system to study regulation of epidermal growth factor (EGF) receptor expression and function in vivo. Using a serum-free defined medium, it has been shown that EGF is a primary mitogen for young but not senescent WI-38 cells [2]. The failure of senescent cells to respond to EGF is not due to lack of expression of the cellular receptor for ligand, since receptor number and affinity are constant throughout the replicative lifespan [3]. Hence, receptor binding of ligand and those functions related to relaying the EGF-induced mitogenic signal become uncoupled during cellular senescence.

Other parameters of receptor expression that remain constant as WI-38 cells senesce include: molecular weight and isoelectric point; ability to be detected at the cell surface by radioimmunoassay, or by immunoprecipitation following radiolabeling of the cell surface by the lactoperoxidase-method; and, post-translational phosphorylation at threonine and serine residues [4]. We have reported previously, however, that the ability of the receptor to catalyze tyrosine-specific autophosphorylation following its immunopurification from NP-40 detergent cell extracts is greatly diminished in senescent but not young cells [4]. This observation holds not only for WI-38, but for several other fetal-lung and adult skin-derived fibroblasts. We now demonstrate that the receptor kinase retains its activity if senescent cells are extracted in the presence of the polar solvent DMSO (Fig. 1). Although a mechanism that would account for the differential susceptibilty of the senescent receptor kinase activity to the various extraction protocols remains unclear, one interpretation is that a regulatory element resides within the membrane microenvironment whose composition changes during cellular senescence, conferring differential solulibilization properties.

Receptor proteins are immunoprecipitated using one of two human receptor-specific antibody reagents: the polyclonal cl 21 antiserum [5]; and the monoclonal antibody EGF-R1 [6]. In the immune complex kinase assay depicted in Fig. 1, EGF-R1 was utilized; identical results are obtained using cl 21 antiserum. When cells metabolically labeled with L[^{35}S]methionine are examined, however, the ability of these reagents to recognize receptor proteins from young versus senescent cells is dependent upon the extraction protocol used. For cells extracted with NP-40 only, cl 21 antiserum recognizes the biosynthetic precursor (MW = 145kD) and the mature form (MW = 165kD) of the receptor in both young and senescent cells, whereas EGF-R1 recognizes both species in young cells, but only the 145kD species in senescent cells. When cells are extracted with NP-40 in the presence of DMSO, however, both antibodies recognize 145kD and 165kD proteins regardless of cell age. Our interpretation is that exposure of the EGF-R1 antigenic determinant in senescent cells is susceptible to conformational constraints that are not at play in the young cell. It is not clear whether the positive correlation between kinase activity and exposure of the EGF-R1 antigenic determinant is fortuitous, or if it reflects a common mechanism. If the latter, it should be possible to exploit the differential reactivity of cl 21 antiserum and EGF-R1 as we manipulate the plasma membrane microenvironment to determine conditions that render the kinase inactive or active in young and senescent cells, respectively. This work was supported by Public Health Serice grants CA 18470 and 10815 from the National Institutes of Health.

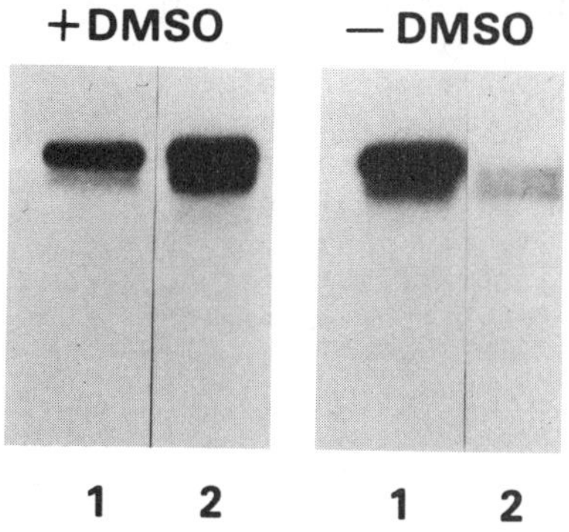

Fig. 1. EGF receptor tyr specific autophosphorylation in an immune complex assay. Cells were extracted with NP-40 in the absence or presence of DMSO. Receptor proteins from young (lane 1) and senescent (lane 2) WI-38 were immunoprecipitated with EGF-R1, allowed to catalyze autophosphorylation, separated by SDS-PAGE, and visualized by autoradiography.

1. Hayflick, L. 1965. Exp. Cell Res. 37: 614.
2. Phillips, P.D. and Cristofalo, V.J. 1981. Exp. Cell Res. 134: 297.
3. Phillips, P.D., et al. 1983. J. Cell. Physiol. 114: 311.
4. Carlin, C.R., et al. 1983. Nature 306: 617.
5. Carlin, C.R. and Knowles, B.B. 1984. J. Biol. Chem. 259: 7902.
6. Waterfield, M.D., et al. 1982. J. Cell. Biochem. 20: 149.

An Antibody that Recognizes an Opiate Receptor on Murine Splenocytes. D.J.J. Carr, K.L. Bost, and J.E. Blalock, Dept. of Microbiology, UTMB, Galveston, TX 77550

In recent years, numerous investigators have demonstrated that hormones (i.e., corticotropin [ACTH], endorphins, and enkephalins) can modulate immune responses (1), presumably by interacting with specific hormone receptors on the immunocytes. We have developed a methodology which allows for the generation of antibodies (Ab) specific for hormone receptor binding sites (2), and these Abs have been used to dissect receptor structure (3). This technology has recently been used to generate anti-opiate receptor Ab by immunizing rabbits with a peptide encoded by the RNA complementary to the mRNA for γ-endorphin (termed "complementary peptide"). The anti-complementary peptide Ab has the ability to bind to endorphin receptors on NG108-15 neuroblastoma x glioma cells, and this Ab can block the binding of a radiolabeled opiate ligand ([^{3}H]-dihydromorphine) to NG108-15 cells. Furthermore, by coupling this anti-opiate receptor Ab to sepharose, opiate receptors were immunoaffinity purified from sonicates of NG108-15 cells. By injecting material eluted from the affinity columns into rabbits, we have produced a second Ab (termed "anti-opiate receptor" Ab) which recognizes an opiate receptor. This α opiate receptor Ab exhibits an agonist activity (enhancement) in the generation of cytotoxic T lymphocytes (CTLs) as compared with β-endorphin in one-way mixed lymphocyte reactions (MLRs). From these results, we have demonstrated additional evidence for the presence of opiate receptors on cells of the immune system by employing Abs which recognize opiate receptors. In addition, the α opiate receptor Ab has biological activity similar to opiate peptide ligands (β-endorphin and Met-enkephalin). Finally, the data supplies additional support for the basis of the inter-relatedness between the immune and neuroendocrine systems through the commonality of their receptors (4).

Fig. 1. Inhibition of [^{3}H]-dihydromorphine by anti-complementary peptide and anti-opiate receptor Abs.

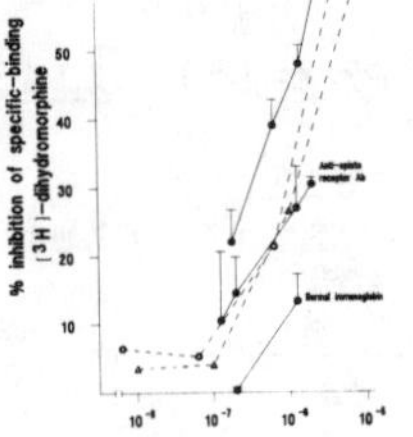

(I) RADIORECEPTOR ASSAY. Splenocytes were obtained from female C57Bl/6 mice (2-4 months old). Cells were placed in wells of a polystyrene, 96-well microtiter plate at a concentration of $1x10^6$ cells/well. Addition of cold ligand or antibodies at various concentrations in a 100 µl volume was next followed by incubation at 4°C for 30 min. After the incubation period, $1x10^{-12}$M [^{3}H]-dihydromorphine (87.7 Curies/mmol) was added to each well followed by an additional 15 min incubation at 4°C. Cells were then washed 3 times

Table I. Enhancement of the generation of CTLs

E/T[a]	Normal Ig	Normal Ig + β-end	α opiate receptor Ab
100:1	8.4±0.6[b]	38.0±4.5	30.4±1.3
50:1	4.1±1.5	25.2±3.1	26.7±1.4
25:1	1.9±1.4	18.7±1.0	15.6±2.5
12:1	2.4±1.5	11.0±0.8	8.6±0.7

[a]Effector to target cell ratio.

[b]± standard deviation.

Table I - Enhancement of the generation of CTLs by anti-opiate receptor Ab. $1x10^6$ irradiated (3000 rads) DBA/2J spleen cells were mixed with $6x10^6$ C57Bl/6 spleen cells in a volume of 2.0 mls of culture medium (RPMI 1640 + 5% [heat inactivated] fetal bovine serum, 100 Units/ml penicillin, and 1mM glutamine) in 24 well microtiter plates. Ab or β-endorphin was added at the initiation of the culture. After 5 days, cells were assayed for the generation of CTLs against the mastocytoma, P815.

with phosphate buffered saline (PBS)-azide + 1.0% fetal bovine serum, placed in scintillation fluid, and then counted. Results indicate that the antibody to the complementary peptide and to the opiate receptor block binding of [^{3}H]-dihydromorphine to its receptor (Fig. 1). The antibody to the complementary peptide inhibited labeled dihydromorphine better than either [D-Ala^2, MePhe^4, Gly-ol^5] enkephalin (DAGO) or [D-Ala^2, D-leu^5] enkephalin (DADLE) and well above the control normal immunoglobulin at the same concentration.

(II) GENERATION OF CTLs IN A MLR. Previous data suggest β-endorphin and Met-enkephalin, through opiate receptors, enhance the kinetics for the generation of CTLs in one-way MLRs in a dose dependent fashion (Carr, D.J.J. and G.R. Klimpel, submitted for publication). We have applied the anti-opiate receptor Ab in this assay to determine if an agonist activity can be observed in CTL generation compared to β-endorphin. The application of 12.5 μg of DEAE-purified anti-opiate receptor Ab to cultures on day 0 of a 5 day MLR produced an enhanced effect similar to β-endorphin-mediated effects and well above normal immunoglobulin alone (Table I). Furthermore, this activity was dose dependent (data not shown).

References

1. Blalock, J.E. and Smith, E.M. (1985) Federation Proc. 44, 108-111.
2. Bost, K.L., Smith, E.M., and Blalock, J.E. (1985). Proc. Natl. Aca. Sci. USA 82, 1372-1375.
3. Bost, K.L. and Blalock, J.E. (1985). Mol. & Cell. Endocrinol. In press.
4. Blalock, J.E. (1984). J. Immunol. 132, 1067-1070.

ENDOTOXIN ALTERS HEPATIC PROLACTIN BINDING IN THE LACTATING MOUSE

Jean K. Carr, Linda M. Keefer, and J. Craig Cohen

Depts. of Biochemistry, Physiology, and Medicine, Louisiana State University Medical Center, 1542 Tulane Ave., New Orleans, LA 70112.

Endotoxin or lipopolysaccharide (LPS) is a component of the outer membrane of gram-negative bacteria which produces profound physiologic changes in most animals. Recent work (1) has shown that both milk production and serum prolactin (PRL) levels are reduced in lactating sows following LPS treatment. We further explored the effects of LPS on lactating animals by examining the binding of ^{125}I-ovine PRL (oPRL) to the PRL receptor in liver membranes of lactating mice. The two mouse substrains used differ genetically at only one locus, the Lps locus, which mediates the response to LPS. Since C3H/HeN mice respond normally to the injection of LPS while C3H/HeJ mice do not respond (2), these mice are a useful model for studying the effects of LPS injection *in vivo*.

METHODS. Midlactation C3H/HeJ and C3HfB/HeN mice, nursing 5 pup litters, were injected with either 2 mg/kg LPS (E.coli strain 0127:B8) or saline intravenously. Mice were sacrificed at varying times after injection and the liver membranes prepared according to Liscia and Vonderhaar (3).

Pituitary oPRL (NIADDK-oPRL-17,AFP-75909826) and crystalline monocomponent porcine insulin (Dr. B. Frank, Eli Lilly) were iodinated with Na^{125}I using adaptations of the stoichiometric Chloramine T procedure of Roth (4) and Keefer *et al*. (5). Approximately 200 μg of liver membranes were incubated (4°C for 20 hrs) with 500 pg of ^{125}I-oPRL and varying amounts of oPRL in a fluid volume of 0.5 ml 25 mM Tris-HCl, pH 7.4, 15 mM $CaCl_2$, 0.5% BSA. Insulin binding was performed identically except that 50 pg of ^{125}I-insulin was incubated with and without 5 μg of insulin. At 20 hours 0.5 ml cold buffer was added, the membranes were pelleted and the excised pellet counted.

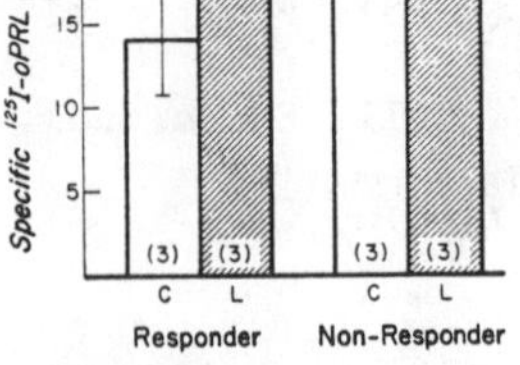

SPECIFIC BINDING OF oPRL INCREASED BY LPS.

C3HfB/HeN mice injected with LPS show a dramatic increase in specific ^{125}I-oPRL binding even as soon as 15 minutes post-injection (Fig. 1). However, the ^{125}I-oPRL binding of C3H/HeJ mice is totally unaffected. This indicates that the LPS effect seen in C3HfB/HeN but not in C3H/HeJ is mediated somehow by the Lps locus. To examine the specificity of this effect we measured insulin binding to the same membranes (Fig.2). No significant change in insulin binding by

Fig. 1: Specific ^{125}I-oPRL Binding to Liver Membranes of C3HfB/HeN and C3H/HeJ Mice treated with Saline (C) or LPS (L) 15 Minutes before Sacrifice. Means, standard deviations and (n) are shown.

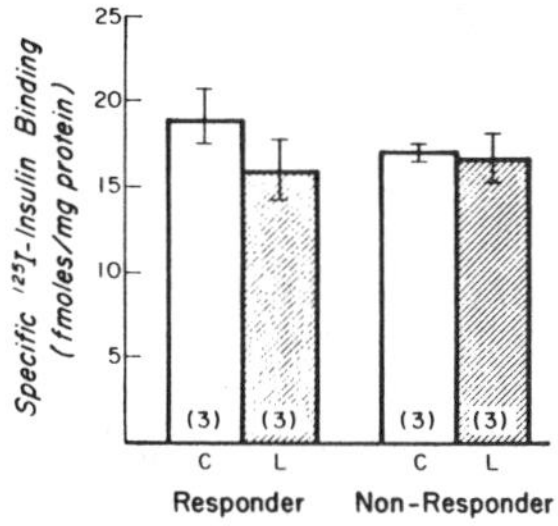

Fig. 2: Specific ^{125}I-Insulin Binding to Liver Membranes from Fig. 1.

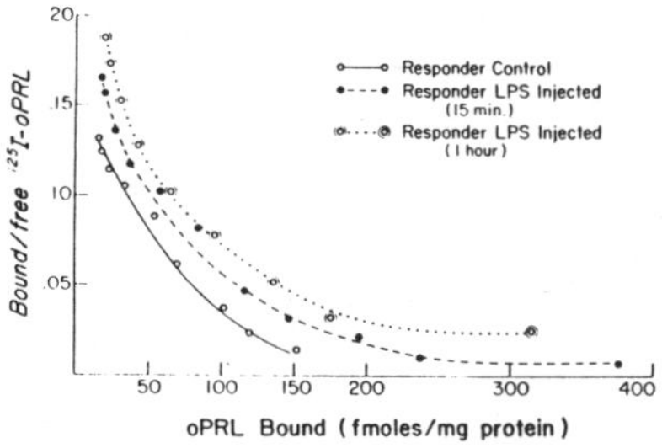

Fig. 3: Scatchard Plots of ^{125}I-oPRL Competitive Binding to Liver Membranes of C3HfB/HeN Mice.

liver membranes from either strain of mouse was detected after LPS injection. This fact suggests that a general effect on membrane fluidity is not responsible for the change in PRL binding.

AFFINITY AND RECEPTOR CONCENTRATION ALTERED BY LPS. Data for competitive equilibrium binding of ^{125}I-oPRL to liver membranes of C3HfB/HeN mice killed at varying times post-injection were analysed according to Scatchard (Fig.3). Analysis of the data with LIGAND (BCTIC MED-59) confirmed that all three Scatchard plots significantly fit two-site models. The initial effect of LPS injection, seen at 15 minutes, is to double the number of high affinity (4 X 10^{9} M^{-1}) sites to 5.8 X 10^{-11} M and to decrease the affinity of the low affinity site 70-fold while increasing the number 40-fold (to 2 X 10^{9} M^{-1}). By 1 hour the low affinity site is returning towards the control but the high affinity site has now increased in affinity to 1.9 X 10^{10} M^{-1} and has half the number of sites as the control.

These extremely rapid and transitory changes in the oPRL binding sites suggest that the receptor response to LPS in a lactating mouse is almost immediate. Several mechanisms, such as unmasking of previously blocked binding sites or recruitment of binding sites from sub-cellular compartments might account for this. In the light of these data and recent reports implicating a role for PRL in immune response, we are investigating these possibilities as well as the possibility that direct interaction of LPS with the PRL receptor is an early event in its action.

REFERENCES

1. Smith, B. and Wagner, W. (1985) Am.J.Vet.Res. 46:175.
2. Watson, J. and Riblet, R. (1975) J. Exp.Med. 140:1147.
3. Liscia, D. and Vonderhaar, B. (1982) Proc.Natl.Acad.Sci.79:5930.
4. Roth, J. (1975) Meth. Enz. 37:223.
5. Keefer, L., Piron, M. and DeMeyts, P. (1981) Proc.Natl.Acad.Sci. 78:1391.

ACKNOWLEDGEMENTS. This work was supported in part by U.S.P.H.S. Grants R01-CA-34823 (JCC) and R23-AM35159-01 (LMK).

EXPRESSION OF A HUMAN INSULIN RECEPTOR FROM A CLONED cDNA IN CHINESE HAMSTER OVARY CELLS

M. Edery[**], Y. Ebina[*], L. Ellis [*], D. Standring [*], J. Beaudoin[γ], R.A. Roth[γ], and W.J. Rutter [*]

[*]Hormone Research Laboratory, University of California, San Francisco, CA 94143, USA ; [**]Present Address : Laboratoire de Physiologie de la Lactation, I.N.R.A., 78350 Jouy-en-Josas, France ; [γ] Department of Pharmacology, Stanford University, School of Medicine, Stanford, CA 94305, USA

Recently the human IR cDNA has been cloned in our laboratory (1) and by Ullrich et al. (2). The nucleotide sequence of the cDNA reveals the primary structure of the single chain IR precursor of 1382 amino acids (154 kd). These remarkable features of the human IR and related Epidermal Growth Factor receptor provide the structural basis for understanding receptor function ; they also intensify the mystery surrounding the specific biological effects associated with these molecules. Here, we demonstrate that the human IR cDNA can be expressed in heterologous cell systems.

I) An expression plasmid, pcDL1-HIR7, containing the entire coding sequence of the human IR cDNA was constructed. In this vector the human IR cDNA is placed under the transcriptional control of the early promoter of SV40. The transcriptional unit is completed with the SV40 late region introns and a polyadenylation signal. We established stable rodent (CHO), rat hepatoma (HTC), and mouse L (LTA) cell lines by cotransfection of the human IR expression plasmid, pcDL1-HIR7, with a plasmid conferring resistance to the neomycin analog, G418). These permanent cell lines were assayed for the presence of the human IR on the cell surface by selective binding of a monoclonal antibody specific for the human IR. We chose for further study one of the CHO clones (designated CHO-HIR3) which showed the highest binding of the monoclonal antibody. Northern blot analysis (Fig. 1, lane 1) of total cellular RNA from CHO-HIR3 cells revealed the presence of a human IR mRNA of about 4.7 kb, a size expected from the receptor cDNA encoded by this expression vector. No cross-hybridizing species were detected in control CHO cell RNA (lane 2).

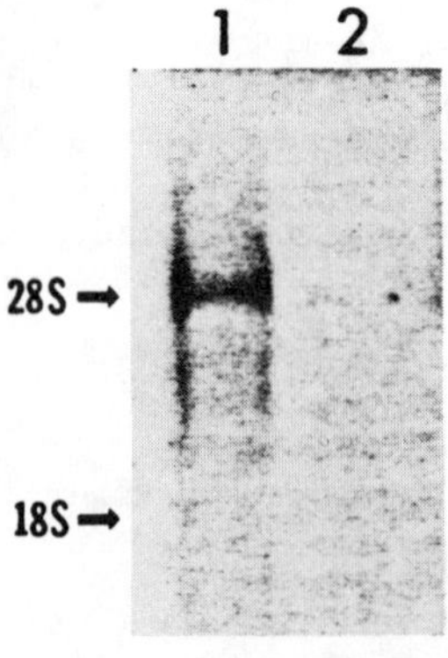

Fig. 1 - Northern blot analysis of human IR mRNA synthesized in CHO-HIR3 cells. Lane 1 : CHO-HIR3 total RNA (12 μg). Lane 2 : CHO total RNA (12 μg).

II) To examine the protein expressed in these cells, we immunoprecipitated metabolically-labeled (^{35}S-methionine) proteins from nonionic detergent extracts of CHO-HIR3 and CHO cells (Fig. 2). Two bands of approximately 135 and 95 kd (corresponding to the α- and β-subunits respectively) were immunoprecipitated by the human IR-specific monoclonal antibody from CHO-HIR3 (lane 4) but not CHO (lane 2) cells. Normal mouse IgG likewise did not immunoprecipitate these bands (lanes 1 and 3). We conclude that the transfected rodent cells,process the IR precursor into mature α- and β-subunits. The ability to express the human IR in this heterologous cell system permits the further analysis of structure/function relationships of the IR molecule and the role it plays in eliciting the various physiological responses of insulin.

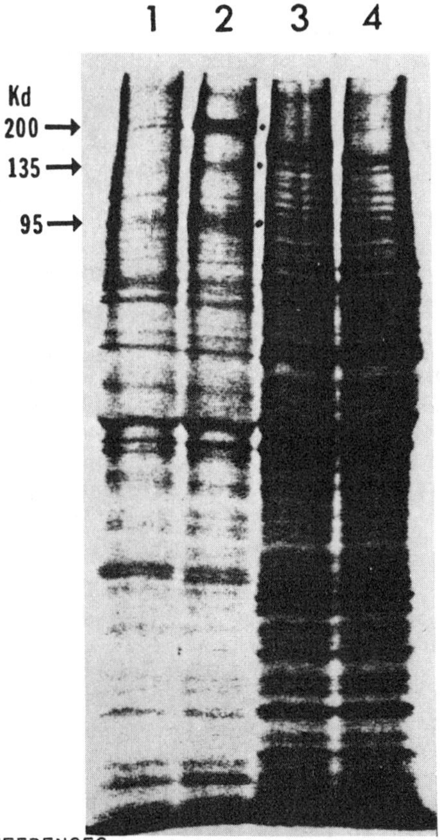

Fig. 2 - Identification of the human IR subunits expressed in CHO-HIR3 cells. Lane 1 : CHO cell extract immunoprecipitated with normal mouse IgG. Lane 2 : CHO, human IR-specific monoclonal antibody (IgG). Lane 3 : CHO-HIR3, normal mouse IgG. Lane 4 : CHO-HIR3 cells, human IR-specific monoclonal antibody (IgG).

REFERENCES

1 Ebina, Y., Ellis, L., Jarnagin, K., Edery, M., Graf, L., Clauser,E. Ou, J.-H., Masiarz, F., Kan, Y.W., Goldfine, I.D., Roth, R.A. and Rutter, W.J.(1985) Cell **40**, 747-758.

2) Ullrich, A., Bell, J.R., Chen, E.Y., Herrera, R., Petruzzelli, L.M. Dull, J.J., Gray, A., Coussens, L., Liao, Y.-C., Tsubokawa, M., Mason, A., Seeburg, P.H., Grunfeld, C., Rosen, O.M. and Ramachandran, J. (1985) Nature **313**, 756-761.

EFFECTS OF MOLYBDATE AND ATP ON THE BINDING ACTIVITY OF THE NUCLEAR T_3 RECEPTOR.

R. Faure, and J.H. Dussault, Unité de Recherche en Ontogénèse et Génétique Moléculaire, Le Centre Hospitalier de l'Université Laval, 2705, boul. Laurier, Québec, G1V 4G2, Canada.

Thyroid hormone action is initiated by the binding of L-Triiodothyronine to high affinity, low capacity chromatin associated binding sites. The localization of the T_3 receptor in the nucleus of target cells is not an hormone dependant process, only binding proteins with much lower affinity for T_3 have been found in the cytosol (1). In this work we have studied the effect of molybdate and ATP on the binding activity of the nuclear T_3 receptor, agents which are widely used for the study of physicochemical properties of steroid receptors (2).

METHODS. T_3 receptors were solubilized from rat liver nuclei by extraction with TEM Buffer (20 mM Tris, 3 mM $MgCl_2$, 5 mM EDTA, ph 8) containing 0.4 M NaCl. Saturation analysis were done by incubation with increasing concentration of L-(^{125}I)-T_3. Non specific binding was measured by adding a 500 fold excess of unlabeled hormone. Bound and free hormone were separated by exclusion chromatography on microcolumns of Sephadex G_{25} fine. DEAE Sephadex A50 chromatography was performed as previously reported (3).

Effects of molybdate and ATP. Scatchard analysis of the data show that in presence of 10 mM molybdate the affinity of the receptor for T_3 was significant decreased ($p < 0.01$) while the maximum binding capacity was not affected. This effect is not due to an alteration of the hormone or protein aggregation during incubation time as assessed by paper chromatography and centrifugation on a linear 5-20% sucrose gradient. Time course of incubation at 37°C indicate that the rate of degradation of the (^{125}I)-T_3 receptor complex was not affected by the molybdate treatment. SDS polyacrylamide gel electrophoresis revealed, after affinity labeling with BrAc-(^{125}I)-T_3 and photoaffinity labeling, two receptor forms of 57,000 daltons and 47,000 daltons which are not affected by adding molybdate in the incubation medium.
DEAE Sephadex column chromatography shows that the L-(^{125}I)-T_3-receptor complex eluted at a lower salt concentration when molybdate is added to the incubation medium (control: 0.21 M NaCl; MoO_4: 0.18 M NaCl). The L-(^{125}I)-T_4-receptor complex eluted in two close peaks in control experiments (0.21 M; 0.4 M NaCl) whereas only one with the molybdate treated preparation (0.21 M).
Other phosphatase inhibitors like G1P and NaF at concentration of 20 and 100 mM have no effects. Conversely when incubations were performed with (^{125}I)-T_4 at tracer concentration instead of (^{125}I)-T_3 the T_4 binding activity was increased. Similarly, binding studies performed with 5 mM ATP in the incubation medium, show a dramatic decrease of the T_3 binding activity ($p < .001$).

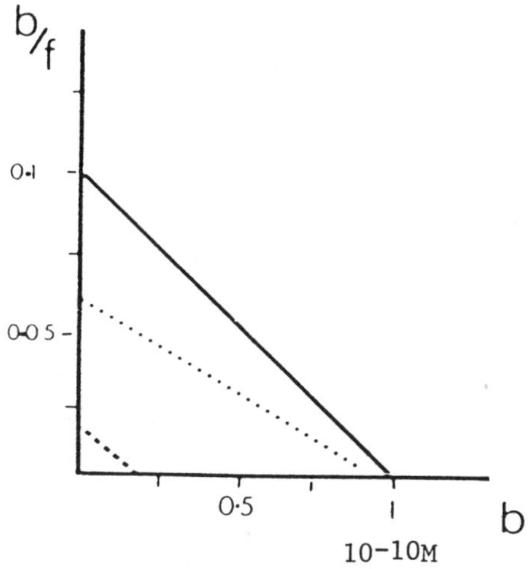

Fig. 1. Scatchard plots of the (^{125}I)-T3 binding to solubilized nuclear receptors from rat liver nuclei:
(——) Control Ka = 0.552 $10^{10}.M^{-1}$
(·····) 10 mM molybdate Ka = 0.324 $10^{10}.M^{-1}$
(---) 5 mM ATP

These results demonstrate that molybdate and ATP at concentration used for others systems are able to induce by an unknown mechanism, modifications in certain molecular properties of the T3 receptor. Thus the modified receptor could be similar to others lower affinity binding sites.

REFERENCES

(1) Oppenheimer, J.H., Samuels, H.H., Eds (1983) Molecular basis of thyroid hormone action, Academic Press, N.Y.

(2) Grody, W.W., Schrader, W.T., O'Malley, B.W. (1982) Activation, transformation, and subunit structure of steroid hormone receptors. Endocrine Reviews 3, 141-163.

(3) Silva, E.S., Astier, H., Thakare, U., Schwartz, L. (1977) J. Biol. Chem. 252, 6799-6805.

IS THE PRIMARY STRUCTURE OF THE INSULIN RECEPTOR TISSUE SPECIFIC?

*H.J.Goren and **C.R.Kahn, M.F.White, and M.Okamoto
*Department of Medical Biochemistry, Universtiy of Calgary, Calgary, AB T2N 4N1 Canada, and **Joslin Diabetes Center, Boston, MA 02215 USA

INTRODUCTION

The primary structure of the human placenta receptor has been reported (1,2). Whether this structure is the same for insulin receptors in other tissues and animals has been investigated. Mild digestion products of phosphorylated-insulin receptor from human and rat tissues and their tryptic phosphopeptides have been compared. The evidence suggests that, minimally, the B-subunit primary structure is different in different tissues.

METHODS

Solubilized (0.1% Triton X-100), wheat germ agglutinin-purified insulin receptors from human placenta, IM9 lymphocytes, rat liver, and rat hepatoma cells (FAO), were autophosphorylated in the presence of 5 mM $MnCl_2$, 10^{-7} M insulin, and 50 uM [γ-^{32}P]ATP (3). Phosphorylated receptors were mildly digested with trypsin, chymotrypsin, elastase or staphylococcal protease V8 (5 ug/ml, 30 min, 20°C). ^{32}P-B-subunit and ^{32}P-B-subunit fragments were seperated by dodecyl sulphate polyacrylamide gel electrophoresis, detected autoradiographically, excised and digested (trypsin 100 ug, 24 h, 37°C). Tryptic-phosphopeptides were seperated, by reverse-phase HPLC (C_{18} column), collected and counted (Cerenkov).

RESULTS

In each receptor preparation, insulin stimulated the phosphorylation of a 95 kDa protein, the B-subunit. Mild trypsin digestion of ^{32}P-receptor produced 90 kDa and 70 kDa ^{32}P-proteins. IM9 lymphocyte receptor, however, also gave a 60 kDa phosphoprotein. Trypsin digestion prior to the phosphorylation reaction, demonstrated that the 90 kDa protein could autophosphorylate. With mildly digested rat liver receptor, however, the 70 kDA B-subunit fragment could also be phosphorylated. Staphylococcal protease V8 digested the ^{32}P-FAO-B-subunit to 85 kDa and the ^{32}P-placenta-B-subunit to 85 kDa and 60 kDa proteins.

HPLC analyses of completely digested phosphorylated B-subunit and its mildly digested fragments demonstrated several phosphopeptides. Insulin-stimulated phosphorylation increased phosphopeptides in 2 regions of 100 min chromatograms (1ml/min); mostly between 10% and 20% acetonitrile (region II) and some between 20% and 30% acetonitrile (reagion III). Placenta receptors, however, demonstrated a more even distribution of tryptic-phosphopeptides than FAO or rat liver receptors. The 90 kDa phosphoprotein from FAO receptor contained little region II phosphopeptides, whereas the 90 kDa placenta phosphoprotein did retain some.

DISCUSSION

This report presents evidence that the insulin receptor B-subunit primary structure is tissue dependent. Mild trypsin digestion of the ^{32}P-IM9 insulin receptor produced 3 ^{32}P-B-subunit fragments, while the other receptors yielded 2 fragments. Similarly, tryptic-B-subunit fragments demonstrated differences in their ability to autophosphorylate, e.g. the 70 kDa fragment of the rat liver receptor autophosphorylated, while similar sized fragments from the IM9 lymphocyte or FAO receptor did not. In addition, the major sites of autophosphorylation in the B-subunit may differ with receptor preparation. Thus, the HPLC chromatograms of digested ^{32}P-B-subunits differed, e.g. human placenta receptor demonstrated region II and region III phosphopeptides while FAO receptor yielded predominantly region II phosphopeptides.

Insulin is a key hormone in the regulation of cell metabolism. Its actions include rapid onset of membrane transport events, slower changes in metabolism and slow tissue growth promoting events. All insulin actions are initiated through its receptor. Since evolution can lead to multiple copies of a gene and tissue differentiation can lead to specific gene expression, then the primary structure of the insulin receptor may be tissue specific. Furthermore, it is tempting to speculate that the primary structure of the receptor may determine the major action of insulin in a cell.

ACKNOWLEDGEMENT

This work was supported by the Medical Research Council of Canada (MA 7271, HJG) and the NIH (AM33201, CRK).

REFERENCES

1. Ullrich, A., Bell, J.R., Chen, E.Y., Herrera, R., Petruzzelli, L.M., Dull, T.J., Gray, A., Coussens, L., Liao, Y.C., Tsubakawa, M., Mason, A., Seeburg, P.H., Grunfeld, C., Rosen, O.M. and Ramachandran, J. (1985) Nature 313, 756-761.
2. Ebina, Y., Ellis, L., Jarnagin, K., Edery, M., Graf, L., Clauser, E., Ou, J., Masiarz, F. Kan, Y.W. Goldfine, I.D., Roth, R.A. and Rutter, W.J. (1985) Cell 40, 747-758.
3. Kasuga, M., White, M.F. and Kahn, C.R. (1984) Meth. Enzymol. 109, 609-621.

ANOMALOUS BINDING OF INSULIN TO RECEPTORS IN LACTATING RAT MAMMARY GLAND

Holness, M., & Coore, H.G. Biochemistry Dept., University of the West Indies, Mona, Kingston 7, Jamaica.

INTRODUCTION

There are only a few reports on the properties of insulin receptors in lactating rat mammary gland (1,2) although it is a major target tissue for insulin (3). These reports describe a concave-upward Scatchard binding curve similar to that of several other tissues (4). However, using a mono-component, mono-iodinated insulin (not used in the earlier studies) we have found a more complex binding curve for lactating mammary gland reminiscent of that described for rat hepatoma (5).

MATERIALS AND METHODS

Unlabelled and labelled porcine insulin and labelled human insulin (^{125}I in tyrosine-A14, 1800-2000 Ci/mmol) were from Nova Research Institute, Denmark and Amersham Radiochemicals, U.K. respectively. Lactating mammary gland acini (LMG), liver plasma membranes (LPM) and washed red blood cells (RBC) were prepared as earlier described (6,7,8).

Equilibrium binding was carried out in a volume of 0.4 ml (LMG) or 0.25 ml (LPM and RBC) in 1.5 ml polyethylene centrifuge tubes at a pH of 7.5 or 8 at 4°C for 18 h (LMG and LPM) or 15°C for 2 h (RBC). Tubes contained 2 mg acinar protein or 0.25 mg protein of LPM or 0.9 x 10^9 RBC and [^{125}I] insulin, 100 pg (LMG) or 50 pg (LPM and RBC), Unlabelled insulin was present in concentrations ranging from 0-10 μg/ml. Separation of bound from free insulin was by centrifugation for 2 or 5 min. Bacitracin (10 mg/ml) was present in 18 h incubations.

RESULTS AND DISCUSSION

Maximum % specific insulin binding was 11% for LMG and RBC and 25% for LPM. Non-specific binding was < 5% of total counts bound.

Scatchard binding curves for LPM and RBC, Fig. 1, were similar to published curves but for LMG a consistent (30 experiments) 'hump' was seen in the region of 0.18-0.85 nM free insulin which is in the physiological range (9). The type of binding curve seen for LPM and RBC has been interpreted either as two classes of non-interacting binding sites of different affinities (10) or as negative cooperativity of a single class of binding sites (11). Neither model fits our data for LMG. Instead, we seem to detect a class of high affinity non-interacting binding sites and another class of low affinity <u>interacting</u> binding sites. Decision on the nature of the interaction requires more experiments. We may note that the shape of the binding curve for insulin to LMG was unaffected by starvation of the donor animal (increasing number of receptors) or by prolactin deprivation (diminishing number of receptors).

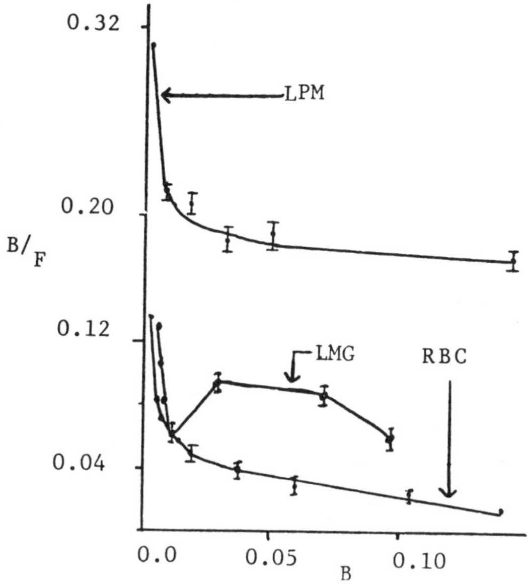

Fig. 1

Segments of Scatchard plots of Insulin binding to 3 tissues. Units: (B) Insulin Bound, pmoles/unit tissue used per ml incubation medium; (F) Free Insulin, pmoles/ml. Each data point was derived from averages of 6-10 preparations. Binding experiments were done in duplicate. Some error bars are omitted for clarity.

ACKNOWLEDGEMENTS

We have received financial support from the Wellcome Trust, U.K., and the Research and Publications Fund (UWI).

REFERENCES

1. O'Keefe, E., and Cuatrecasas, P. (1974). Biochim. Biophys. Acta. 343, 64-77.
2. Flint, D.J. (1982) J. Endocrinol. 93, 279-285.
3. Anderson, R.R. (1974) In Lactation, A Comprehensive Treatise, Larson, B.L., and Smith, V.R., eds. Vol. 1, New York and London: pp 97-140
4. Gammeltoft, S. (1984) Physiological Reviews 64, 1321-1378.
5. Marsh, J.W., Westley, J., and Steiner, D.F. (1984) J. Biol. Chem. 259, 6641-6649.
6. Threadgold, L., Coore, H.G., and Kuhn, N.J. (1982) Biochem. J. 204, 493-501.
7. Neville, D.M. Jr. (1968) Biochim. Biophys. Acta. 154, 540-551.
8. Gambhir, K.K., Archer, J.A., and Bradley, C.J. (1978) Diabetes 27, 701-708.
9. Collier, S.A. (1983) Proc. Natl. Acad. Sci., U.S.A. 80, 1068-72.
10. Kahn, C.R., Freychet, P., Roth, J., and Neville, D.M. Jr. (1974) J. Biol. Chem. 249, 2249-2257.
11. DeMeyts, P., Roth, J., Neville, D.M. Jr., Gavin, J.R. III Lesniak, M.A. (1973) Biochem. Biophys. Res. Comm. 55, 154-161.

EXPRESSION OF EPIDERMAL GROWTH FACTOR RECEPTOR IN VARIOUS HUMAN TUMORS.

David L. Hwang, Shu S. Lin, Yee-Chaw Tay and Arye Lev-Ran.
Dept of Endocrinology, City of Hope Medical Center,
Duarte, CA. 91010

INTRODUCTION

Epidermal growth factor (EGF) is a polypeptide (M.W. 6000) which stimulates proliferation and differentiation of a great variety of cell types (1). The activities of EGF are mediated through its specific receptor which is a 170 KD glycoprotein located on the cell surface membrane. Receptors for EGF, insulin, platelet-derived growth factor, insulin-like growth factor-I as well as retroviral transforming proteins (2) are characterized by their tyrosine-specific protein kinase activity and ligand-stimulated receptor autophosphorylation. Furthermore there are sequence homologies between the growth factors receptors and certain virus-derived oncogene proteins. For instance, EGF receptor has certain structural similarities to the avian erythroblastosis virus (AEV) v-erb-B transforming protein (3). On the other hand, EGF itself has also an extensive sequence homology with the transforming growth factor (TGFα) which functions via the EGF receptor (4). Recently, several reports showed that the binding activity of EGF to the receptor was either decreased or increased in transformed cells and malignant tumors (5-8). We studied the EGF receptor binding and autophosphorylation activities in various human tumor tissues.

METHODS

Human normal and tumor tissues of colon, breast, lung, kidney, ovary and liver obtained during surgery were used for the studies on the expression of epidermal growth factor receptor (EGF-R). Adjacent histologically normal tissues of the same patient served as control. The Triton X-100 solubilized, wheat germ agglutinin affinity column purified receptors ($\sim$50 ug) were immunoprecipitated with anti EGF-R antibody (IgG)-protein A-sepharose beads followed by autophosphorylation with [γ-^{32}P]ATP. The ^{32}P-phosphorylated EGF-R (170KD) was separated by SDS-PAGE and excised from the dried gel to measure the ^{32}P incorporation. The same receptor preparations were also used for receptor binding with ^{125}I-EGF.

RESULTS AND DISCUSSION

The main results are summarized in the Table.

TABLE: EGF receptor autophosphorylation and receptor binding in human tumor tissues. (median)

Specimen	Receptor Phosphorylation (^{32}P incorporated into 170 KD band, cpm)		Receptor binding (EGF bound, p mol/mg protein)	
	Control	Tumor	Control	Tumor
Colon (N=10)	173	170	0.94	0.92
Breast (N=6)	171	186	0.66	0.67
Lung (N=5)	213	400	0.96	1.83
Kidney (N=3)	174	160	1.05	0.80
Ovary (N=3)	191	180	0.97	0.85
Liver (N=2)	357	190	1.47	0.63

Of the specimens studied, colon and breast showed no difference between control and tumor tissues. The lung tumors had an average of 2-fold increase (range 1.3-3.5) in EGF receptor binding and autophosphorylation as compared to control tissues. On the other hand liver tumors had 50-100% decrease in EGF-R activities. The tumors of kidney and ovary showed a 12-24% decrease in EGF receptor binding without significant changes in receptor autophosphorylation.

The increase or decrease in EGF-R in human tumors may indicate that EGF or EGF-R has some regulatory mechanisms during the process of tumogenesis. The changes of EGF-R activities may be used as a marker for certain types of tumors.

ACKNOWLEDGMENTS

The authors thank the Dept of Surgical Pathology of the City of Hope Medical Center (Dr. H. Battifora and his staff) for the supply of human tissues. We also thank Dr. J. Schlessinger of the Weizmann Institute of Science for providing us with the anti-A431 membrane antibodies.

REFERENCES

1. Carpenter, G. and Cohen, S. (1979) Annu. Rev. Biochem 48:183-216
2. Bishop, J.M. (1983) Annu. Rev. Biochem 52:301-354
3. Downward, J. et al (1984) Nature, 307:521-527
4. Marquardt, H. et al (1983) Proc. Natl. Acad. Sci. 80:4684-4688
5. DeLarco, J.E. and Todaro, G.J. (1978) Proc. Natl Acad. Sci. 75:4001-4005
6. Liberman, T.A. et al (1984) Cancer Res. 44:753-760
7. Cowley, G. et al (1984) Cancer Cells 1:5-10

EGF-STIMULATED TYROSINE KINASE ACTIVITY IN PLASMA MEMBRANES FROM AS-30D RAT HEPATOMA. THE POSSIBLE ROLE OF LONIDAMINE IN INHIBITING GROWTH FACTORS RECEPTORS PHOSPHORYLATION

M.G. Paggi, A.Floridi, R. Falcioni, C.Nervi°, B.Silvestrini* and A.Caputo

Regina Elena Institute for Cancer Research, Viale Regina Elena 291 00161 ROME ITALY; °Institute of Histology and General Embriology, and *Institute of Pharmacology and Pharmacognosy "La Sapienza" University, Rome,

INTRODUCTION AS-30D rat hepatoma (1) has already been characterized as far as it concerns its preferential glucose utilization and high lactate production (2). It features, moreover, high percentage of mitochondrially-bound hexokinase (HK) activity (3). Because of its high amount of ATP production and consumption, protein phosphorylation was investigated in the absence and in the presence of the phorbol ester TPA. As a control TPA stimulation in human fibroblasts is reported. ATP-dependent protein phosphorylation in hepatoma plasma membranes was also investigated. Moreover, it is under investigation how drugs able to specifically interfere with tumor energy metabolism can modulate this ATP-dependent tyrosine-kinase activity. Lonidamine (LND) is shown to selectively inhibit tumor glycolysis (4) at the level of the mitochondrially-bound HK (5). The effect of (LND) was tested on AS-30D energy metabolism and ATP production.

METHODS AS-30D cell line was mantained as in Ref. 2. Human fibroblasts were cultured as in Ref. 6. Cells were washed 3 times in a Phosphate-free buffer and incubated in the presence of 0.2mCi of 32P-ortophosphate for 45 min + 15 min in the presence of TPA at 37°C. Cells were then washed and lisated. Electrophoresis was run according to Laemmli (7) in a 10% acrylamide concentration. Plasma membranes from AS-30D cells were prepared according to Ref. 8 and phosphorylation was carried out in the presence of 32P-gamma ATP (2.3 uCi). Plasma membranes were then precipitated with a policlonal anti-phosphotyrosine antibody (9) and the immunoprecipitate was run in a 7.5% acrylamide gel.

RESULTS AND DISCUSSION As previously reported for chicken fibroblasts (6), TPA is able to increase protein phosphorylation also in human fibroblasts. AS-30D cells are less sensitive to TPA stimulation, due to its high basal rate of phosphorilation. The presence of a high appearent m.w. protein (140Kd) was interpreted as a receptor membrane protein. AS-30D plasma membranes were purified and

ATP-dependent protein phosphorylation was assayed in basal conditions and in the presence of 45 uM EGF or 100 uM insulin. Phosphorylated proteins were precipitated using a policlonal antibody against phosphotyrosine where precipitation was specifically inhibited by free phosphotyrosine. In this case a major band ranging between 135 and 140Kd was evidentiated, thus indicating the presence in the hepatoma plasma membranes of a receptor with a basal tyrosine-kinase activity barely sensitive to insulin and highly stimulable by EGF.

Because LND was proposed as a regulator of cellular differentiation (10) and because there is a very well known relationship between oncogenes and growth factors receptors with tyrosine-kinase activity, the effect of LND on the energy cell metabolism of AS-30D hepatoma cells was investigated, showing a dramatic decrease in the ATP production (50%). The role of LND in interfering with growth factors receptors phosphorylation is currently under investigation.

REFERENCES

1. Smith DF et al., Cancer Res 30, 2306-2309, 1970
2. Nakashima RA et al., Cancer Res 44, 5702-5706, 1984
3. Paggi et al. in "Cell Membranes and Cancer" (Galeotti T et al. eds.), 203-208, Elsevier 1985
4. Floridi A et al., J Natnl Inst 66, 497-499, 1981
5. Floridi A et al., Cancer Res 41, 4661-4666, 1981
6. Bouchè M et al., Carcinogenesis 5, 559-563, 1984
7. Laemmli UK, Nature 227, 680-685, 1970
8. Thom D et al., Biochem J 168, 187-194, 1977
9. Ek B and Heldin CH, J Biol Chem 259, 11145-11152,1984
10. Caputo et al, Chemioter Oncol 4, 276-281, 1979

Work supported by the CNR project "Oncologia" grant n° 85.02159.44 and by A.I.R.C.

CHARACTERIZATION OF THE DETERGENT-SOLUBILIZED RECEPTOR FOR ATRIAL NATRIURETIC PEPTIDE FROM CULTURED VASCULAR SMOOTH MUSCLE CELLS

D.B. Schenk, M.N. Phelps, R. Scarborough, K. Johnson and J. Lewicki
California Biotechnology Inc., 2450 Bayshore Frontage Road,
Mountain View, California 94043 USA

Atrial natriuretic peptide (ANP) is known to have biological effects on several target organs such as kidneys, adrenals and blood vessels. Specific ANP binding sites have been characterized in some of these tissues (1, 2). Recently, several of the putative receptors have been identified by ^{125}I-ANP crosslinking studies (3, 4). One such protein of 66,000 M_r (after ANP crosslinking) was identified in cultured vascular smooth muscle cells (4). Here we describe the solubilization and partial characterization of this ANP receptor protein.

(I) SOLUBILIZATION OF THE ANP RECEPTOR. Cultured bovine aortic smooth muscle cells (BASM) were grown to confluence in Dulbecco's Modified Eagle's medium and membranes were prepared. Appropriate concentrations of a purified component of Triton X-100 were used to solubilize ^{125}I-ANP binding activity from the membranes. The 100,000 X g supernatant was then characterized for its ability to bind ^{125}I-ANP in a concentration-dependent manner (Fig. 1). Scatchard analysis of the binding data revealed a single class of sites with a K_d=1.77 X 10^{-10} moles/liter and a B_{max}=34.6 pmol/mg protein. The binding activity was stable for 14 days at 4°C or 2 months at -70°C. The binding parameters of the solubilized ANP receptor are essentially identical to those of the cell-associated receptor (K_d=0.1 - 2.0 X 10^{-9} moles/liter, B_{max}=250,000 sites/cell, ref. 4).

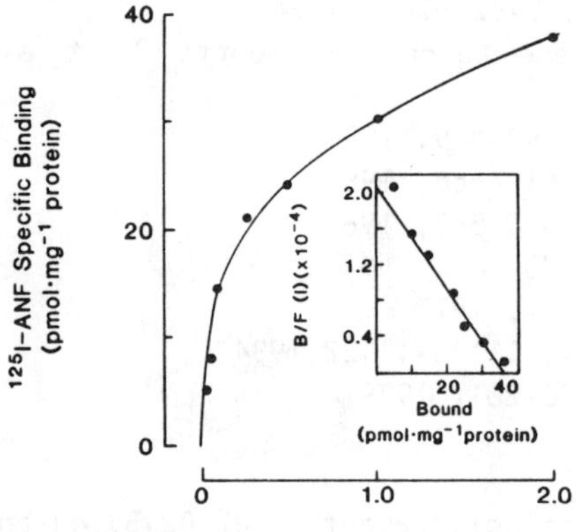

Fig. 1

(II) CHARACTERIZATION OF THE SOLUBILIZED ANP RECEPTOR. The physiochemical properties of the solubilized ANP receptor were further investigated by specifically labeling the protein with ^{125}I-ANP via disuccimidyl suberate (4).

Chromatography of the labeled ANP receptor on wheat germ agglutinin (WGA) agarose showed that it bound and could be eluted only at high concentrations of α-acetyl glucosamine (.30 M, data not shown). This finding demonstrates that the solubilized-labeled receptor is a glycoprotein and contains accessible glucosamine moieties.

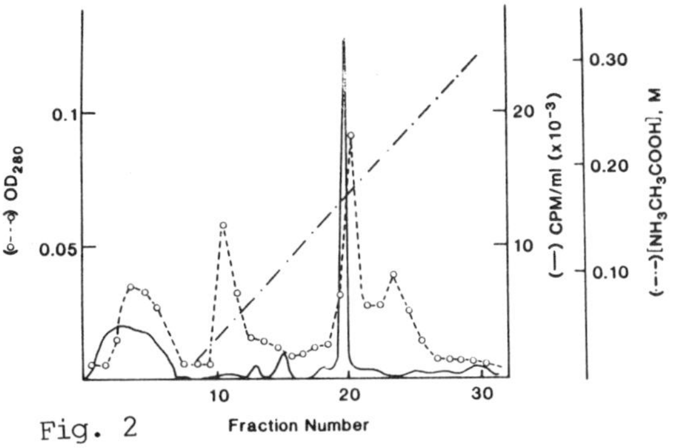

Fig. 2

Further characterization of the ^{125}I-labeled ANP receptor by chromatography on CM-cellulose is shown in Fig. 2. Material specifically eluted from the WGA column was dialyzed and loaded onto CM-cellulose at pH 4.1, 0.01M NH_3COOH (AmAc) followed by a linear gradient to 0.3 M AmAc pH 6.0. A sharp peak of radioactivity eluted at fractions 18-20 (Fig. 2). Autoradiography of this pooled peak, analyzed by SDS-PAGE, revealed the presence of a 66,000 M_r protein. Silver stain protein analysis of the SDS-PAGE gel suggested that the 66,000 M_r protein constituted 30-40% of this material.

(III) CONCLUSIONS. These findings show that the ANP receptor in cultured vascular bovine smooth muscle cells can be solubilized in a stable manner with binding parameters equivalent to that of the membrane-bound receptor. Furthermore, preliminary characterization of the receptor suggests that it is a glycoprotein that is slightly basic in nature. Hopefully the initial characterization of the ANP receptor will be useful for further purification and characterization of the protein-leading ultimately to an understanding of its role in hypertension.

ACKNOWLEDGEMENT
This work was supported by the Biotechnology Research Partners Ltd.

REFERENCES

(1) Napier, M.A., Vandelen, R.L., Albers-Schonberg, G., Nutt, R.F., Brady, S., Lyle, T., Winquist, R., Faison, E.P., Heind, L.A. and Blaine, E.H. (1984) Proc. Natl. Acad. Sci. USA 81, 5946-5950.

(2) Schenk, D.B., Johnson, L.K., Schwartz, K., Sista, H., Scarborough, R.M. and Lewicki, J. (1985) Biochem. Biophys. Res. Commun. 127, 433-442.

(3) Yip, C.C., Laing, L.P. and Flynn, T.G. (1985) J. Biol. Chem. 260, 8229-8232.

(4) Schenk, D.B., Phelps, M.N., Porter, J.G., Scarborough, R.M., McEnroe, G. and Lewicki, J. (1985) J. Biol. Chem. 261, in press.

Glycoprotein Hormones

STRUCTURE AND EXPRESSION OF HUMAN PLACENTAL HORMONE GENES. Irving Boime, Mark Boothby, Susan Daniels-McQueen, Robert Darnell, Makoto Hoshina, and Paul Policastro. Departments of Pharmacology and Obstetrics and Gynecology, Washington University School of Medicine, St. Louis, Missouri, U.S.A. 63110

Introduction

One of the important functions of the human placenta is to produce peptide hormones during pregnancy; e.g., human chorionic gonadotropin (hCG) and human placental lactogen (hPL). The appearance of these hormones in maternal serum during pregnancy is quite different. Whereas hCG peaks in the first trimester, hPL reaches maximal levels at term. Since the levels of these hormones differ during the course of gestation, it is apparent that the factors controlling their synthesis are not the same. Thus, the human placenta represents a convenient and unique tissue for studying expression of human hormonal genes during development.

Placental lactogen is a single non-glycosylated polypeptide chain which shares greater than 90% homology with human growth hormone. Chorionic gonadotropin consists of two non-identical glycosylated subunits (alpha and beta) linked non-covalently. The amino acid sequence of hCGα is identical to that of the α-subunits contained in human pituitary gonadotropins, and in thyrotropin (1). The β-subunit confers the unique biologic action on each hormone (1).

Expression of chorionic gonadotropin is evoked in tumorigenesis. A significant number of non-trophoblastic tumors secrete hCG subunits. This is referred to as ectopic hCG production. Cell lines from some of these cancers and from choriocarcinomas -- the malignant tumors of trophoblastic cells -- produce hCG *in vitro* (2) and change production levels in response to physiologic effects. In addition, most such lines produce more alpha subunit than beta (2), reminiscent of the subunit imbalance of placenta (see below).

A unique feature of the human placenta is its continued differentiation during gestation. Progeny of mitotically active mononucleated cytotrophoblasts fuse to form mitotically inactive syncytiotrophoblast (3). Gestational abnormalities of trophoblast development such as choriocarcinoma and hydatidiform mole occur at different stages of trophoblast differentiation. Such changes in patterns of differentiation lead to alterations in the expression of hCG and hPL (4).

Despite the extensive information regarding these hormones, the factors regulating their synthesis are obscure. This point will be addressed here by dealing with the following issues:

(1) Structure and organization of the hCGα and β subunit genes in normal placenta and in trophoblast and non-trophoblast derived tumors.
(2) What are the mechanisms by which net hCG subunit production is regulated during pregnancy? Are there translational and/or transcriptional controls operative during subunit synthesis?

(3) Expression of chorionic gonadotropin during tumorigenesis.
(4) The linkage between trophoblast differentiation and placental hormone production.

Structure of hCG subunit genes

hCGα

That the amino acid sequence of the hCGα subunit is identical to that of the α subunits contained in the pituitary hormones LH, FSH, and TSH raises the question of whether or not the α subunits are encoded by more than one gene. In humans, only one gene bearing hCGα sequences could be detected per haploid complement (5,6). The structure of this gene is the same in DNA from first trimester and term placenta (Fig. 1).

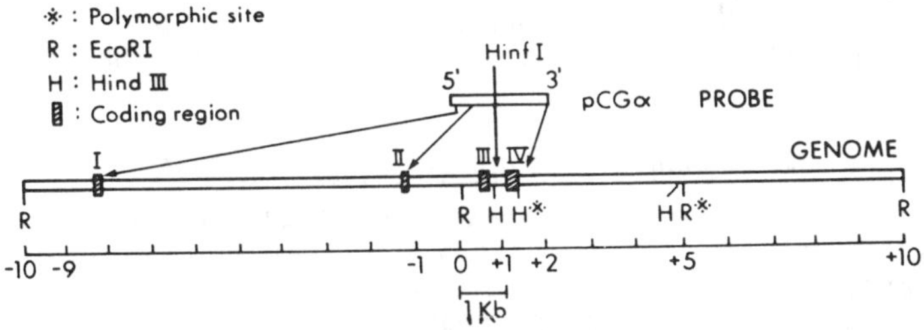

Polymorphisms were observed for the presence of a HindIII site in exon 4 and an EcoRI site at position +5 in the 3' flanking sequence of the gene (Fig. 1). These polymorphic sites were used as markers of tissue genotype in normal placenta and trophoblastic disease (7). The first 140 bp of 5' flanking sequence contains a 9 bp DNA sequence homologous to a concensus viral enhancer sequence. This may be significant, since tissue-specific expression of many genes are thought to be dependent on such sequences.

hCGβ

The hCGβ subunit is encoded by a multigene family (7,8), comprised of six genes (or pseudogenes) and the single LH-β gene (Fig. 2)

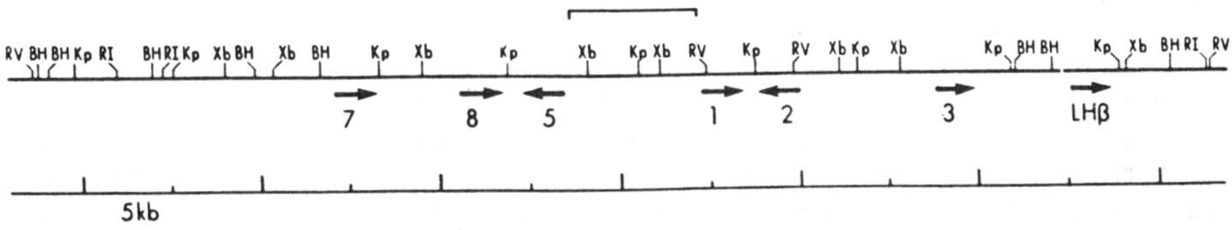

To date there is evidence for the in vivo expression of only two hCGβ genes, CGβ3 and CGβ5 (9) while CGβ1, CGβ2 and CGβ7 are nonfunctional or poorly expressed genes (10). The reason for the multiplicity of β subunits is not clear. Though LHβ and hCGβ apparently evolved from the same ancestral coding sequence, there are undoubtedly differences in regulatory sequences which account for the differential hCGβ and LHβ expression in placenta and anterior pituitary. Analogous to globin gene switching, the hCGβ gene family may be a developmentally regulated system that is sequentially expressed from embryogenesis to a fully developed placenta at term. Alternatively, a different β subunit gene may be activated in tumorigenesis.

Expression of chorionic gonadotropin during tumorigenesis

In choriocarcinoma cells, (eutopic) hCGα production is induced by cyclic AMP, whereas in HeLa (ectopic) cells, it is induced by sodium butyrate (2). Using plasmid expression-vector systems, the role of 5'-flanking hCGα sequences in the differential expression of the gene in these cell types was examined. Deletion mutants revealed that cell specific induction of the α gene was dependent on 140 bp of α 5' flanking DNA. This is the same stretch of DNA that contains the concensus enhancer sequence.

Regulation of net hCG subunit production during pregnancy

Previous studies have demonstrated an imbalance in placental levels of hCG subunits. Free α subunit was present in first trimester placenta, and the α:β ratio was increased as gestation approached term. Labeling nascent chains of polysomes derived from first-trimester and term placenta and quantitation of mRNA showed that at first trimester, the α:β ratio was 1.8:1, whereas at term this ratio was greater than 10:1. The data demonstrated that the progressive rise in production of free α subunit during gestation must for the most part be attributed to independent regulation of mRNA accumulation. Translational control is not the major determinant for subunit production in vivo; rather, the ratio of peptide production is comparable to the ratio of the corresponding mRNA and thus subunit mRNA levels are the major determinant of the imbalance of hCG subunits during gestation.

Relationship of trophoblast differentiation to hormone production

As discussed above, mitotically active cells, cytotrophoblasts are progenitors to the differentiated syncytiotrophoblast layer. Using in situ hybridization and tissue sections from normal and neoplastic tissue, we showed that the hCG subunit and hPL genes were activated at different stages of placental differentiation. Expression of hCG subunit genes occurs at an earlier step in the differentiation pathway than hPL. To investigate this issue, a cell culture system employing normal cytotrophoblasts, which would allow an examination of their differentiation in vitro, is essential. To isolate differentiating cytotrophoblasts, first trimester placenta was disaggregated with trypsin and DNAse to release cells. Cytotrophoblasts were cultured on fibronectin-coated plates to obtain efficient plating of cells. Fibroblast contamination was prevented using media containing D-Valine. Initially, the cytotrophoblasts appeared as discrete epithelial cells and then formed closely knit colonies containing multinucleated syncytial-like cells. That these were epithelial cells was confirmed by immunohistochemistry using antibodies (provided by C. Loke) directed against 44-55 Kd cytokeratins from HeLa cells. Only the epithelial-like cells were stained; macrophages and fibroblasts were negative. Use of serum-free media containing epidermal growth factor supported the differentiation for a longer time than serum-supplemented medium. As a functional test, we examined hCG subunit synthesis in cultures labeled with [^{35}S]cysteine. Initially, hCG dimer and free α subunit were observed. Over 3 weeks in culture, synthesis of β subunit was reduced to background and only free α subunit was seen. This is similar to that observed *in vivo* where hCG declines during pregnancy and free α subunit increases.

We have identified at least one step in the differentiation pathway: The data support the hypothesis that mature syncytium is not required for hCG production and β subunit synthesis occurs in a transitory trophoblast intermediate.

Bibliography

1. Pierce, J. and Parsons, T. (1981). Ann. Rev. Biochem. 50, 465-495.
2. Hussa, R. (1980). Endocrine Rev. 1, 268-294.
3. Enders, A. (1965). Obstet. Gynecol. 25, 378-384.
4. Hoshina, M. *et al.* (1983). J. Cell Biol. 97, 1200-1206.
5. Boothby, M. *et al.* (1981). J. Biol. Chem. 256, 5121-5127.
6. Fiddes, J. and Goodman, H. (1981). J. Molec. Appl. Genet. 1, 3-18.
7. Boorstein, W. *et al.* (1982). Nature 300, 419-422.
8. Policastro *et al.* (1983). J. Biol. Chem. 258, 11492-11499.
9. Talmadge, K. *et al.* (1984). Nucleic Acids Res. 12, 8415-8426.
10. Policastro, P. *et al.* J. Biol. Chem., in press.

STRUCTURE AND EXPRESSION OF THE GONADOTROPIN GENES

J.H. Nilson, R.G. Goodman, J.B. Virgin, M.T. Nejedlik, A. Milsted and B.J. Silver

Case Western Reserve University, School of Medicine
Cleveland, OH 44106

Overview. Luteinizing hormone (lutropin, LH) and chorionic gonadotropin (CG) are heterodimeric glycoproteins composed of noncovalently associated α and β subunits (1). Like all glycoprotein hormones, LH and CG contain identical α subunits. Their β subunits are unique but share an amino acid sequence homology of 80% (1,2); the major difference is an an extension of 24 amino acids on the carboxyl terminus of CGβ. LH and CG can bind to the same gonadal receptor and stimulate both steroidogenesis and gametogenesis, yet LH is synthesized in the pituitary, while synthesis of CG occurs only in the placenta of primates and horses (1,2). This difference in tissue distribution suggests that the two gonadotropins may be regulated via different hormonal pathways. For example, hypothalamic releasing hormones and gonadal steroids regulate synthesis and secretion of pituitary LH (2,3), while a physiological regulator of CG synthesis and secretion has not been identified (4).

Despite appreciable progress in identifying hormones and intracellular mediators which regulate secretion of the pituitary gonadotropins (3), little is known about the regulation of their synthesis. Regulation of intracellular gonadotropin levels could occur coordinately through balanced synthesis of both subunits, or through the regulated synthesis of one subunit which is limiting with respect to assembly of the α/β complex. The latter possibility is consistent with several reports (4) of free α subunit in pituitary and placental tissue. With the recent identification and characterization of gonadotropin cDNA clones from several species, regulation of gonadotropin synthesis can now be approached directly at the level of gene expression. Consequently, we initiated our studies by isolating and characterizing the bovine genes encoding the α subunit and the β subunit of LH.

Structure of the α Subunit and Gonadotropin β Subunit Genes. The α subunit gene is present as a single copy in both the bovine (5) and human (6,7) genome. Expression of the bovine α subunit gene is restricted to the pituitary, whereas the human α subunit gene is expressed in pituitary and placenta (1,2). The lack of α subunit gene expression in bovine placenta is consistent with the absence of gonadotropins in ruminant placenta. Both the bovine and human α subunit genes contain 4 exons and 3 introns, encoding an mRNA of approximately 750 nucleotides. The mature α subunit in ruminants contains 96 amino acids. However, the human α subunit contains 92 amino acids (1,2), the result of a 4 codon deletion near the amino-terminal coding sequence of the human gene (2,6). When an allowance is made for this deletion, the position of the exons and introns in the bovine and human α subunits genes appear to be precisely conserved. However, the sizes of the introns vary, with the greatest difference occurring in intron A (13.4 kbp in the bovine gene versus 6.4 kbp in the human gene). Intron A accounts for most of the size of the α subunit gene in both species, 16 kbp and 10 kbp for bovine and human, respectively. It remains to be demonstrated whether the difference in intron A size is functionally significant.

Comparison of the nucleotide sequence information available for the bovine and human α subunit genes reveals a high degree of homology (82%) which is maintained in the coding region, the 3'-untranslated region, and the proximal 100 bp of 5'-flanking sequence. The strong conservation of nucleotide sequence in non-coding regions of the bovine and human α subunit genes may reflect a functional role for these sequences.

We have also characterized the unique bovine LHβ gene and found no other closely related sequences in the bovine genome (8). A similar result has also been reported for the rat (9). Additional studies indicate that the bovine LHβ gene is not expressed in the placenta. The unique LHβ gene found in cattle and rats stands in contrast to the human gene family which consists of 7 CGβ genes and 1 LHβ gene sharing greater than 90% homology in nucleotide sequence (10). We have used selective oligodeoxynucleotide hybridization probes to confirm that that LHβ and CGβ genes are expressed exclusively in pituitary and placenta, respectively. The high level of nucleotide sequence homology between the human LHβ and CGβ genes and the lack of CGβ genes in the cow and rat suggest that the CGβ genes have evolved recently from an ancestral LHβ gene via a series of duplications (8-10).

Both the structure and length of the gonadotropin β subunit genes is highly conserved in humans, cattle and rats. Yet, there is a surprising difference in the transcription start site for bovine and rat LHβ compared to human CGβ. The bovine and rat genes transcribe LHβ mRNAs with very short 5'-untranslated regions of 6-11 nucleotides, while the human CGβ mRNAs have 5'-untranslated regions in excess of 350 nucleotides (8-10). We have mapped the transcription start site of the human LHβ gene and found that it also starts at a position analogous to the bovine and rat LHβ genes. The short 5'-untranslated region of the human LHβ gene is of interest because the human CGβ genes (350 bp) are virtually identical (>90% nucleotide homology) to the proximal 350 bp of 5'-flanking sequence of the human LHβ gene (10). The presence of two different promoters may lead to tissue-specific differences in hormonal regulation of LHβ and CGβ gene expression.

Regulation of Gonadotropin Gene Expression. As mentioned earlier, unbalanced accumulation of α and β subunits is consistent with the notion that synthesis of the β subunit may be the rate limiting step regulating heterodimer formation. We have explored this possibility by using a sheep animal model. Chronic treatment of ovariectomized ewes with estradiol leads to a marked suppression in serum and tissue LH (2,11). Through the use of cDNA probes specific for the α and β subunits of bovine LH, we found that estradiol treatment of castrate ewes leads to a 98% decrease in LHβ mRNA and an 86% reduction in α subunit mRNA (11). The reduction in tissue and serum LH was approximately 99%, suggesting a strong correlation between the concentration of both gonadotropin mRNAs and tissue content of LH. No changes were observed in levels of mRNAs encoding prolactin or growth hormone. These results suggest that the mRNAs for α subunit and LHβ are coordinately regulated by estradiol.

Synthesis and secretion of α and CGβ subunits can be regulated in several human trophoblastic and non-trophoblastic cell lines by either cAMP or butyrate (4). To further pursue whether α subunit and gonadotropin β subunit mRNAs are regulated by these chemical agents, we have used two human cell lines, HeLa and BeWo. Under standard conditions of growth, HeLa S3 cells normally synthesize and secrete α subunit whereas CGβ subunit is undetectable. We have found that short-term exposure of HeLa cells to butyrate leads to an increase in α subunit mRNA levels (>7-fold) and the appearance of CGβ mRNA (12). Messenger RNAs for both gonadotropin subunits accumulate with essentially the same kinetics and are induced to maximal levels with the same concentration of butyrate, suggesting that their regulation is coordinated.

When HeLa cells are treated with 8-bromo cAMP, α subunit mRNAs increase only slightly (approximately 2-fold), while CGβ mRNA remains undetectable. This is consistent with other studies (4) which indicate that cAMP has little or no effect on α subunit secretion in non-trophoblastic cell-lines. To determine whether cAMP can regulate expression of gonadotropin mRNAs in trophoblastic cells, we have used a human choriocarcinoma cell-line (BeWo) which secretes high levels of α and CGβ subunits. Treatment of these cells with 8-bromo cAMP leads to at least a 10-fold increase in both α and CGβ mRNA levels; the magnitude of the responses are dose-dependent. Both mRNAs accumulate with the same kinetics and are maximally induced by the same concentration of 8-bromo cAMP, again suggesting their regulation is coordinated. In addition, treatment with either forskolin or cholera toxin stimulates accumulation of both mRNAs, confirming that intracellular generation of cAMP can efficiently regulate gonadotropin mRNA levels in trophoblastic cells.

Tissue specific factors may be required for a maximal cAMP response since the response of α subunit mRNA to the cyclic nucleotide is attenuated in HeLa versus BeWo cells (2-fold and 10-fold, respectively). In addition, the inability of cAMP to induce expression of detectable CGβ mRNA levels in HeLa cells suggests that cAMP can regulate only genes which are transcriptionally active. Preliminary results from experiments in progress indicate that at least part of the effect of cAMP is due to an increase in transcription of both the α subunit and CGβ genes.

Summary. Structurally, the glycoprotein hormones are among the most complex of all polypeptide hormones (1). Their biological activity becomes manifest only after heterodimer formation. Even though the common α subunit and gonadotropin β subunit genes are located on different chromosomes (2), our data suggest that expression of their mRNAs can be coordinately regulated, either negatively by estradiol or positively by cAMP. Consequently, gonadotropin synthesis appears to be regulated prior to translation, either through alterations in transcriptional activity, subsequent post-transcriptional events, or a combination of both. Since the α subunit and gonadotropin β subunit genes of bovine or human do not share any obvious regions of nucleotide sequence homology, it will be of particular interest to define the nature and location of specific nucleotide sequence elements which mediate the actions of estradiol and cAMP.

Acknowledgments. This work was supported by grants awarded by NSF (PCM-8309164) and NIH (AM-28559). JHN is the recipient of an NIH Research Career Development Award (AM-01316).

References

1. Pierce, J.G. and Parson, T.F. 1981. Ann. Rev. Biochem. 50:465-495.
2. Chin, W.W. 1985. in "The Pituitary Gland" (H. Imura, ed.) Raven Press, New York. pp. 103-125.
3. Conn, P.M. 1984. In "Biochemical Actions of Hormones" (G. Litwack, ed.) Vol XI, Academic Press, New York. pp. 68-92.
4. Hussa, R.O. 1980. Endocrine Rev. 1:268-294.
5. Goodwin, R.G., Moncman, C.L., Rottman, F.M. and Nilson, J.H. 1983. Nucleic Acids Res. 11:6873-6781.
6. Fiddes, J.C. and Goodman, H.M. 1981. J. Mol. Appl. Genet. 1:3-18.
7. Boothby, M., Ruddon, R.W., Anderson, McWilliams, D. and Boime, I. 1981. J. Biol. Chem. 256:5121-5127.
8. Virgin, J.B., Silver, B.J., Thomason, A.R., and Nilson, J.H. 1985. J. Biol. Chem. 260:7072-7077.
9. Jameson, L., Chin, W.W., Hollenberg, A.N., Chang, A.S. and Habener, J.F. 1984. J. Biol. Chem. 259:15474-15480.
10. Fiddes, J.C. and Talmadge, K. 1984. Recent Prog. in Hormone Res. 40:43-78.
11. Nilson, J.H., Nejedlik, M.T., Virgin, J.B., Crowder, M.E., and Nett, T.M. 1983. J. Biol. Chem. 258:12087-12090.
12. Milsted, A., Silver, B.J., Cox, R.P. and Nilson, J.H. 1985. Endocrinology 117:2033-2039.

HORMONAL REGULATION OF LUTROPIN AND THYROTROPIN GENE EXPRESSION

William W. Chin, Margaret A. Shupnik, Susan L. Naylor*, Soheyla D. Gharib, Frances E. Carr, and †E. Chester Ridgway

Lab of Molecular Genetics, Dept of Medicine, Brigham and Women's Hospital and Howard Hughes Medical Institute Labs, Harvard Medical School, Boston, MA 02115; *Dept of Cellular and Structural Biology, Univ of Texas Health Sciences Center, San Antonio, TX 78284; and †Div of Endocrinology, Dept of Medicine, Univ of Colorado Health Sciences Center, Denver, CO 80262

Lutropin (LH) and thyrotropin (TSH) are glycoprotein hormones that contain two different subunits, α and β, associated in a non-covalent manner. The protein backbone of the α subunit is identical among hormones within a species whereas the β subunits are varied and contribute biologic specificities (1). In addition, it is known that each subunit is encoded by separate mRNAs and hence separate genes (2). LH along with follicle-stimulating hormone represent the pituitary gonadotropins which regulate gonadal function whereas TSH controls thyroid gland function. The ultimate products of the gonads and thyroid gland are sex steroid and thyroid hormones, respectively, which regulate the production and secretion of LH and TSH in a classic endocrine negative-feedback fashion. Although much insight has been gained over the past several decades in the hormonal regulation of LH and TSH secretion, relatively little information has been obtained for the regulation of synthesis of these hormones and their subunits at the pre-translational level. The recent success in several laboratories in the molecular cloning of cDNAs and genes encoding the subunits of the glycoprotein hormones has accelerated the pace of work in this area. This abstract reviews briefly the data concerning the hormonal control of expression of the LH and TSH subunit genes at the transcriptional level.

MOLECULAR CLONING OF cDNAs and NATURAL GENES ENCODING THE SUBUNITS OF LUTROPIN AND THYROTROPIN

Over the past several years, our group and others including several participants in this Symposium have been successful in the molecular cloning of cDNAs and genes encoding the subunits of the glycoprotein hormones (for review, see ref. 2 and 3). The availability of these molecular reagents have permitted a detailed analysis of the regulation of LH and TSH biosynthesis at the pre-translational level. In addition, they will allow the dissection of the critical DNA elements involved in the mediation of hormonal effects on these genes.

This work also indicates that, except for hCGβ, the subunits are encoded by single copy genes. The structures of the genes between species suggest conservation of the basic architecture of the subunit genes so that the α gene in man and cow is large with a size of approximately 9--15 Kb and contains three introns (3-5), and the LHβ and TSHβ genes in man, cow, and rodent are smaller with sizes of approximately 1--2 Kb and contain two introns (6-10).

We have recently isolated and partially characterized the gene encoding the β subunit of rat TSH (10). The rat TSHβ gene is ~2.0 Kb in size and contains two introns. One is located one bp 5′ of the translational start signal and the other between codons +33--+34 of the TSHβ subunit apoprotein. The locations of the introns in the rat TSHβ gene are non-homologous with those of the rat LHβ gene.

CHROMOSOMAL LOCALIZATION OF THE α, LHβ, AND TSHβ GENES IN MAN AND MOUSE

Using these molecular probes and somatic-cell hybrids that segregate specific human and mouse chromosomes, the genomic localization of the glycoprotein hormone subunit genes has been determined. The genes are located on separate loci on different chromosomes (11-13) (Table 1). In addition, the chromosomal localization of these genes in the two species is syntenic with several other gene clusters. For instance, the TSHβ gene is imbedded in a linkage group containing the genes for amylase 1 and 2, nerve growth factor and the proto-oncogene, Nras (13). Hence, the coordinate regulation of the subunit genes does not occur in tandem pairs but rather among genes that are not linked but yet evidently share common regulatory DNA elements that likely respond to trans-acting intracellular regulatory factors.

	chromosome #	
	mouse	human
α subunit	6	4
LHβ subunit	19	7
TSHβ subunit	1	3

Table I. Chromosomal localization of the genes encoding the LH and TSH subunit genes in man and mouse.

HORMONAL REGULATION OF LUTROPIN GENE EXPRESSION

Recently, Nilson <u>et al</u> have shown that long-term treatment of ovariectomized ewes with estradiol results in suppression of LH mRNAs (14). These data and others (15-18) indicate that estrogen indeed regulates LH mRNAs level <u>in vivo</u>. We have examined the regulation further and have studied the short-term regulation of LH mRNAs by gonadal sex steroids in the rat anterior pituitary gland (18) using two experimental paradigms: (a) gonadectomy, and (b) hormone-replaced castrate male and female rats. Using blot hybridization analysis, we have shown that the α and LHβ mRNAs increase gradually after gonadectomy in parallel with the increase in serum hormone levels. After four weeks after operation, the α and LHβ mRNAs have increased 9--10-fold and 7--12-fold, respectively, in males and females. In the other set of experiments, gonadectomized males and females, three-week post-operative, were treated with testoserone propionate (100μg/100g bw/d) and 17-β-estradiol 3-benzoate (10μg/100g bw/d), respectively. Analysis of pituitary mRNAs showed that α decreased to 26% and 19%, and LHβ declined to 12% and 10% of control levels in male and female rats, respectively, after 48 h of replacement. In fact statistically significant decreases were first observed at 24 h. Also, the effects of hormones appeared greater for the LHβ than α mRNAs. Thus, these data indicate that the gonadal sex steroid hormones regulate the biosynthesis of LH at the pre-translational level. It is not clear however whether these effects are produced at the transcriptional or post-transcriptional levels.

HORMONAL REGULATION OF THYROTROPIN GENE EXPRESSION

Recent studies from our laboratories and others (19-22) have established that thyroid hormones regulate the synthesis of TSH in part at the pre-translational level. In particular, thyroid hormone administration to normal and hypothyroid rats, and to mice bearing thyrotropic tumors results in rapid decreases in TSH subunit mRNAs with an effect that is greater for the TSHβ than the α mRNAs. Further studies (23-24), using nuclear run-off assays in the thyrotropic tumor system, indicate that there is a rapid effect (<15 min) of thyroid hormones on the transcriptional activities of the TSH subunit genes, again with an effect that is more pronounced for the TSHβ gene. These effects are dependent on nuclear T3-receptor occupancy and are observed in the presence of protein synthesis inhibitors such as cycloheximide. Hence, thyroid hormones regulate TSH synthesis at least in part at the transcriptional level.

The dominant regulation of the β subunit genes compared to the α gene may reflect the constitutive synthesis of the α subunit in several cell types in the pituitary. However, the lack of complete suppression of the α subunit mRNA in the thyrotropic tumor which contains no gonadotropes suggests that such regulation of the α gene may be a fundamental property of each glycoprotein-hormone-producing cell.

Future focus will concern the roles of regulation DNA regions of the α, LHβ, and TSHβ genes in the mediation of thyroid and gonadal-steroid-hormone effects in the gonadotrope and thyrotrope. Such studies will involve <u>in vitro</u> mutagenesis of these DNA regions and DNA transfection techniques.

REFERENCES

(1) Pierce, J.G., Parsons, T.F. (1981) Annu. Rev. Biochem. 50, 465-495
(2) Chin, W.W. (1985) in The Pituitary Gland (Imura, H, ed.) pp. 164-184, Raven Press, New York.
(3) Fiddes, J.C., Talmadge, K. (1984) Recent Prog. Horm. Res. 40, 43-78.
(4) Goodwin, R.G., <u>et al</u>. (1983) Nucleic Acids Res. 11, 6873-6882.
(5) Boothby, M., <u>et al</u>. (1982) J. Biol. Chem. 256, 5121-5127.
(6) Virgin, J.B., <u>et al</u>. (1985) J. Biol. Chem. 260, 7072-7077.
(7) Jameson, J.L., <u>et al</u>. (1984) J. Biol. Chem. 259, 15474-15480.
(8) Whitfield, G.K., <u>et al</u>. (1985) 9th Intl. Thyroid Cong., Sao Paulo, Brazil Abstract #14.
(9) Hayashizaki, Y., <u>et al</u>. (1985) FEBS Lett 188, 394-400.
(10) Carr, F.E., <u>et al</u>. (1985) 9th Intl. Thyroid Cong., Sao Paulo, Brazil, Abstract #13.
(11) Naylor, S.L., <u>et al</u>. (1983) Somatic Cell Genet. 9, 757-770.
(12) Kourides, I.A., <u>et al</u>. (1984) Proc. Natl. Acad. Sci. USA 81, 517-519.
(13) Naylor, S.L., <u>et al</u>. (1986) Som. Cell. Genet. (submitted).
(14) Nilson, J.H. <u>et al</u>. (1983) J. Biol. Chem. 258, 12087-12090.
(15) Counis, R., <u>et al</u>. (1983) Biochem. Biophys. Res. Commun. 114, 65-72.
(16) Tepper, M.A., <u>et al</u>. (1985) 7th Con. Endo. Quebec City, Canada. Abstract #2293.
(17) Landefeld, T., Kepa, J. (1984) Biochem. Biophys. Res. Commun. 122, 1307-1313.
(18) Gharib, S.D., <u>et al</u>. (1986) J. Clin. Invest. (in press).
(19) Gurr, J.A., Kourides, I.A. (1983) J. Biol. Chem. 258, 10208-10211.
(20) Croyle, M.L., Maurer, R.A. (1984) DNA 3, 231-236.
(21) Carr, F.E., <u>et al</u>. (1985) Endocrinology 117, 1272-1278.
(22) Chin, W.W., <u>et al</u>. (1985) Endocrinology 116, 873-878.
(23) Shupnik, M.A., <u>et al</u>. (1985) J. Biol. Chem. 260, 2900-2903.
(24) Shupnik, M.A., <u>et al</u>. (1986) in Mechanism of Action of Thyroid Hormone (Tolman and DeGroot, eds.), in press.

SULFATION OF THE HUMAN CHORIONIC GONADOTROPIN α SUBUNIT IN PLACENTAL EXPLANTS

M. Bielinska,* S. Birken** and I. Boime*
*Department of Pharmacology, Washington University School of Medicine, St. Louis, MO 63110 and **Department of Medicine, Columbia University, New York, NY 10032

The asparagine-linked oligosaccharides of bovine lutropin terminate with sulfate while the oligosaccharides of human chorionic gonadotropin contain terminal sialic acid (1-3). Using a cell-free system to study sulfation of gonadotropins we unexpectedly observed that asialo hCG or its subunits could serve as substrates for in vitro sulfation (4).

To investigate a possible physiological role of sulfate in the expression of hCG, first trimester placental explants were incubated with $[^{35}S]O_4$ in Krebs-Ringer-bicarbonate solution. The media were immunoprecipitated with antisera against α or β subunits of hCG and the proteins were subjected to SDS-polyacrylamide gel electrophoresis. Both free and dimer α subunits contained sulfate. No detectable sulfation of β subunit occurred under our labelling.

Digestion of sulfated α subunit with pronase and subsequent paper electrophoresis of the digest revealed that in both free and dimer α subunits, sulfate is attached to tyrosine. There are four tyrosine residues in hCGα distributed in three tryptic peptides (5). To identify which of the tyrosine peptides were sulfated, placental explants were incubated in the presence of various labels and the tryptic peptides of immunoprecipiated α subunit were subjected to reverse-phase HPLC (6). Based on labelling pattern seen with $[^{35}S]O_4$, $[^{3}H]$tyrosine, $[^{3}H]$glucosamine, $[^{3}H]$proline and $[^{35}S]$cysteine, sulfate is confined to a single tryptic peptide which appears to correspond to the penultimate carboxyterminal tryptic peptide with the following structure: -Val-Glu-Asn(CHO)-His-Thr-Ala-Cys-His-Cys-Ser-Thr-Cys-Tyr-Tyr-His-Lys-.

The above data indicate that the α subunit is sulfated in first trimester placental explants. In contrast to that observed with the related pituitary glycoprotein hormones, sulfate is attached to protein rather than carbohydrate. This difference in posttranslational modification may reflect the use of different routes of secretion in trophoblast and pituitary.

REFERENCES

(1) Pierce, J. and Parsons T. (1981) Ann. Rev. Biochem. 50, 465-495.

(2) Hortin, G., Natowicz, M., Pierce, J., Baenziger, J., Parsons, T. and Boime, I. (1981) Proc. Natl. Acad. Sci U.S.A. 78, 7468-7472.
(3) Green, E., Van Halbeek, H., Boime, I. and Baenziger, J. J. Biol. Chem. in press.
(4) Green, E., Gruenebaum, J., Bielinska, M., Baenziger, J. and Boime, I. (1984) Proc. Natl. Acad. Sci. U.S.A. 81, 5320-5324.
(5) Morgan, F., Birken, S. and Canfield, R. (1975) J. Biol. Chem. 250, 5247-5258.
(6) Corless, C. and Boime, I. (1985) Endocrinology 117, 1699-1706.

PROCESSING AND SECRETION OF GLYCOPROTEIN HORMONE SUBUNITS IN TRANSFECTED C-127 AND AtT-20 CELLS

C.L. Corless,* T.V. Ramabhadran, B.A. Reitz, D.C. Tiemeier, and I. Boime*
*Department of Pharmacology, Washington University School of Medicine, St. Louis, Missouri 63110 and Monsanto Company.

The family of glycoprotein hormones includes chorionic gonadotropin (hCG) of the placenta and lutropin (LH), follitropin, and thyrotropin of the pituitary. These hormones share a dimeric structure consisting of noncovalently bound α and β subunits. Whereas the β subunit of each hormone is unique, the α subunit is identical in all four hormones (1). In addition to dimer, both pituitary and placenta secrete excess, uncombined α subunit that has a larger apparent molecular weight than dimer α. Free α from bovine pituitary fails to combine with β subunit due to the presence of a threonine-linked oligosaccharide that is not present on dimer α (2). To explore the role of subunit combination in determining the processing and secretion of glycoprotein hormone subunits, we used gene transfer experiments in which α and β subunits may be expressed and analyzed independently or together within the same cell type. Mouse mammary tumor cells (C-127) and mouse pituitary tumor cells (AtT-20) were used as host cells.

METHODS. 1) Expression of α and hCG-β subunits in C-127 cells. The expression of a cDNA for human α subunit in C-127 cells has been described (3). The mouse metallothioneine-I (MT) promoter used to express the α subunit was placed in front of a genomic fragment bearing a copy of the hCG-β gene. Both the α and hCG-β constructs were put into bovine papilloma virus (BPV) vectors and introduced, either singly or together, into C-127 cells by calcium phosphate precipitation. Transformed colonies were isolated and screened for the secretion of either or both subunits by RIA.

2) Expression of α, hCG-β and hLH-β subunits in AtT-20 cells. Both the MT-α and MT-hCG-β constructs described above were inserted into the plasmid pSV2neo (see Fig.). Expression of the neo gene in transfected cells confers resistance to the toxic antibiotic G418. To express hLH-β subunit, a fragment bearing exons 2 and 3 was excised from the MG-hCG-β construct and a homologous fragment of the hLH-β gene was inserted. Although this MT-hLH-β construct retained exon 1 of the hCG-β gene, four out of the five amino acids (all part of the signal sequence) encoded by this exon are common to both β subunits. Each

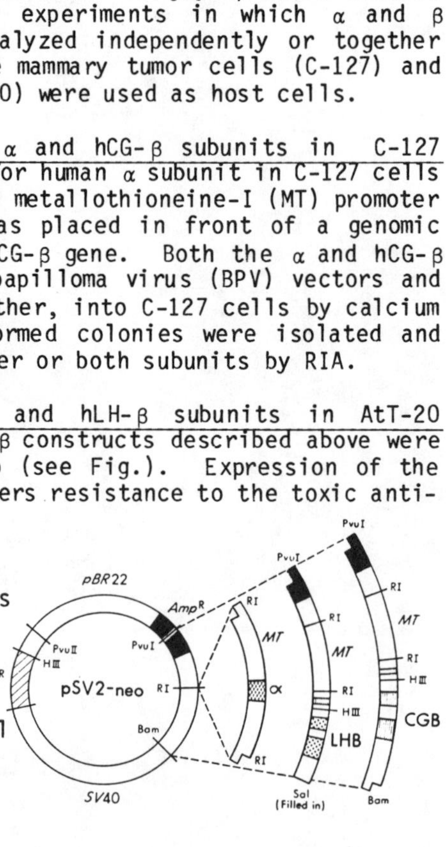

of the above plasmids was transfected into AtT-20 cells and G418 resistant colonies were isolated as described (4). Clones expressing both α and hLH-β or hCG-β subunits were obtained by transfecting with pSV2neo/MT-α plasmids bearing inserted MT-hLH-β or MT-hCG-β constructs.

RESULTS. 1) C-127 cells. Transfection of C-127 cells with the BPV constructs yielded clones expressing detectable levels of α or hCG-β subunit, as measured by RIA. Although the subunit levels were variable among the clones, expression of hCG-β subunit was consistently greater than that of α subunit. Clones transfected with both the α and hCG-β subunit constructs secreted hCG dimer that is bioactive in a rat luteal cell progesterone stimulation assay (T.V. Ramabhadran, manuscript in preparation). To compare subunits expressed individually with subunits from dimer secreting clones we used SDS-polyacrylamide gel electrophoresis. Subunits were immunoprecipitated from the media of [^{35}S]cysteine-labeled clones using either an antiserum to hCG-α or a monoclonal antibody to hCG-β subunit. Both the α antiserum and the β antibody were fully cross-reactive with hCG dimer. There was no detectable difference in the migration of dimer-derived and uncombined hCG-β subunits secreted from C-127 clones. In contrast, α subunit secreted from clones in the absence of transfected hCG-β migrated as a diffuse band of larger molecular weight than α from dimer-secreting clones. Thus, the post-translational processing of α subunit is altered by combination with hCG-β subunit. We are further characterizing the free and dimer forms of α from the C-127 clones to identify the difference(s) in their processing. 2) AtT-20 cells. AtT-20 clones transfected with the pSV2neo plasmids have been isolated. As in C-127 cells, the yield of hCG-β subunit in AtT-20 cells is much greater than that of α subunit, and clones transfected with both subunits secrete bioactive hCG dimer. Expression of hLH-β subunit is detected in appropriate clones using antiserum to hCG-β subunit. The rate of secretion of subunits varies: α subunit exits the cell faster than hCG-β, while hLH-β is secreted very slowly. Further experiments should reveal whether there are differences in the processing of free α and hCG- or hLH-dimer α.

ACKNOWLEDGEMENTS. Antisera to hCG-α and hCG-β were the gift of S. Birken and R. Canfield. The hCG-β monoclonal antibody was provided by Gijs vanDedem at Organon and A. Krichevsky, Dept. of Medicine, Columbia University

REFERENCES

(1) Pierce, J.G. and Parsons, T.F. (1981) Ann. Rev. Biochem. 50, 465-495.
(2) Parsons, T.F. and Pierce, J.G. (1984) J. Biol. Chem. 259, 2662-2666.
(3) Ramabhadran, T.V. et al. (1984) PNAS 81, 6701-6705.
(4) Moore, H.-P. H., et al. (1983) Cell 35, 531-538.

PROTEIN KINASE C ACTIVATORS UNCOUPLE GONADOTROPIN-STIMULATED INOSITOL PHOSPHOLIPID HYDROLYSIS IN ISOLATED BOVINE LUTEAL CELLS

JOHN S. DAVIS, W. ALLEN CONWAY, and LEIGH A. WEST
J. A. HALEY VETERANS HOSPITAL and DEPARTMENT OF INTERNAL MEDICINE, UNIVERSITY OF SOUTH FLORIDA COLLEGE OF MEDICINE, TAMPA, FLORIDA 33612 USA

Phosphoinositide metabolism may play an important role in the regulation of cellular growth and metabolism. Several hormones, growth factors , and oncogene products are reported to stimulate phosphoinositide hydrolysis (1, 2), producing diacylglycerol (DAG) and inositol trisphosphate (IP_3). Both products are second messengers serving to stimulate protein kinase C and mobilize calcium, respectively. Tumor-promoting phorbol esters by-pass this second messenger system and directly activate protein kinase C, providing a selective and sensitive probe to study the effects of protein kinase C in intact cells. It has recently been proposed that protein kinase C may have a bidirectional role in cellular activation; it may mediate as well as terminate agonist-induced cellular responses (3). The following experiments were conducted to determine whether the effects of activation of protein kinase C by phorbol esters leads to alterations in gonadotropin receptor function. Our results indicate that phorbol esters uncouple luteinizing hormone (LH)-receptor-mediated stimulation of phosphoinositide hydrolysis in bovine luteal cells.

RESULTS and DISCUSSION. The preparation of bovine luteal cells (4) and quantification of inositol phosphates (5) were as previously described. The stimulatory effect of LH on phosphoinositide hydrolysis in bovine luteal cells

TABLE 1. Effect of LH on inositol phosphate accumulation.

TREATMENTS		IP	IP_2	IP_3
		($cpm/10^6$ cells)		
Control	2 min	3034 ± 38	285 ± 13	339 ± 1
LH	2 min	3419 ± 98	334 ± 8	442 ± 1
Control	5 min	3354 ± 26	299 ± 5	366 ± 2
LH	5 min	3624 ± 69	525 ± 19	512 ± 22
Control	15 min	3462 ± 58	301 ± 1	347 ± 18
LH	15 min	5014 ± 58	752 ± 32	648 ± 14
Control	30 min	3949 ± 42	293 ± 8	382 ± 2
LH	30 min	8114 ± 56	1158 ± 6	902 ± 19

Bovine luteal cells were prelabeled with ^{3}H-inositol for 3 h, washed, and incubated in the absence or presence of LH (1 µg/ml). Mean ± SEM, n=3.

TABLE 2. Effect of TPA on LH-stimulated $^{3}H-IP_3$ accumulation in bovine luteal cells.

LH (ug/ml)	-TPA	TPA (50 nM)
	IP_3 (cpm/10^6 cells)	
0	256 ± 38 (100)	253 ± 22 (100)
0.01	333 ± 29 (130)	234 ± 29 (90)
0.10	592 ± 3 (231)	285 ± 16 (113)
1.00	1117 ± 21 (436)	490 ± 11 (194)
10.00	1155 ± 11 (451)	589 ± 43 (232)

Luteal cells were pretreated with TPA for 60 min and were further incubated for 30 min in the presence of various concentrations of LH. Mean ± SEM, n=3; (% control).

is shown in Table 1. Under control conditions, the levels of inositol phosphates were relatively unchanged. LH provoked significant increases in IP_3 levels within 2 min of incubation. Increases in levels of inositol phosphate (IP) and inositol bisphosphate (IP_2) were observed after 5 min and further increases in the levels of all inositol phosphates were observed throughout 30 min of incubation. The effect on IP_3 was concentration dependent, with maximal increases occurring at 1 ug/ml of LH. The results indicate that one of the early responses to LH is the formation of second messengers derived from phosphoinositide hydrolysis.

To examine the effects of protein kinase C activation on LH-induced phosphoinositide hydrolysis, groups of cells were treated with the tumor promoting phorbol ester, 12-O-tetradecanoylphorbol 13-acetate (TPA). Incubation with 50 nM TPA inhibited LH-stimulated IP_3 accumulation (Table 2). The inhibition was dose-dependent (not shown) and could not be overcome by maximally effective concentrations of LH. In other experiments TPA increased (2-3 fold) progesterone levels when present alone, but markedly decreased LH-stimulated progesterone production.

The results demonstrate that LH stimulates phospholipase C activity and point to the involvement of protein kinase C in the action of LH. The results also demonstrate that activation of protein kinase C may be part of a negative feedback mechanism in the regulation of gonadotropin action.

REFERENCES

(1) Berridge, MJ and Irvine, RF (1984) Nature 312, 315-321
(2) Nishizuka, Y (1984) Science 225, 1365-1370
(3) Drummond, AH and MacIntyre DE (1985) Trends Pharm Sci 6, 233-234
(4) Davis, JS, Farese, RV, and Marsh, JM (1981) Endocrinology 109, 469-475
(5) Farese, RV, Davis, JS, Barnes, DE, Standaert, ML, Babischkin, JS, Hock, R, Rosic, NK, and Pollet, RJ (1985) Biochem. J. 231, 269-278

HUMAN CHORIONIC GONADOTROPIN (hCG) REGULATES LOW DENSITY LIPOPROTEIN RECEPTOR (LDL-R) EXPRESSION IN CULTURED HUMAN GRANULOSA CELLS

T.G. Golos and J.F. Strauss III
Departments of Obstetrics and Gynecology and Pathology and Laboratory Medicine, University of Pennsylvania, Philadelphia, PA. 19104

We demonstrated previously that hCG, through the intermediacy of cAMP, stimulates metabolism of LDL by cultured human granulosa cells (1), enabling enhanced steroidogenesis utilizing lipoprotein-delivered cholesterol as substrate (2). This increased metabolism of LDL is, at least in part, due to a specific hormone-induced increase in LDL-R synthesis (3). In this report we describe the dynamics and mechanism(s) of hormone-regulated expression of the LDL-R in this steroidogenic cell.

TIME COURSE OF INDUCTION OF LDL-R SYNTHESIS. We previously observed a significant (3-5 fold) induction of LDL-R synthesis within 6 h of hCG or cAMP treatment (3). We further investigated LDL-R synthesis in human granulosa in cells pulse-labeled with [35S]methionine for 1 h after 0.5 to 6 h of hCG treatment. Figure 1A demonstrates that LDL-R synthesis was increased by 50% within 3.5 h of exposure to hCG, and was further increased 5-7 h after treatment. This elevated rate of LDL-R synthesis was maintained for at least 14 h.

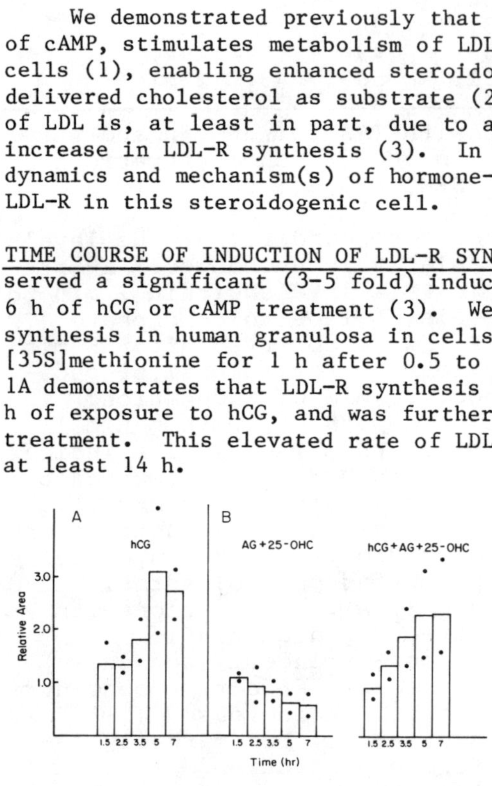

Fig. 1A. Time course of response to hCG. Human granulosa cells, cultured as previously described (1), were treated with 500 mIU/ml hCG or control medium for the indicated period of time, which includes a 1 h labeling with [^{35}S] methionine. LDL-R was immunoisolated from samples containing equal amounts of TCA-precipitable radioactivity. Results represent the relative area under the densitometric tracing of the LDL-R band as identified in fluorograms of SDS-polyacrylamide gels from two separate experiments. 1B. Cells were exposed to 25-hydroxycholesterol (10 ug/ml) and aminoglutethimide (AG) (100 ug/ml) in the presence or absence of hCG. Experiments were conducted as described for Fig. 1A. None of the treatments significantly altered the specific activities of total cell protein.

To learn how rapidly increased LDL-R synthesis is reflected in increased content of receptor, granulosa cells were exposed to hCG for 6, 14, or 24 h, scraped from dishes and analyzed by immunoblotting as described by Bieseigel et al (4). Consistent with previously published data on the surface-binding activity and metabolism of $[^{125}I]$LDL (1), immunoblot analysis of a separate experiment revealed that the hCG-induced elevation in LDL-R synthesis resulted in a 3-fold increase in cellular LDL-R content within 6 h, and that by 24 h, hCG-treated cells exhibited a 6-fold increase in LDL-R content.

MECHANISM OF INDUCTION OF RECEPTOR SYNTHESIS. Gonadotropin-induced depletion of cellular cholesterol stores for steroidogenesis could possibly lead to an increase in LDL-R expression via the cholesterol feedback pathway (5). To further characterize the regulation of LDL-R expression, granulosa cells were pulse-labeled with $[^{35}S]$methionine after exposure to 25-hydroxycholesterol (25-OHC) and aminoglutethimide (AG) with or without hCG. Fig. 1B, demonstrates that 25-OHC (in combination with AG to block cholesterol side-chain cleavage) suppresses LDL-R synthesis by approximately 40% within 5 h of exposure to these agents; hCG, on the other hand, increases LDL-R synthesis by nearly 50% within 2.5-3.5 h despite the presence of 25-OHC, indicating that hCG rapidly and specifically stimulates LDL-R expression by a mechanism not dependent on, and indeed, apparently superceding regulation by cellular cholesterol balance.

To determine whether active synthesis of cellular RNA is required for the stimulation of LDL-R expression by hCG and cAMP, granulosa cells were treated for 6 h with hCG and cAMP in the presence or absence of actinomycin D (2 ug/ml). Whereas LDL-R synthesis was increased 4.5 or 3.2-fold, respectively, by hCG or cAMP, in the presence of actinomycin D, synthesis of the LDL-R was identical to that in control incubation, supporting the view that hCG and cAMP stimulate LDL receptor synthesis by effects primarily at the level of mRNA transcription.

We conclude that hCG, through the intermediacy of cAMP, increases expression of the LDL-R in cultured human granulosa cells, most likely by increasing transcription of the gene for the receptor. This is one mechanism by which gonadotropins act to stimulate steroidogenesis in target cells.

REFERENCES

(1) Golos, T.G., Soto, E.A., Tureck, R.W. and Strauss, J.F. III. (1985) J. Clin. Endocrinol. Metab. 61, 633-637.
(2) Soto, E.A., Silavin, S.L., Tureck, R.W. and Strauss, J.F. III (1984) J. Clin. Endocrinol. Metab. 58, 831-837.
(3) Golos, T.G., and Strauss, J.F. III (1985) J. Biol. Chem. 260, in press.
(4) Beisiegel, U., Schneider, W.J., Brown, M.S., and Goldstein, J.L. (1982) J. Biol. Chem. 257, 13150-13156.
(5) Goldstein, J.L. and Brown, M.S. (1977) Annu. Rev. Biochem. 46, 897-930.

CHARGE HETEROGENEITY OF PARTIALLY PURIFIED OVINE LH SUBUNITS AND THE NATIVE HORMONE

B.A. Keel* and H.E. Grotjan, Jr.**
*Dept. Ob/Gyn, University Kansas School of Medicine-Wichita, 550 N. Hillside, Wichita, KS 67214, **Dept. of Physiology & Pharmacology, University South Dakota School of Medicine, Vermillion, SD 57069.

INTRODUCTION. The contribution of individual subunits to the isoelectric profile of pituitary gonadotropins remains to be fully established. Further, the isoelectric pattern of uncombined α and β subunits is currently unknown. Therefore, we have utilized gel filtration to resolve native oLH from its uncombined subunits followed by chromatofocusing to define the isohormones of native oLH and the subunits in an attempt to address these questions.

METHODS. Pituitary extracts were prepared from sexually mature, castrate sheep. Native oLH was resolved from uncombined subunits by gel filtration essentially as described previously (1). Chromatofocusing of crude tissue extracts, partially purified native oLH, and uncombined subunits was performed as described previously (2). Subunit RIA's were performed using NIH kits while oLH RIA's were performed using reagents kindly provided by Drs. L.E. Reichert Jr., D.N. Ward, and G.D. Niswender.

RESULTS. When crude extracts of anterior pituitaries from wethers were subjected to chromatofocusing at least eight isohormones of oLH were observed (Fig.1). Six of the isohormones focused within the defined limits of the pH gradient and exhibited apparent pI's ranging from 9.33 to 8.83; one isohormone eluted in the void volume of the column (apparent pI$>$9.8) and one isohormone was bound to the column but could be eluted with 1 M NaCl (apparent pI$<$7.0). The relative distribution pattern, shown in Table 1, demonstrated that isohormones E and F were the major forms observed representing nearly 50% of immunoreactive oLH recovered from the column. When the native oLH peak from gel filtration was chromatofocused a similar pattern of at least eight isohormones was observed. As with the oLH isohormones in the crude pituitary extract, the majority ($>$67%) of the partially purified immunoreactive oLH focused as isohormones D through G (Table 1).

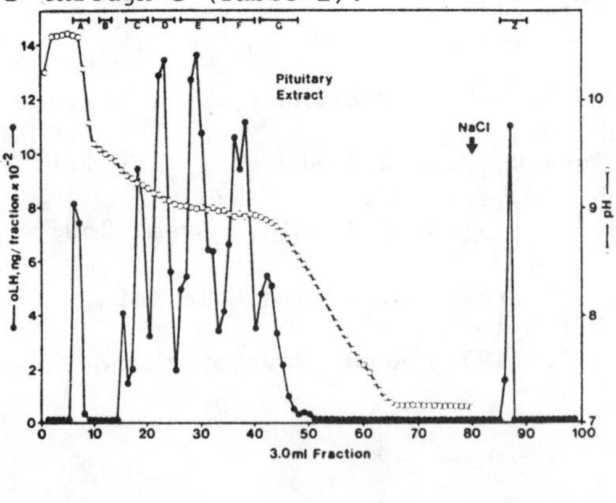

Fig. 1 Representative chromatofocusing elution profile of immunoreactive oLH in the extract of an anterior pituitary obtained from a wether. The fractions summed to calculate the relative distribution of oLH among its isohormones (Table 1) are denoted by bars. Components bound to the column were eluted with 1M NaCl.

Table 1. Distribution of oLH and its uncombined subunits into various isohormones as defined by chromatofocusing.

Isohormone	Apparent pI	Percentage in each Isohormone			
		oLH in Pituitary Extracts	Samples Derived from Gel Filtration		
			Native oLH	Uncombined oLHα	Uncombined oLHβ
A	>9.80	3.9 ± 1.9*	2.0 ± 1.3	1.1 ± 0.8	12.9 ± 3.6
B	9.33	2.7 ± 0.2	5.1 ± 0.9	0.3 ± 0.3	2.0 ± 0.9
C	9.22	5.5 ± 1.4	11.4 ± 2.3	6.8 ± 1.4	7.2 ± 1.8
D	9.11	15.6 ± 1.4	22.9 ± 3.1	10.3 ± 1.6	4.4 ± 1.2
E	9.01	18.9 ± 3.0	21.0 ± 1.9	7.9 ± 1.4	4.0 ± 1.6
F	8.95	29.3 ± 4.0	17.0 ± 4.3	21.3 ± 1.9	6.4 ± 1.6
G	8.83	14.5 ± 1.8	6.8 ± 3.1	14.4 ± 1.0	6.3 ± 1.7
Z	<7.00	9.6 ± 3.0	13.7 ± 3.7	37.0 ± 3.2	56.7 ± 7.0

* Mean ± SE, n = 4 (pituitary extracts) or 6 (pools from gel filtration).

Uncombined oLHα obtained from gel filtration exhibited a preponderance of acidic components. Particularly apparent was the 3-fold increase in the relative amount of the most acidic species (isohormone Z) of oLHα compared with oLH. When uncombined (free) oLHβ was chromatofocused, more than half of the immunoreactive oLHβ was bound to the chromatofocusing column indicating an acidic species (apparent pI<7.0). In addition, a significant amount of the highly basic species of oLHβ (isohormones A; apparent pI>9.8) was also observed. The remaining 30% of the immunoreactive oLHβ was more or less uniformly distributed across the pH gradient corresponding to the pI's of the other six isohormones.

DISCUSSION. The pI's and relative distribution of oLH isohormones are markedly different from those of rLH (2). Identical isohormones are observed when native oLH is separated from uncombined subunits by gel filtration prior to chromatofocusing. These findings suggest that contamination of native oLH with uncombined subunits (as in crude extracts) does not significantly alter the isoelectric pattern of the native hormone.

Uncombined oLHα in the subunit pool from gel filtration was composed predominately of acidic components (apparent pI's<7.0) and exhibited a distinctly different chromatofocusing profile from native oLH. Due to its acidic characteristics, it is conceivable that a significant portion of the uncombined oLHα in the subunit pool from gel filtration could be O-glycosylated as has been previously shown for LH free α subunit in bovine pituitaries (3). In a recent study in which an assay was developed to measure the O-glycosylated form of free LHα, it was discovered that under basal conditions 75% of secreted uncombined bovine subunit is in the O-glycosylated form (4). These findings (4) suggest that the majority of free α subunit secreted by the pituitary contains an O-linked oligosaccharide (4) which is acidic and is incapable of combining with a β subunit to form the native hormone (3). The acidic nature of the uncombined oLHα in the subunit pool from gel filtration may be the result of O-glycosylation, which would render the subunit incapable of forming an α - β dimer.

REFERENCES

1. Grotjan, Jr. H.E., Leveque, N.W., Berkowitz, A.S. and Keel, B.A. (1984) Mol Cell Endocrinol 35:121.
2. Keel, B.A. and Grotjan, Jr., H.E. (1984) Anal Biochem 142:267.
3. Parsons, T.F., Bloomfield, G.A. and Pierce, J.G. (1983) J Biol Chem 258:240.
4. Corless, C.L. and Boime I. (1985) Endocrinology 117:1699.

DISCORDANT EFFECTS OF TRH ON PRE- AND POST-TRANSLATIONAL REGULATION OF TSH BIOSYNTHESIS IN RAT PITUITARY

S. S. Lippman, S. Amr, and B. D. Weintraub
Molecular, Cellular and Nutritional Endocrinology Branch, NIADDK, National Institutes of Health, Bethesda, MD 20892

INTRODUCTION. To investigate whether TRH regulates TSH production through a pre- or post-translational mechanism, the pituitary levels of mRNA for the TSH subunits were determined in male Sprague Dawley rats given chronic TRH in the presence or absence of thyroid hormones and/or hypothalamic influence.

METHODS. Groups of 8-12 animals three weeks old were implanted sc with osmotic minipumps (model 2001 or 2002, Alza Corp.) under diethyl ether anesthesia. These minipumps were filled with TRH at a concentration that delivered 1 mg/kg body weight/day of the hormone. The control groups were given normal saline. T_4 was given by daily sc injection at a dose of 15 ug/kg body weight.

Serum samples were radioimmunoassayed for T_3, free T_4, and TSH; the latter was expressed in ng of the rat standard RP-2. The pituitaries were individually processed for RNA extraction (1), and measurement of DNA and TSH content. A dot blot hybridization assay was used to determine mRNA levels. Full length cDNAs for the mouse TSH beta and common alpha glycoprotein hormone subunits (2-4) were provided by Dr. W. Chin. Plasmids were constructed to synthesize ^{32}P-labeled cRNA probes and ^{3}H-labeled mRNA-like strands. The latter served as standards to calculate the amounts of pituitary mRNA for alpha and TSH beta subunits (5). The assay was validated by gel electrophoresis of glyoxal denatured RNAs.

Fig. 1

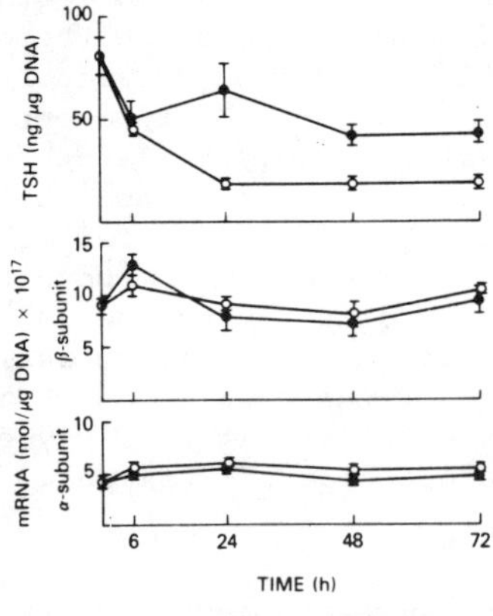

Fig. 2

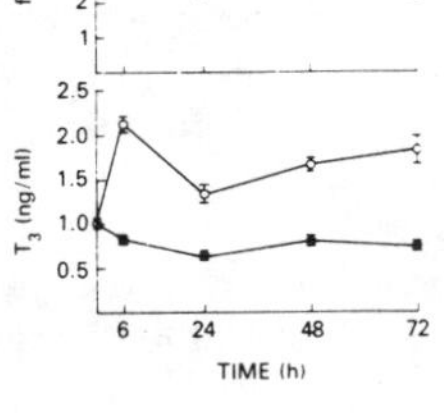

RESULTS. Figs. 1 and 2 show pituitary and serum parameters, respectively, in normal rats killed at intervals following implantation of osmotic minipumps that were filled with either saline (●) or TRH (o). Each point represents the mean ± SEM of 8 samples.

In thyroidectomized rats, the serum TSH level was 31 times the level observed in normal animals. The pituitary content of mRNA for TSH beta and alpha subunits were 75 and 27 times, respectively, the content measured in normal rats. TRH infusion did not further stimulate TSH release or change the levels of mRNA for either subunit (data not shown).

TABLE 1. Effects of TRH, infused for one week, on serum and pituitary parameters of male rats, thyroidectomized, hypophysectomized, and with their own pituitary gland transplanted under the renal capsule in the presence or absence of exogenous thyroid hormone.

			mRNA	
	n	Serum TSH	TSH beta subunit	alpha subunit
None	12	64[¶]	54	31
Normal saline	12	65 ┐**	70 ┐NS	31 ┐NS
Normal saline + 1.5 ug/d T_4	10	┌<45	┌62	┌31
TRH (1 mg/kg/d)	10	* 295 ┘	NS 66 ┘	NS 49 ┘
TRH (1 mg/kg/d) + 1.5 ug/d T_4	8	└109	└93	└43

¶ The data are expressed as percents of values in normal rats.
* p <.05, ** p <.01 (2-sided t-test).
NS, not significant.

CONCLUSION. In the presence or absence of thyroid hormones and/or hypothalamic influence, TRH failed to increase the rat pituitary levels of mRNA for both TSH subunits, despite persistent enhancement in TSH release. Therefore, we found no evidence of pre-translational regulation of TSH production by TRH. Although a translational regulation cannot be completely excluded, the present data, in conjunction with the literature (6), support the hypothesis that TRH regulates TSH biosynthesis primarily by stimulating its carbohydrate processing and release of this hormone.

REFERENCES

(1) Cathala, G., Savouret, J. F., Mendez, B., West, B. L., Karin, M., Martial, J. A., and Baxter, M. D. (1983) DNA 2, 329-335.

(2) Chin, W. W., Shupnik, M. A., Ross, D. S., Habener, J. F., and Ridgway, E. C. (1985) Endocrinology 116, 873-878.

(3) Chin, W. W., Kronenberg, H. M., Dee, P. L., Maloof, F., and Habener, J. F. (1981) Proc. Natl. Acad. Sci. U.S.A. 78, 5329-5333.

(4) Kourides, I. A., Gurr, J. A., and Wolf, O. (1984) Rec. Prog. Horm. Res. 40, 79-120.

(5) Melton, D. A., Krieg, P. A. Rebagliati, M. R., Maniatis, T., Zinn, K., and Green, M. R. (1984) Nuc. Acid Res. 12, 7035-7056.

(6) Ronin, C., Stannard, B. S., and Weintraub, B. D. (1985) Biochemistry 24, 5626-5631.

USE OF A CYCLIC AMP ANALOG WHICH INHIBITS CYCLIC AMP DEPENDENT PROTEIN KINASE (A-KINASE) TO STUDY THE ROLE OF CYCLIC AMP AND A-KINASE AS MEDIATORS OF hCG AND FSH INDUCED STEROIDOGENESIS.

Kelly M. McMasters*, Donna M. Anderson, Lynne H. Parker Botelho**, Gordon J. Macdonald* & Wm. R. Moyle. Molecular Endocrinology and Immunology Laboratory, OBGYN & *Anatomy Departments, UMDNJ-Rutgers Medical School, Piscataway, NJ 08854 and **Sandoz Research Institute, Sandoz, Inc., East Hanover, NJ 07936.

Human chorionic gonadotropin (hCG) and follicle stimulating hormone (FSH) are known to induce formation of cyclic AMP and to initiate steroidogenesis in Leydig and granulosa cells. Since cyclic AMP and several analogs can mimic the effect of the hormones, cyclic AMP is usually presumed to mediate the hormonal response by activating one or both A-kinases isozmyes. Although the relationship between cyclic AMP accumulation and steroidogenesis has strong support, two observations raise the possibility that this nucleotide is not the only mediator or even the primary mediator of the effects of FSH and hCG. First, the concentrations of hormones needed to stimulate cyclic AMP accumulation are usually much higher than those needed to stimulate steroidogenesis (1). Second, cyclic AMP independent mechanisms which can stimulate steroidogenesis have been reported (2). Indeed, some hormones can induce steroid formation although they inhibit adenyl cyclase (3). Since the major actions of cyclic AMP almost certainly involve activation of A-kinase, the role of this nucleotide could be tested using inhibitors of A-kinase subunit dissociation. (Rp)-adenosine cyclic 3',5'phosphorothioate (Rp-cAMPS) has been shown to bind to A-kinase and prevent its activation by cyclic AMP (4). This analog inhibits glucagon induced glycogenolysis and has been used to evaluate the role of A-kinases during glucagon action (5). We report here that Rp-cAMPS inhibits FSH and hCG stimulated steroidogenesis.

METHODS: Granulosa cells were isolated from ovaries of rats (aged 23-27 days) which had been implanted with sialastic capsules containing diethylstilbestrol. Granulosa cells were expressed from the follicles and cultured in DMEM:F12 (1:1) containing 0.1 uM androstenedione and varying amounts of FSH or 8-Br-cyclic AMP for 24, 48, or 72 hours at 37°. Progesterone and estradiol were measured by radioimmunoassay using specific antisera (6). Leydig cells were isolated from testes of immature rats using collagenase digestion and incubated for 2 hours at 37° in the presence of varying amounts of hCG and 8-Br-cyclic AMP. Testosterone secretion was measured using an antiserum which also cross-reacted with dihydrotestosterone (1).

RESULTS and DISCUSSION: Rp-cAMPS (.01 mM) inhibited FSH induced steroidogenesis (Fig. 1a,b). Inhibition was evident at 24 hours, the earliest time studied, and continued for at least 3 days. High concentrations of FSH were able to reverse inhibition of aromatase synthesis (i.e., assayed by conversion of androstenedione to estradiol). Similar concentrations of FSH were able to at least partially reverse the inhibition of cholesterol side chain cleavage (i.e., measured by progesterone formation). Rp-cAMPS also inhibited the ability of 8-Br-cAMP to induce estradiol and progesterone formation (not shown). The influence of Rp-cAMPS on hCG stimulation of Leydig cell testosterone formation was more difficult to assess. Concentrations of inhibitor less than 0.1 - 1 mM were usually without effect. High concentrations of Rp-cAMPS were always inhibitory (Fig. 2), however, the inhibition was not readily reversed by high concentrations of either hCG or 8-Br-cAMP. Thus, although the inhibition of testosterone synthesis is consistent with the ability of Rp-cAMPS to prevent induction of Leydig cell A-kinase activity, we

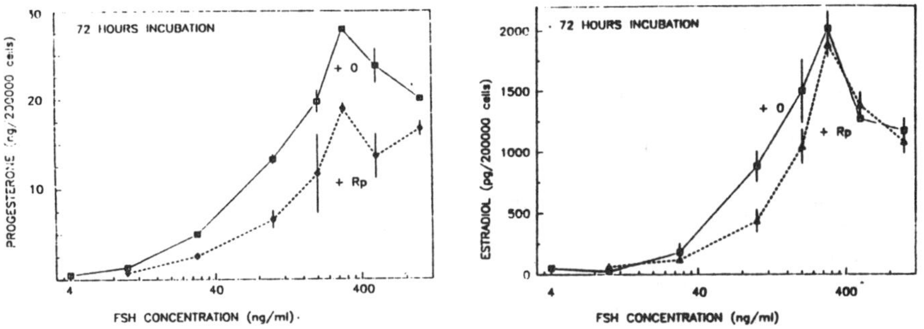

Fig 1. Effect of Rp-cAMPS on progesterone formation (panel A) and estradiol synthesis (panel B) in cultured granulosa cells. Cells were placed in culture and steroidogenesis measured as described (6). Progesterone formation was also measured at 24 and 48 hours (not shown) and results similar to those illustrated at 72 hours were observed.

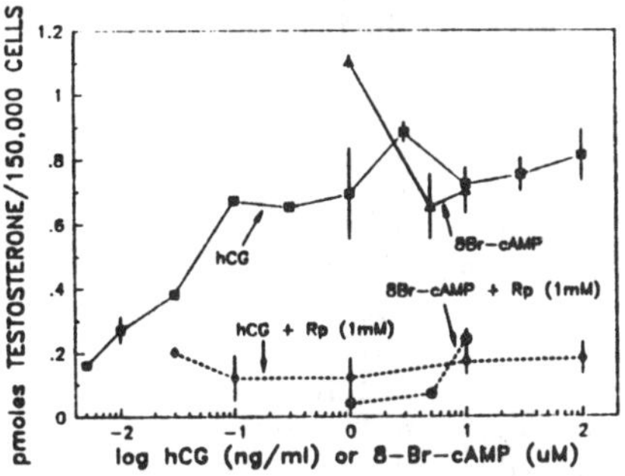

Fig 2. Effect of Rp-cAMPS on testosterone formation in isolated Leydig cells (1). Cells were incubated with 1mM Rp-cAMPS for 30 min at 37° and for an additional 2 hours with hCG or 8-Br-cAMP.

cannot exclude the epossibility that high concentrations Rp-cAMPS have other effects. An action of the analog to inhibit protein synthesis would also explain the ability of Rp-cAMPS to inhibit testosterone formation. The differences in the ability of Rp-cAMPS to inhibit granulosa cell and Leydig cell steroidogenesis are not readily apparent and may be related to the preparation of the cells and the length of time that the cells are incubated.

CONCLUSION: Rp-cAMPS, an analog of cyclic AMP which inhibits A-kinase activity in liver cells, inhibits hormone induced steroidogenesis in Leydig cells and cultured granulosa cells. Although the mechanism of inhibition has not been elucidated in either cell type, use of this analog is likely to provide information concerning the role of cyclic AMP in hCG and FSH induced steroid and protein synthesis.

REFERENCES:

1. Moyle WR, Bahl OP, Marz L 1975 J Biol Chem 250:9163
2. Hsueh AJW, Adashi EY, Jones PBC, Welsh TH 1985 Endocrine Rev 5:76
3. Woodcock EA, Johnston CI 1984 Endocrinol 115:337
3. Rothermel JD, Perillo NL, Marks JS, Botelho LHP 1984 J Biol Chem 259:15294
4. Rothermel JD, Jastorff B, Botelho LHP 1984 J Biol Chem 259:8151
5. Skaf RA, Macdonald GJ, Shelden RM, Moyle WR 1985 Endocrinol 117:106

EFFECTS OF SWAINSONINE ON PROCESSING AND TURNOVER OF LYSOSOMAL GLYCOPROTEINS.

J.E. Tropea*, R.T. Swank**, and H.L. Segal*
*Dept. of Biol. Sci., SUNY, Buffalo, N.Y. 14260 and **Dept. of Cell and Molec. Biol., RPMI, Buffalo, N.Y. 14263

Swainsonine (SW), an α-mannosidase inhibitor originally isolated from the Australian plant, *Swainsona canescans*, has been shown to inhibit the carbohydrate processing of a number of glycoproteins via its inhibitory effect on Golgi α-mannosidase II (for ref., see (1)) and to inhibit the lysosomal degradation of endocytosed glycoproteins, but not nonglycoproteins, via its inhibitory effect on lysosomal α-mannosidase (2,3). Results from the laboratory of one of us (RTS) has shown that the lysosomal enzymes, β-galactosidase (β-gal) and β-glucuronidase (β-gluc), from murine macrophages could be detected in both precursor and mature forms and that the former were found only in the light membrane fraction while the latter were found only in the lysosomal fraction (4,5). The purpose of the present study has been to determine the effects of SW on the conversion of precursor to mature forms of these two glycoproteins and on their turnover.

RESULTS

Fig. 1 is an SDS-PAGE fluorograph from a pulse-chase experiment showing the conversion of precursor to mature forms of both enzymes in the presence and absence of SW. As can be seen, there was only a small decrease in the M_r of β-gluc in the precursor to mature form conversion (from 73 kd to 71 kd) and any effect of SW on the M_r of the mature form was difficult to detect. On the other hand, there was a substantial decrease in the M_r of β-gal in the precursor to mature form conversion (from 85 kd to 63 kd) and a distinct effect of SW on the M_r of the mature form of this enzyme (60 kd) was observed. The mature forms produced in the presence of SW were more clearly distinguished from the normal forms on the basis of their susceptibility to endo H (Fig. 2). With both enzymes maturation in the absence of SW led from endo H-susceptible precursor forms to mature forms only slightly susceptible to endo H, while maturation in the presence of SW yielded mature forms fully susceptible to endo H.

There was no effect of SW during a 1 hour labeling period on the incorporation of labeled methionine or labeled mannose into the precursor forms of either enzyme nor on their susceptibility to endo H.

Turnover of the enzymes was measured during a 4 day period in the presence and absence of SW subsequent to a pulse labeling with radioactive methionine. Counts were lost from both β-gluc and β-gal at a somewhat slower rate in the presence of SW and there was a corresponding increase in the total enzymatic activity in both cases.

ACKNOWLEDGEMENTS

This work was supported by a grant from the NIH (GM-33559) to RTS and from the NSF (DMB-8417805) to HLS.

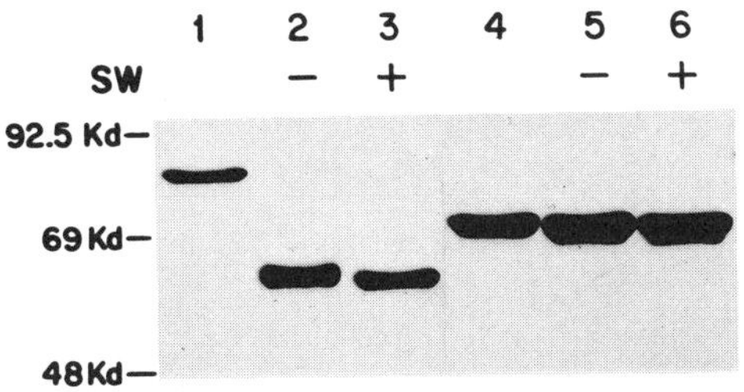

Fig. 1. Conversion of precursor forms to mature forms of β-gluc and β-gal. Lanes 1 and 4 are precursor forms of β-gal and β-gluc, resp., produced during a 1 hour labeling period. Lanes 2, 3 and 5, 6 are the mature forms of β-gal and β-gluc, resp., after a 6 hour chase. Pluses and minuses in the row marked "SW" indicate the presence or absence of SW during the 6 hour chase period in which precursors were converted to mature forms. The presence of SW during the 1 hour labeling period had no effect on the precursor forms produced.

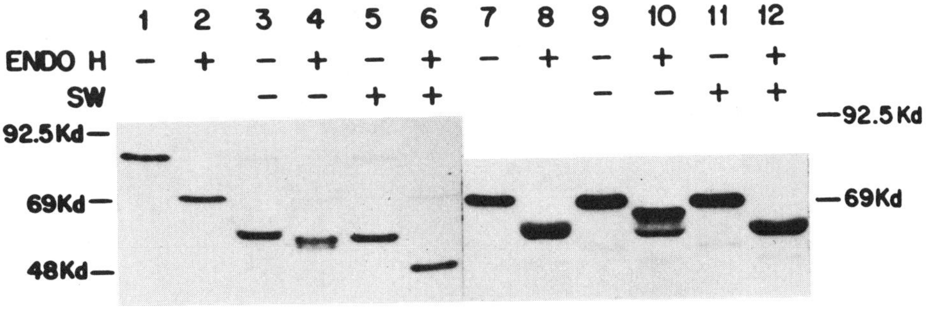

Fig. 2. SDS-PAGE fluorograph of endo H-treated enzymes. Lanes 1-6 represent β-gal and lanes 7-12 represent β-gluc. Pluses in the row marked ENDO H" indicate treatment with endo H prior to electrophoresis. Endo H treatment was modified from refer. 6.

REFERENCES

(1) Yeo, T.-K., Yeo, K.-T., Parent, J.B., and Olden, K. (1985) J. Biol. Chem. 258, 15323-15328.

(2) Winkler, J.R., and Segal, H.L. (1984) J. Biol. Chem. 259, 1958-1962.

(3) Winkler, J.R., and Segal, H.L. (1984) J. Biol. Chem. 259 15369-15372.

(4) Skudlarek, M.D., and Swank, R.T. (1981) J. Biol. Chem. 256 10137-10144.

(5) Brown, J.A., and Swank, R.T. (1983) J. Biol. Chem. 258 15323-15328

(6) Brown, J.A., Novak, E.K., and Swank, R.T. (1985) J. Cell Biol. 100, 1894-1904.

Steroid Receptors and Gene Regulation

RECEPTORS AND THEIR ACTIONS

Bert W. O'Malley, M.D.

Baylor College of Medicine
One Baylor Plaza
Houston, Texas 77030

Over the past decade, work from many laboratories has led to a generally accepted hypothesis for the primary synthetic events involved in steroid hormone action. Although no universal agreement exists for the specific molecular details, the overall steps in the pathway have been elucidated.

In the chick oviduct, a series of investigations designed to define the pathway for progesterone (and estrogen) effects on egg-white protein (e.g., ovalbumin, ovomucoid, avidin, etc.) synthesis has led us to postulate the specific sequence of events shown summarized above and shown in Figure 1.

It has been postulated that hormones act primarily at the level of DNA transcription from the following lines of evidence. Hormone-receptor complexes accumulate in the nuclear compartment and bind to chromosomal DNA with high affinity. Steroid regulatable genes contain sequences in their 5'-flanking regions which preferentially bind receptors with an affinity greater than average DNA. Removal of these 5'-flanking sequences prevents induction of gene expression by steroid hormones. Precursor mRNA and mature mRNA both accumulate in response to steroid hormone action. Following accumulation of steroid hormone receptors on the nuclear chromosomes, radio-labeling experiments demonstrate that synthesis of nascent pre-mRNA is stimulated. Thus, although steroids can have an effect on mRNA half-life under certain conditions, their primary action appears to occur at the DNA or transcription level.

In chick oviduct cells, we have reported the existence of a receptor complex composed of 2 hormone-binding peptides (Fig. 1). Subunit A (MW=79,000) which binds to deproteinized DNA with high affinity (KD 10^{-10}M) is considered to be the "effector" subunit. Subunit B (MW=105,000) which binds to interphase chromosomes (Kd 5×10^{-9}M), has been postulated to play a "specifier" or catalytic role in chromosomal localization of hormone-receptor complex. The structural proof and structure-function speculations have been published in details previously. It is noteworthy that a similar subunit structure has been reported recently for the progesterone receptors for human tissues but not in the rabbit.

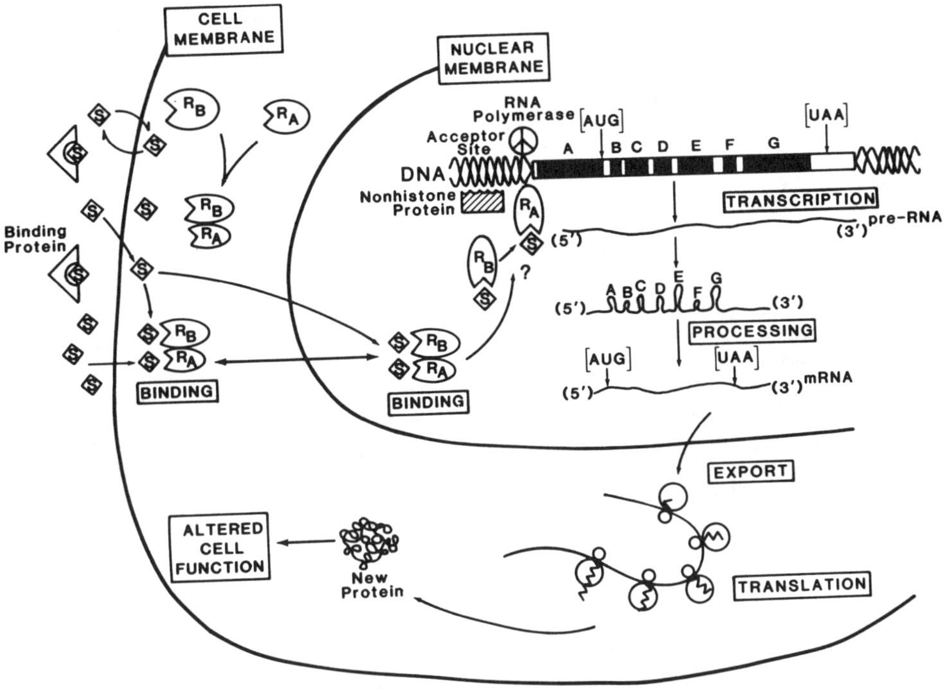

FIGURE LEGENDS

Figure 1. Schematic representation of the pathway for steroid hormone action in a eucaryotic cell (e.g., chicken oviduct. In this scheme, progesterone binds to the receptor complex and it interacts with interphase chromosomes, presumably at or near the 5'-flanking DNA of regulatable genes. Gene activation occurs and a large precursor mRNA is synthesized. This precursor is spliced and processed (introns removed) and the mature mRNA is transported to the cytoplasm where it is translated on ribosomes, producing the designated protein.

In order to assess the peptide structure of functional domains of steroid receptor in the avian species, we set out to clone the cDNAs for a variety of steroid hormones and to determine their sequence. We have attempted cloning of the progesterone receptor "family", the estrogen receptor, the glucocorticoid receptor and the receptor for vitamin D. The data to date reveal the following structural characteristics: (1) receptors in the same species show moderate homology between molecules which bind different hormones; (2) receptors for the same hormone are highly conserved among species; (3) certain receptors have limited homology with viral oncogenes; (4) the progesterone receptor shares certain homologies with a family of proteins, some of which appear to be other DNA-binding regulatory proteins and some of which are "heat shock" proteins; (5) the mRNAs for steroid receptors are surprisingly large due to extensive 3'-untranslated sequences; and (6) tissue specificity and hormonal regulation of receptor mRNA levels can be demonstrated in the avian species.

In the chick oviduct, we have characterized four genes (ovablumin, X, Y, and ovomucoid) in terms of their primary structure and inducibility in response to hormone administration. The ovalbumin gene has been sequenced completely together with its surrounding genomic regions. Our more recent evidence suggests that the ovalbumin gene contains certain sequences in its adjacent 5'-flanking region which are considered to be important for both accurate and efficient expression. Accurate initiation of transcription of the ovalbumin gene appears to be influenced primarily by the TATATAT box located at -32 base pairs upstream from the first nucleotide (+1) of the structural gene.

Sequences located slightly further upstream from theTATA box (-95 to -48) form an important part of the basal promoter. The "hormone control" region, however, appears to be structurally separate and is located further upstream (-222 to -95). Finally, in vivo regulation of the ovalbumin gene may be even more complicated due to the proposed existence of a negative regulatory sequence located upstream of -250 and perhaps even more distally located transcription "enhancer" sequences.

It is fair to speculate that the cellular forces involved in steroid hormone induction of gene expression are complex indeed. These paprameters are summarized in Figure 2. At the present time, our best guess on the major structural determinants for induction are as follows: (1) steroid receptor is the obligatory and active intermediate to transduce the informational signal inherent in the hormone to the regulatable gene; (2) the linear sequence of the gene itself is of obvious importance since it not only contains the inherited structural code for the protein, but it appears to contain structurally distinct "promoter" and "regulatory" sequences, the latter of which both binds receptor and determines the maximal rate of hormone induced gene expression; (3) inducible genes are contained within large structurally distinct (DNase I-sensitive) domains which are an index of molecular differentiation and which are likely to maintain the capacity of genes to respond to inductive influences; and (4) the chromatin itself undergoes a specific attachment to the nuclear matrix so that actively expressed regions of these domains appear to be more firmly bound, and perhaps, more easily transcribed by the nuclear transcriptive apparatus. This picture is only complicated further by consideration of other potentially important levels of substructure such as modification of primary DNA sequence (e.g., methylation and Z-DNA) and chromatin fine structure (DNase hypersensitivity).

It appears safe to speculate that only by obtaining more precise structural and functional information on each of these levels of regulation can we understand completely the molecular mechanism of steroid hormone action. To accomplish this task, a continued application of the combined technologies of molecular biology and cell biology will most certainly be required.

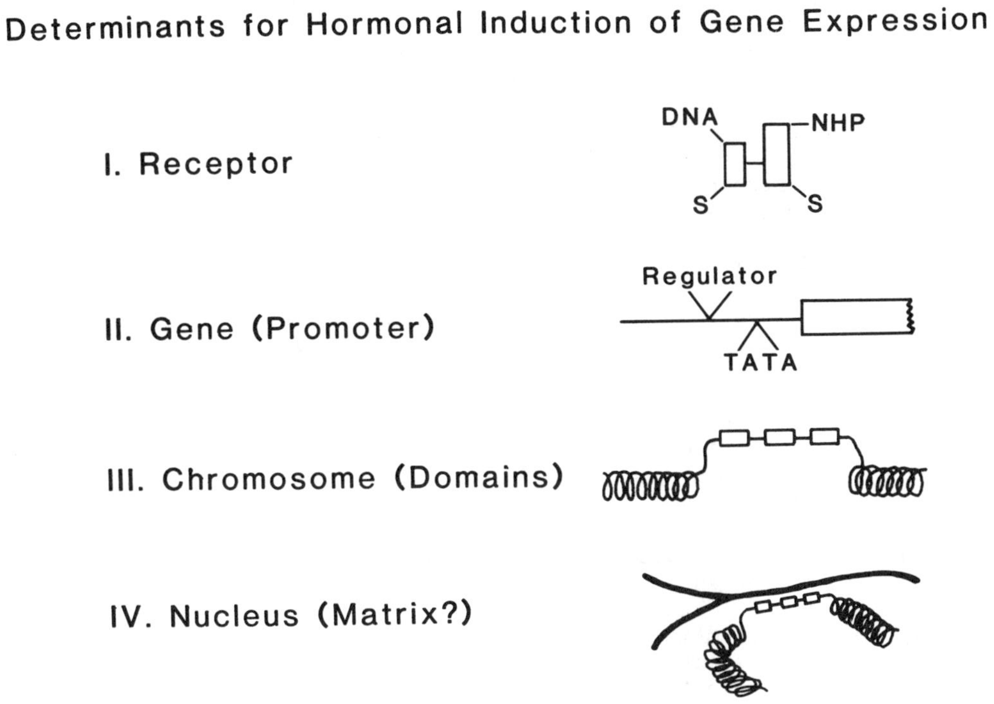

Figure 2. Schematic representation of the structural determinants for hormonal induction of gene expression. These include the steroid hormone receptor, the gene and its regulatory elements, the chromosomal domain and the nuclear matrix.

PURIFICATION, OLIGOMERISM, REGULATION AND LOCALIZATION OF THE GLUCOCORTICOID RECEPTOR

J.-Å. Gustafsson, O. Bakke, J. Carlstedt-Duke, K. Fuxe*, A. Härfstrand*, S. Okret, L. Poellinger and A.-C. Wikström.

Department of Medical Nutrition, Karolinska Institute, Huddinge University Hospital, S-141 86 Huddinge, and *Department of Histology, Karolinska Institute, Stockholm, Sweden

Immunoaffinity purification of the glucocorticoid receptor. The glucocorticoid receptor (GR) is a 94K protein that exists in low abundance, i.e. approximatively 0.01% of the total cytosolic protein. Glucocorticoids exert their action via binding to GR. The hormone-GR complex interacts with chromatin, and stimulates transcription of specific genes.

Monoclonal antibodies to rat liver GR (1) were used to purify GR. A monoclonal GR-specific IgG2a antibody was purified on a protein A-Sepharose column. The antibody was then coupled to cyanogen bromide activated Sepharose 4B (Pharmacia AB, Uppsala, Sweden), 5 mg antibody per g gel, according to the procedure recommended by the manufacturer.

Rat livers from either normal 8-week-old Sprague-Dawley rats or rats adrenalectomized 48-72 h before sacrifice, were perfused with ice-cold EPG (20 mM phosphate, 1 mM EDTA, 50 mM NaCl, 2 mM DTT and 10 % [w/v] glycerol, pH 7.0). All further procedures were performed in the cold. Cytosol was prepared and then either incubated with 100 nM ^{3}H-triamcinolone acetonide or directly applied on a 20 ml phosphocellulose column. The flow-through was chromatographed on a cyanogen bromide activated Sepharose, to which 5 mg of protein A-purified ascites from mice injected with SP 2/0 cells was coupled. The flow-through from this column was applied to the anti-GR specific column. After washing with PBS, (20 times the column volume), bound GR was eluted stepwise with 10 ml each of 0.5 M, 1.25 M, and 2.5 M sodium thiocyanate in PBS. The fractions were collected and precipitated with a final concentration of 20% trichloroacetic acid. The precipitate was dissolved in SDS buffer, and then run on a 10% SDS-PAGE gel, according to Laemmli. A high degree of enrichment of proteins with molecular weights of 94K, 91K, 79K, 72K, 50K, 32K and 28K was observed. Under the different elution conditions these bands were equivalent to 40-100% of the total protein, as determined by densitometric scanning of a silver stained gel. The 94K, 91K, 79K, 50K and 28K were shown to react with the other GR-specific monoclonal antibodies (for ref. see above) on Western immunoblotting. Proteolytic fragments of rat GR have earlier been shown to appear in similar sizes (2). The 72K protein is not a proteolytic fragment of GR, but copurifies with GR on sequential DNA-cellulose chromatography (2).

The above method has made it possible to purify unliganded GR for the first time. The method will be a potent tool for studying proteins copurifying with the receptor in the transformed and untransformed state, as well as for studies of receptor phosphorylation.

On the role of a 72K glucocorticoid receptor subunit. The purified and activated GR complex contains a 94K hormone-binding polypeptide in association with a 72K non-hormone-binding polypeptide (2). GR binds selectively to discrete regions of DNA of mouse mammary tumor virus (3). Such GR-binding DNA fragments were used to measure the stoichiometry of GR to DNA. Quantitative DNaseI-protection "footprinting" analysis was used to control that saturation conditions for specific DNA-binding were achieved. Glycerol density gradient centrifugation was used to quantitate binding of 94K GR to specific and non-specific DNA-sites. Such experiments showed that one 94K entity bound per specific DNA-site. Furthermore the use of a faster GR purification procedure resulted in increased amounts of 72K polypeptide (1.6:1, 94K:72K molar ratio), compared to previous GR preparations. Glycerol gradient centrifugation followed by SDS-polyacrylamide gel electrophoresis showed that the specific GR·DNA complex contained similar amounts of 94K and 72K polypeptides and that the interaction of these polypeptides seemed to be stabilized by the presence of DNA. The data suggests that the activated GR is a heterodimer containing one 94K hormone-binding subunit and one 72K non-hormone-binding subunit.

Regulation of the glucocorticoid receptor. A cDNA clone for the rat GR was used to study levels of GR mRNA by RNA blot hybridization after various endocrine manipulations. Growing rat hepatoma culture cells in the presence of 0.5 μM dexamethasone causes a 5-10 fold reduction of the GR mRNA level after 24 h of incubation. A similar reduction in rat liver GR mRNA was seen after treatment *in vivo* with dexamethasone. Preliminary data indicate that inhibition of protein synthesis by cycloheximide increases the concentration of GR mRNA in both glucocorticoid-treated and non-treated rat hepatoma culture cells. Using an immunoprecipitation assay, we could demonstrate that the GR specifically interacts with a GR cDNA-clone representing 2.6 kb of the 3' end of the GR mRNA. It is also possible to demonstrate the presence of internal specific receptor binding regions in the GR cDNA by nuclease protection experiments.

Intracellular localization of GR. Using a monospecific, monoclonal antibody against GR, an immunocytochemical study was performed to investigate the intracellular location of the receptor in both the presence and absence of ligand. Several fixation and permeabilization procedures were used. A rat Rueber hepatoma (H-II-4-E) and a human uterus carcinoma (NHIK 3025) cell line were used as well as normal rat hepatocytes. A specific GR stain was obtained with the indirect peroxidase-anti peroxidase

(PAP) technique or with fluorescein isothiocyanate (FITC) labelled second antibodies, both in the cytoplasm and in the nucleus. Staining in all cellular compartments was abolished (PAP) or diminished (fluorescence) if the monoclonal antibody was pre-incubated with a 90% pure GR preparation. Furthermore, GR was translocated from the cytoplasm to the nucleus of H-4-II-E cells following addition of dexamethasone to the medium. These findings are not in line with recently reported results from immunocytochemical studies showing strict nuclear existence of the estrogen and progesterone receptors. Consequently, generalizations regarding intracellular localization of steroid receptors should be avoided.

Localization of GR in the central nervous system. By means of a monoclonal antibody against rat liver GR and antibodies against tyrosine hydroxylase (TH), α-phenylethanolamine-N-methyl transferase (PNMT) and 5-hydroxytryptamine (5-HT) in combination with indirect immunoperoxidase technique using immunocytochemistry, strong GR immunoreactivity has been demonstrated in large numbers of central monoamine nerve cell bodies of the male rat. A vast majority of the noradrenaline (NA) cell bodies of groups A1 to A7 and of the 5-HT cell bodies of groups B1 to B9 were demonstrated to contain strong GR immunoreactivity in the nuclei (stained brown by means of diaminobenzidine, as a substrate for the peroxidase). Among the hypothalamic dopamine (DA) cell groups a vast majority of the DA cell bodies of group A12 were found to be GR immunoreactive, while about 50% of the DA cell bodies of the peri- and paraventricular hypothalamic DA systems were GR immunoreactive, and none of the DA cell bodies of zona inserta (group A13) was GR immunoreactive. Among the midbrain DA cell groups large numbers of GR immunoreactive DA cell bodies were found within group A10 especially in its medial parts, while no GR immunoreactivity was demonstrated in most of the PNMT immunoreactive nerve cell bodies of group C2 (rostral part of dorsal motor nucleus of the vagus) and group C3 (dorsomedial reticular formation of the medulla oblongata).

In view of the strong GR immunoreactivity present in several brain stem monoamine neurons it is suggested that a large number of DA and adrenaline (A) nerve cell bodies and a vast majority of the NA and 5-HT cell bodies represent major targets for glucocorticoid action in the central nervous system. Thus, stress induced increases of glucocorticoid serum levels may via long loop feedback regulate biochemical events in the DA, NA, A and 5-HT neurons known to be stress responsive and to control sleep-wakefulness cycle, emotional behaviour and mood.

ACKNOWLEDGEMENTS

This work was supported by a grant from The Swedish Medical Research Council (No. 13x-2819), O. Bakke is a fellow of the Norwegian Cancer Society.

REFERENCES

(1) Okret, S., Wikström, A.-C., Wrange, Ö., Andersson, B. and Gustafsson, J.-Å. (1984) Proc. Natl. Acad. Sci. USA 81, 1609-1613.

(2) Wrange, Ö., Okret, S., Radojćić, M., Carlstedt-Duke, J. and Gustafsson, J.-Å. (1984) J. Biol. Chem. 259, 4534-4541.

(3) Payvar, F., DeFranco, D., Firestone, G.L., Edgar, B., Wrange, Ö., Okret, S., Gustafsson, J.-Å. and Yamamoto, K.R. (1983) Cell 35, 381-392.

STRUCTURAL ANALYSIS OF HUMAN GLUCOCORTICOID RECEPTOR: DNA BINDING INTERACTIONS*

John A. Cidlowski*, Corinne M. Silva, Leslie A. Petch, Douglas B. Tully, Deborah L. Bellingham, Patricia P. Scheible, Mark M. Compton, Victoria E. Allgood, Christine M. Jewell

Depts. of Physiology, Biochemistry and Pharmacology
University of North Carolina at Chapel Hill
Chapel Hill, North Carolina

*To whom inquiries should be addressed.

Glucocorticoids, like other steroid hormones, regulate many important biological processes in both developing and differentiated tissues and are vital in the adaptation of animals to stress. Glucocorticoid effects that have been clearly established _in vivo_ are primarily catabolic actions in lymphoid tissue, skin, bone and liver, where a limited set of enzymes active in cellular metabolism are up- or down-regulated to alter cellular function (for review, Munck and Leung 1977). This regulation appears to involve an increase or decrease in the rate of transcription of certain mRNAs (for review Rousseau 1984), although reports of additional post-transcriptional effects such as mRNA stabilization have been found to occur (Hynes et al 1982).

Glucocorticoid-responsive cells contain specific receptor proteins whose presence is required in order to transduce the signals carried by the steroid molecule to the genetic machinery. The finding by many laboratories that the hormone-receptor complex binds strongly to DNA sequences upstream and within affected genes (Payvar et al 1983, Govindan et al 1982, Pfahl 1982, Scheidereit et al 1983) suggests a direct role of the receptor in regulating mRNA transcription. These DNA sequences share homology with a region of the long terminal repeat in the glucocorticoid-regulated mouse mammary tumor virus (Huang et al 1982, Lee et al 1981, Majors and Varmus 1983, Buetti and Diggelman 1983, Karin et al 1984) and confer hormone responsiveness upon heterologous genes in transfection experiments. Definition of these sequences, collectively known as glucocorticoid regulatory elements, has enabled the development of new strategies to analyze the microanatomy of glucocorticoid receptors. Additionally, recent developments in receptor purification, affinity labelling and monoclonal antibody production have led to the cloning of both rat and human glucocorticoid receptor genes (Meisfeld et al 1985, Weinberger et al 1985). Despite this progress, a great many unanswered questions remain concerning steroid receptor structure relative to the physiological significance of DNA interactions. The principal emphasis in our laboratory over the past year has been the development of new technologies which permit simultaneous receptor structural analysis and sequence-specific DNA recognition with crude receptor preparations.

Our strategy combines the use of site-specific techniques of receptor affinity labelling with protein blotting and binding of specific cloned DNA probes corresponding to cellular and synthetic glucocorticoid regulatory elements. Recent efforts in our laboratory have permitted selective affinity labelling of human glucocorticoid receptors (Cidlowski and Richon 1984) with the site-specific reagent dexamethasone mesylate developed by Simons and Thompson (1983). This approach permits structural analysis of receptor under denaturing conditions and has led to the discovery that isoelectric polymorphism occurs in the steroid binding subunit of the human glucocorticoid receptor. This heterogeneity is not generated by receptor proteolysis and exists in unactivated, activated and nuclear receptor forms (Silva and Cidlowski, submitted). This surprising diversity suggests several interesting possibilities including post-transcriptional receptor modification, multiple receptor genes or perhaps specific receptor forms which can either induce or repress genes. At present, there is no experimental evidence to support any of these hypotheses.

We have recently begun to explore the possibility that these polymorphic forms of glucocorticoid receptor may differ in their ability to recognize cellular glucocorticoid regulatory elements. These studies result from the development of new DNA binding techniques which permit recognition of steroid receptor-DNA interactions in unpurified receptors. Historically, site-specific DNA-protein interactions have been addressed by nitrocellulose filter assays (Riggs et al 1968), hypersensitivity of chromatin to DNase I (Emerson and Felsenfeld 1984), or footprinting analysis (Scheidereit et al 1983). However, these approaches, which frequently require extensive protein purification, fail to identify the interactive proteins. Several years ago, Bowen et al (1980) developed a procedure to detect DNA-protein interactions after separation of proteins on $NaDodSO_4$/PAGE gels and blotting to nitrocellulose. As introduced, this protocol does not appear to provide sufficient resolution to evaluate selective interactions. We report here however, that with minor modifications and the inclusion of "Blotto Binding Buffer" (Johnson et al 1984), selective glucocorticoid receptor-DNA interactions can be obtained.

Several lines of evidence indicate that the DNA-protein interactions observed reflect glucocorticoid receptor-DNA interaction. These include: 1) co-migration of DNA binding and [^{3}H] dexamethasone mesylate on both one- and two-dimensional gels; 2) the absence of steroid and DNA binding in receptor prepared from down-regulated cells; 3) the ability of partially purified receptor to recognize DNA. Receptor preparations will bind either procaryotic or eukaryotic DNA but preferentially associate with DNA fragments which contain glucocorticoid regulatory elements. Unexpectedly, DNA binding occurs in the absence of hormone and is apparently not influenced by prior receptor activation. The presence of steroid in whole cells results in a predominantly nuclear localization of the binding protein whereas in the absence of steroid, selective DNA binding is detected in both cytoplasmic and nuclear compartments. Our preliminary finding using specific DNA probes on two-dimensional gel blots suggests that the polymorphic forms of receptor may differ in DNA interaction. Furthermore, ongoing studies indicate that the protocols developed may have sufficient sensitivity to detect single base mutations in glucocorticoid regulatory elements (Hutchison et al, in press). In conclusion, these new approaches offer exciting tools to expedite and to enhance the analysis of steroid receptor-DNA interactions.

Acknowledgement studies performed in our laboratory have been supported by NIH Grants AM 23459, AM 32460 and AM 32078.

We thank Kathy Thompson and Janet Leach for excellent clerical assistance.

REFERENCES

(1) Munck, A. and Leung, K., (1977) In Receptors and Mechanisms of Action of Steroid Hormones. J.R. Paggualinir ed. (Marcel/ Deker, New York 11 311-397).
(2) Rousseau, G., (1984) Biochem J. 224, 1-12.
(3) Hynes, N., van Ooyen, A.J.J., Kennedy, N., Herrlich, P., Ponta, H., and Groner, B., (1983) Proc. Natl. Acad. Sci. 80, 3637-3641.
(4) Payvar, F., DeFranco, D., Firestone, G.L., Edgar, B., Wrange O., Okret, S., Gustafsson, J.A., and Yamamoto, K.R., (1983) Cell 35, 381-392.
(5) Govindan, M.V., Speiss, E., and Majors, J. (1982) Proc. Natl. Acad. Sci. 79, 5157-5161.
(6) Pfahl, M. (1982) Cell 31, 475-482.
(7) Scheidereit, C., Geisse, S., Westphal, H.M. and Beato, M. (1983) Nature 304, 749-752.
(8) Huang, A.L., Ostrowski, M.C., Berard, D., Hager, G.L., (1981) Cell 27, 245-255.
(9) Lee, F., Mulligan, R., Berg, P., Ringold, G. (1981) Nature 294, 228-232.
(10) Majors, J. and Varmus, H.E. (1983) Proc. Natl. Acad. Sci. USA 80, 5866-5870.
(11) Buetti, E. and Diggelman, H. (1983) EMBO J. 2, 1423-1429.
(12) Karin, M., Haslinger, A., Holtgreve, H., Richards, R.I., Knauter, P., Westphal, H.M. and Beato, M. (1984) Nature 308, 513-519.

(13) Miesfeld, R., Okret, S., Wikstrom, A., Wrange, O., Gustafsson, J., Yamamoto, K. (1984) Nature 312, 779-781.
(14) Weinberger, C., Hollenberg, S.M., Ong, E.S., Harmon, J.M., Brower, S.T., Cidlowski, J., Thompson, E.B., Rosenfeld, M.G., Evans, R.M. (1985) Science 228 740-742.
(15) Cidlowski, J.A. and Richon, V. (1984) Endocrinology 115, 1588-1597.
(16) Simons, Jr., S.S. and Thompson, E.B. (1981) Proc. Natl. Acad. Sci. 78, 3541-3546.
(17) Silva, C.M. and Cidlowski, J.A. (1985) submitted.
(18) Riggs, A.D., Bourgeois, S., Newby, R.F. and Cohn M. (1968) J. Mol. Biol. 34, 365-368.
(19) Emerson, B.M. and Felsenfeld, G. (1984) Proc. Natl. Acad. Sci. 81, 95-99.
(20) Bowen, B., Steinberg, J., Laemmli, J.K. and Weintraub, H. (1980) Nucl. Acids Res. 8, 1-20.
(21) Johnson, D.A., Gautsch, J.W., Sportsman, J.R., Elder, J.H. (1984) Gene Anal. Tech. 1, 3-8.
(22) Hutchison, D.A., Nordeen, S.K., Vogt, K., Edgell, M.H., Proc. Natl. Acad. Sci. In Press.

STEROID HORMONE RECEPTOR GENES : CLONING, ORGANIZATION AND EXPRESSION.

P. Chambon[1], S. Green[1], P. Walter[1], V. Kumar[1], A. Krust[1], J.M. Bornert[1] and D. Banner[2]
1. LGME/CNRS et U.184/INSERM, Institut de Chimie Biologique, Faculté de Médecine, 67085 - Strasbourg Cédex, France
2. EMBL, Postfach 1022.09, Heidelberg, Germany

We have previously isolated cDNA clones corresponding to the human oestrogen (1) and glucocorticoid (2) receptors present in the breast cancer cell line MCF-7. We have now obtained a full length cDNA clone of the oestrogen receptor (ER) and sequenced it (3). We summarize here the salient features of the ER mRNA and of the corresponding protein, which exhibits an interesting homology with the v-erbA protein of the oncogenic avian erythroblastosis virus (AEV). We also report that the expression of the ER cDNA in HeLa cells produces a protein that has the same molecular weight and binds oestradiol with the same affinity as the MCF-7 ER.

(I) THE MCF-7 ER mRNA. The human ER mRNA is 6322 nucleotides in length, with a 5' untranslated region of 232 nucleotides. The most 5' ATG codon, at position +119, is followed 20 codons downstream by a TGA termination codon. A second ATG codon (at position +233), in the same translational reading frame as the first, represents the start of an open reading frame of 1785 nucleotides which codes for a 595 amino acid protein of 66,182 daltons, in good agreement with the known size of the ER (1). It is unknown whether the first 20 codon open reading frame is expressed and plays any physiological role. The ER mRNA contains a very long (4305 nucleotides) 3'-untranslated region. Other receptor mRNAs (4, 5), including the human glucocorticoid receptor (GR) (2) have a similar structure, the significance of which is unknown.

(II) EXPRESSION OF THE ER cDNA IN HeLa CELLS. The ER-coding segment of the ER cDNA was inserted into the expression vector pKCR2 (6) downstream from the SV40 early promoter. This recombinant (pKCR2-ER) was introduced into HeLa cells and its ability to direct the synthesis of ER molecules was tested in transient expression experiments. Fig. 1A shows that the expression of pKCR2-ER results in the appearance of a protein (lane 3, arrowhead) which has the same molecular weight as the ER present in the breast cancer cells MCF-7 (lane 4). This protein is not present in HeLa cells (lane 1) nor in HeLa cells transfected with the parent pKCR2 vector (lane 2).

The function of the protein synthesized into HeLa cells following transfection with pKCR2-ER was studied by investigating its ability to bind oestradiol (Fig. 1B). HeLa cells transfected with the pKCR2 vector had only background binding activity (open squares). On the other hand, significant amount of oestradiol-binding activity (triangles) were found in HeLa cells transfected with pKCR2-ER. The corresponding protein exhibited an affinity for oestradiol (KD = 0.4 nM) very similar to that of the MCF-7 ER (KD = 0.5 nM) (Fig. 1B, inset). Thus, the expression of the ER cDNA in HeLa cells yields a protein which, using these criteria, is indistinguishable from the MCF-7 ER.

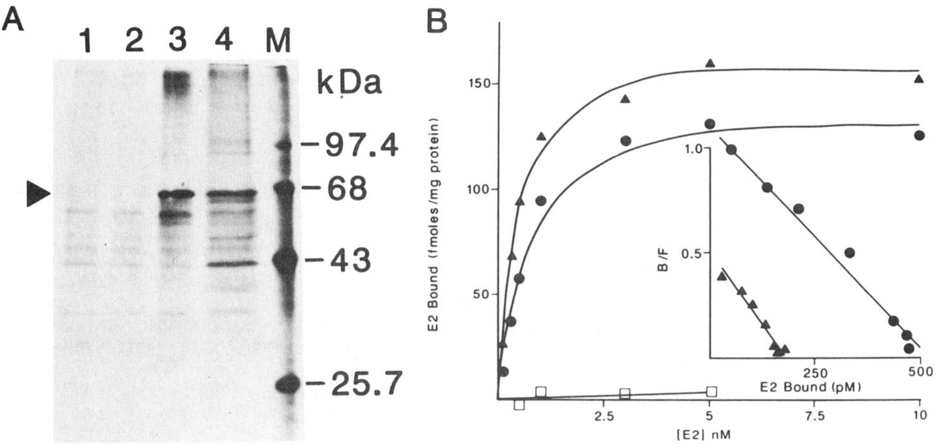

Fig. 1. Expression of the oestrogen receptor cDNA in HeLa cells. A. The size of the protein coded by the cloned ER cDNA is identical to that of the MCF-7 ER. The ER cDNA sequence was inserted into the eucaryotic expression vector pKCR2 (6), yielding pKCR2-ER which was transfected into HeLa cells and the proteins were labelled with [^{35}S] methionine. Cytoplasmic proteins were immunoprecipitated with ER antibodies, separated by SDS-PAGE (7%) and revealed by fluorography. Lane 1, wild type HeLa cells; lane 2, HeLa cell transfected with pKCR2; lane 3, HeLa cells transfected with pKCR2-ER; lane 4, wild type MCF-7 cells. The arrow shows the position of the 65 kDa protein. Lane M, [^{14}C]-labelled protein markers : phosphorylase-b (97.4 kDa), bovine serum albumin (68 kDa), ovalbumin (43 kDa), α-chymotrypsinogen (25.7 kDa). B. The ER cDNA-encoded protein binds oestradiol with the same affinity as the MCF-7 ER. Cytosol extracts, prepared from MCF-7 cells (●) or HeLa cells transfected with pKCR2 (■) or pKCR2-ER (▲), were incubated overnight at 0°C in the presence of [^{3}H]-17β-oestradiol (E2) with or without a 100-fold excess of unlabelled 17β-oestradiol. The unbound steroid was removed using dextran-coated charcoal and the receptor-bound steroid counted in a scintillation counter. The number of moles of steroid bound per milligram of cytosolic protein was calculated after substraction of the non-specific binding. Each point was performed in duplicate and line fitting was by computer. The inset shows a Scatchard plot of these same data (see Ref. 3 for further experimental procedures).

(III) HOMOLOGY BETWEEN OESTROGEN RECEPTOR AND v-erbA PROTEIN SEQUENCES. The ER amino-acid sequence was compared with the sequences present in the NBRF protein database. Very significant homology was found with the avian erythroblastosis virus (AEV) gag-erbA fusion protein (7) (Fig. 2). This homology begins at amino acid 150 of the ER and extends to the carboxy-terminal end of the two proteins. The homology is particularly striking in the cysteine-rich region of the ER between amino acids 180 and 250, where each of the 9 cysteine residues in this region is conserved in the erbA protein.

The homology between the human ER sequence and the erbA gene of the oncogenic AEV, which contains two cell-derived genes, termed v-erbA and v-erbB (see Ref. 8 for a review), is extremely interesting. The v-erbA protein, which is a fusion between the viral gag

```
ER    146 PPAFYRPNSDNRRQGGRERLASTNDKGSMAMESAKETRYCAVCNDYASGYHYGVWSCEGCKAFFKRSIQG--HNDYMCPA
ERBA    1 EDTRW-LDGKHKRKSSQCLVKSSMS-GYIPSCLDKDEQ-CVVCGDKATGYHYRCITCEGCKSFFRRTIQKNLHPTYSCTY

ER    224 TNQCTIDKNRRKSCQACRLRKCYEVGM-MKGGI---------------RKDRRGGRMLKHKRQRDDGEGRGEVGSAGDMR
ERBA   78 DGCCVIDKITRNQCQLCRFKKCISVGMAMDLVLDDSKRVAKRKLIEENRERRRKEEMIKSL-QHRPSPSAEEWELIHVVT

ER    288 AANLWPSP-LMIKRSKKNSLALSLTADQMVSALLDAEPPILYSEYDPTRPFSEASMMGLLTNLADRELVHMINWAKRVPG
ERBA  157 EAHRSTNAQGSHWKQRRKFLLEDIGQSPMASML-------------DGDKVDLEAFSE--FTKIITPAITRVVDFAKNLPM

ER    367 FVDLTLHDQVHLLECAWLEILMIGLVWRSMEHPVKLLFAPNLLLDRNQGKCVEGMVEIFDMLLATSSRFRMMNLQGEEFV
ERBA  199 FSELPCEDQIILLKGCCMEIMSLRAAVRYDPESETLTLSGEMAVKREQLKN-GGLGVVSDAIFDLGKSLSAFNLDDTEVA

ER    447 CLKSIILLNSGVYTFLSSTLKSLEEKDHIHRVLDKITDTLIHLMAKAGLTLQQQHQRLAQLLLILSHIRHMSNKGMEHLY
ERBA  302 LLQAVLLMSSD-RTGLICVDK--IEK---------------------------CQES-----YLLAFEHYINYRKHNIPHFW

ER    527 SMKCKNVVPLYDLLLEMLDAHRLHAP-TSRGGASVEETDQSHLATAGSTSSHSLQKYYITGEAEGFPATV (COOH)
ERBA  349 S-K---------LLMKVADLRMIGAYHASRFL---------HMKVECPTEL-PPRRCRALQILGSILPFV (COOH)
```

Fig. 2 : Homology between ER and v-erbA proteins sequences. The alignment between the sequence of the MCF-7 ER and v-erbA protein was determined using a search procedure based on the amino acid physical characteristics (12, 13). There are 378 aligned residues for the ER and v-erbA proteins of which 27% are identical and 41% conserved according to the following scheme : (P,G), (M,C), (Y,W,F,H), (L,V,I,A), (K,R), (E,Q,N,D) and (S,T). The average correlation coefficient, using 6 amino acid physical characteristics, was 0.37. The mean correlation, maximum correlation and standard deviation for control protein sequences (see below) was 0.00, 0.20 and 0.04 respectively. The ER/v-erbA correlation was 9.2 standard deviations above the control mean and 4.2 standard deviations above the control maximum. The control protein sequence consisted of a group of 63 proteins of unrelated tertiary structure, whose sequence was expanded to contain 1000 residues. Segments of 378 amino acids were randomly selected (using a random generator seeded with a number based on the time of day) and an average correlation coefficient calculated. This procedure was repeated at 10 different times and the mean standard deviation and maximum correlations were calculated for the resulting 19,530 average correlations over 6 amino acid characteristics. In order to determine if the homology between the ER and v-erbA is significant throughout the entire v-erbA sequence, the ER sequence was subdivided into three regions (I residues 146-255; II residues 256-467; III residues 468-595) and each aligned with v-erbA. The correlation coefficients were 5.8, 6.2 and 3.2 standard deviations above the control mean, respectively.

protein and the cellular erbA protein, is not in itself oncogenic. However, it increases the oncogenicity of v-erbB, which is homologous to the epidermal growth factor (EGF) receptor (9). It seems highly unlikely that c-erbA could be the chicken ER receptor, since the chicken ER sequence is more homologous to the human ER than to v-erbA (our unpublished data). In addition, the human c-erbA maps to chromosome 17 and is far more homologous to v-erbA than the human ER which maps to chromosome 6 (1). The human genome contains several erbA-related genes; at least two of these map to chromosome 17 (10, 11). Thus the ER appears to belong to a multigene family. It is likely that the conserved cysteine-rich domain which is common to the human ER and v-erbA proteins has some important function. Site-directed mutagenesis of the ER cDNA sequence in the expression vector pKCR2-ER should be helpful in identifying this function and in locating the amino acid sequences involved in the multiple functions of the ER. In this respect it will also be interesting to compare the ER and v-erbA sequences with that of the human glucocorticoid receptor recently cloned in our laboratory (2).

REFERENCES

(1) Walter, P., Green, S., Greene, G, Krust, A, Bornert, J.M., Jeltsch, J.M., Staub, A., Jensen, E., Scrace, G., Waterfield, M. and Chambon, P. (1985) Proc. Natl. Acad. Sci. USA, in press.
(2) Govindan, M.V., Devic, M., Green, S., Gronemeyer, H. and Chambon, P. (1985) Nucleic Acids Res., in press.
(3) Green, S., Walter, P., Kumar, V., Krust, A., Bornert, J.M., Argos, P. and Chambon, P., submitted for publication.
(4) Yamamoto, T., Davis, C.G., Brown, M.S., Schneider, W.J., Casey, M.L., Goldstein, J.L. and Russell, D.W. (1984) Cell 39, 27-38.
(5) Schneider, C., Owen, M.J., Banville, D. and Williams, J.G. (1984). Nature 311, 675-678.
(6) Breathnach, R. and Harris, B.A. Nucl. Acids Res. (1983) Nucl. Acids Res. 11, 7119-7136.
(7) Debuire, B., Henry, C., Benaissa, M., Biserte, G., Claverie, J.M., Saule, S., Martin, P. and Stehelin, D. (1984) Science 224, 1456-1459.
(8) Graf, T. and Beng, H. (1983) Cell 34, 7-9.
(9) Ullrich, A., Coussens, L., Hayflick, J.S., Dull, T.J., Gray, A., Tam, A.W., Lee, J., Yarden, Y., Libermann, T.A., Schlessinger, J., Downward, J., Mayes, E.L.V., Whittle, N., Waterfield, M.D. and Seeburg, P.H. (1984) Nature 309, 418-425.
(10) Jansson, M., Philipson, L. and Vennström, B. (1983) EMBO J. 2, 561-565.
(11) Spurr, N.K., Solomon, E., Jansson, M., Sheer, D., Goodfellow, P.N., Bodmer, W.F. and Vennström, B. (1984) EMBO J. 3, 159-163.
(12) Argos, P., Hanei, M., Wilson, J.M. and Kelley, W.N. (1983) J. Biol. Chem. 258, 6450-6457.
(13) Argos, P. (1985). EMBO J. 4, 1351-1355.

STEROID HORMONE RECEPTORS AS GENE REGULATORS

M. Beato
Institut für Molekularbiologie und Tumorforschung, Philipps-Universität, 3550 Marburg, F.R.G.

INTRODUCTION

The mechanism by which steroid hormones modulate the expression of particular genes in their target cells has been intensively investigated during the past two decades. The emerging view is that the hormones influence gene expresion through their interaction with specific receptor proteins that upon binding the ligand are modified to become DNA regulatory proteins. According to this concept the main function of the hormones would be to "activate" the receptor proteins into a conformation that permits their functional interaction with the regulatory information stored in the genome. Therefore, in order to understand the molecular mechnanism of steroid hormone action two questions have to be answered: how do the hormones activate their receptors, and how do the activated receptors modulate gene expression. The first question is being investigated in several laboratories with the classical techniques of protein chemistry with the aim to detect conformational and/or covalent modifications of the receptor proteins following binding of the hormone. The recent success in cloning the cDNA and the genes for some of the hormone receptors (1,2) may greatly facilitate these studies.

In this paper I will focus on our attempts to answer the second relevant question, namely: how do the activated receptors modulate gene expression.

HORMONE REGULATORY ELEMENTS.

Work during the past few years has led to the identification in the neighborhood of hormonally regulated promoters of DNA sequences that are recognized by the activated hormone receptors. In the following I will first summarize what is known about the location, nucleotide sequence and function of these hormone regulatory elements (HRE). Based on the effects of receptor binding on the topology of plasmids containing HREs, and on the DNaseI sensitivity of regulated genes, I will then formulate an hypothesis as to how binding of the receptors to the HRE could influence transcriptional efficiency.

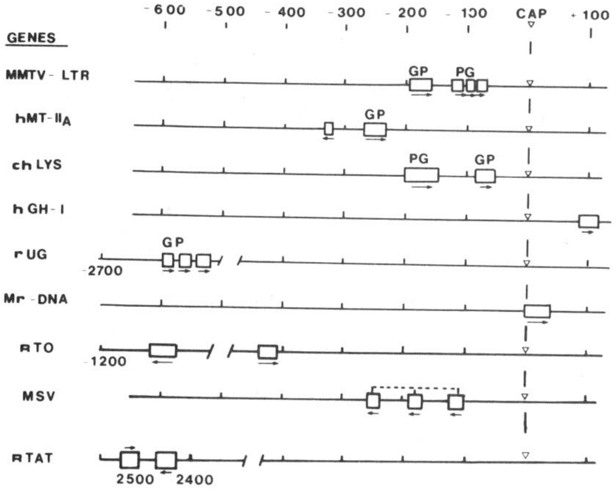

Fig.1. Location and orientation of the HREs. The HREs are indicated by boxes and the orientation is given by the horizonal arrows. The initiation of transcription is labelled "cap", and the numbers refer to the distance from "cap" in nucleotides. The HREs that are labelled with G and P are recognized by both the glucocorticoid and the progesterone receptor. The abbreviations are as follows: MMTV-LTR, the long terminal repeat region of mouse mammary tumor virus; hMTIIA, human metallothionein gene; chLYS, chicken lysozyme gene; hGHI, human growth hormone gene; rUG, rabbit uteroglobin gene; MrDNA, mouse ribosomal gene; rTO, rat tryptophan oxygenase gene; MSV, mouse sarcoma virus (the enhancer region is marked by the broken line); rTAT, rat tyrosine aminotransferase gene.

```
(A)                             10  12  14  16
              1 2 3 4 5 6 7 8 9   11  13  15
              . . . . . . . . . . . . . . . .
                *                   *
MTV I         G G T T A C A A A C T G T T C T
                * *     ^           *     ^
HMTVIIa I     C G G T A C A C T G T G T C C T
                  *     ^           *     ^
RUG I         C T G T T C A C T C T G T T C T
                        ^           *     ^
RUG II        C C G G A C A C G G A G T C C T
                        ^           *     ^
MRib          A C T G A C A C G C T G T C C T
                        ^           *     ^
RUG III       G T G T C A G T C T T G T T C T
                                    *     ^
MTV IIa       T G G T A T C A A A T G T T C T
                                    *     ^
DSC7          C G A T T T G A T C T G T T C T
                *                   *     ^
CLYS I        T G A C A A C T G T A G A A C A
                    ^             *       ^
CLYS II       A A A T T C C T C T G T G G C T
                *       ^           *     ^
rTAT I        T G T A A C A G G A T G T T C T
                                    *
rTAT II       A G G A C T T G T T T G T T C T
                      ^                   ^
B)

HGH I         G G G C A C A A T G T G T C C T
CVIT II       G G G A T C A A T G T G T T C T
rTO I         A T G C A C A G C G A G T T C T
rTO II        C C T T T C A T G A T G T C C T
MSV I         G G G G A C C A T C T G T T C T
MSV II        C T G T T C C A T C T G T T C T
MSV III       G C T G T C T C T C T G T T C C
COV I         G T T T T C T G C C T G T T C T
COV II        G G T C A C G T C T T G T T C T
HMTIIa II     C C C T C C C T C C T G T C C T

              1 2 3 4 5 6 7 8 9   11  13  15
              . . . . . . . . . . . . . . . .
CONSENSUS:    N G G T A C A N N N T G T T C T
              . . . . . . . . . . . . . . . .
(22 SITES)    -  11  11  10 - - -18  20  22
               11  11  17          21  20  20

PROHIBITED BASES:  - a c - G G - - - - C C C A G G
                                       g A a a A a
                                         t g g   c
```

Fig.2. Nucleotide sequence of 22 binding sites for the glucocorticoid receptor. The sequences are aligned according to the hexanucleotide motive. The abbreviations are as in Fig.1; DSC7, is a Drosophila gene for a polypeptide of the salivary gland; cVIT, chicken vitellogenin gene; cOV, chicken ovalbumine gene. A), sites studied by methylation protection. The contacted Gs are marke *, and the Cs corresponding to protected Gs in the lower strand are indicated by . B), sites that have not been analyzed by methylation protection. A consensus sequence is shown at the bottom with the center of symmetry at position 9 indicated. The numbers bellow each position of the consensus indicate the degree of conservation of the corresponding base.

The location and orientation of the HREs in nine genes we have studied is shown in Figure 1. All these sites have been identified in binding studies with purified receptors and have been shown to be needed for hormonal regulation in at least one functional test. The results with the rat tyrosine aminotransferase gene (rTAT) are from U. Strähler, B. Gloss, W. Schmid and G. Schütz, Heidelberg (umpublished). As can be seen the location of the HREs varies between 2,900 bp upstream (rUG) and 100 bp downstream (hGHI) of the transcription start point, and both orientations are found. Thus, the HREs function relatively independent of orientation and distance as do the classical enhancer elements, their peculiarity being that they are dependent on hormones.

The nucleotide sequence of 22 receptor binding sites, including most of those shown in Fig.1 and three other sites for which we do not have functional data, are listed in Figure 2. The right half of the binding sequence, with the hexanucleotide motive 5'-TGTYCT-3', is better conserved than the left half, but even here certain bases never occur (Fig.2, bottom). In the 12 binding sites that have been analyzed by methylation protection (Fig.2A) contact points with the DNA were found at the N-7 position of guanines in the major groove of the double helix. Of these, the G at position 15 (lower strand) was protected in all cases, and the G at position 12 in 91% of the binding sites. In the left half of the regulatory element the best conserved base is the C at position 6 (77%). The corresponding G in the lower strand was contacted by the receptor in 50% of the cases studied. The Gs at positions 2 and 3 were found only in 50% of the binding sites, but were contacted by the receptor in the most active regulatory elements (MTVIa, hMTIIA).

The consensus sequence derived from these 22 sites exhibits a limited inverted symmetry: 5'**GNACANNNTGTNC**3'. This structure is compatible with binding of two receptor monomers in a head to head orientation. Since the distance between the receptor contact points along the DNA is 10 bases in the upper strand and 9 bases in the lower strand, the two blocks of contact points are located on the same face of the DNA double helix separated by a little less than a turn of the helix. A plausible model could involve the high affinity binding of a receptor monomer to the major groove containing the hexanucleotide TGTYCT, followed by binding o a second monomer to the upstream sequence GGTACA in the adjacent major groove. This later interaction will exhibit lower affinty but would be stabilized by protein-protein contacts.

Interestingly we found that the progesterone receptor binds to the same DNA regions that are recognized by the glucocorticoid receptor, and that these sites can mediate progesterone regulation of adjacent promoters (3-5). Within the regulatory elemnt of the cLYS promoter each receptor appears to approach the DNA from a different angle, and to recognize distinct features of the same DNA sequence (6).Thus, the regulatory signals utilized by both hormone receptors may be degenerated.

MECHANISM OF TRANSCRIPTIONAL REGULATION

How could binding of the receptor to the HRE influence the transcription initiation rate? Any attempt to answer this question has to take into consideration that the HREs can act at variable distance and in both orientations. In principle two mechanisms can be envisaged: protein-protein interaction or signal transmission along the DNA. In the first model the receptor bound to the HRE would interact directly with other proteins of the transcriptional machinery and thus modulate transcriptional efficiency. The second model assumes that binding of the receptor to the HRE results in conformational changes of the DNA double helix, that can be propagated along the DNA and translated into local structural changes in other relevant regions of the promoter. These local changes will be recognized by proteins of the transcriptional apparatus and eventually result in modulation of promoter efficiency.

Support for the last model comes from our observation that binding of the purified glucocorticoid receptor to the HRE of MMTV-LTR, introduces topological changes in close circular plasmids (7). A relationship between these topological changes and local alterations of promoter structure and effciency remains to be established. The fact, however, that hormonal administration to rabbits results in the appearance in endometrial chromatin of DNaseI hypersensitive sites near the HRE of rUG that is located 2.6 kb upstream of the transcription start point (umpublished), supports the existance of such DNA structural changes in vivo.

Aknowledgements. The experimental work reported here has been supported by the Deutsche Forschungsgemeinschaft and the Fond der Chemischen Industrie.

REFERENCES

1.Miesfeld,R.; Okret,S.; Wikstrom,A.C.; Wrange,O.; Gustafsson, J-A. and Yamamoto,K.R. (1984) Nature 312, 779-781.

2.Weinberger,C.;Hollenberg,S.M.;Ong,E.S.;Harmon,J.M.; Brower, S.T.;Cidlowski,J.;Thompson,E.B.;Rosenfeld,M.G. and Evans,R.M. (1985) Science 228, 740-742.

3.Ahe,D.von der;Janich,J.;Scheidereit,C.; Renkawitz,R.; Schütz,G. and Beato,M. (1985) Nature 313, 706-709.

4.Renkawitz,R.; Schütz,G.; Ahe,D. von der and Beato,M. (1984) Cell 37, 503-510.

5.Cato,A.C.B.; Miksicek,R.; Schütz,G. and Beato,M., submitted.

6.Ahe,D.von der; Renoir,J.M.; Buchou,T.; Baulieu,E-E.; and Beato,M., Proc.Natl.Acad.Sci.USA, in press.

7.Carballo,M. and Beato,M., submitted

MECHANISMS OF GROWTH REGULATION OF HUMAN BREAST CANCER.

M.E. Lippman, R.B. Dickson, E.P. Gelmann, A. Kasid, S. Bates, C. Knabbe, S.M. Swain, M. McManaway, G. Wilding, N. Davidson, K. Huff, and D. Bronzert
Medicine Branch, National Cancer Institute, Bldg. 10, Room 12N226, Bethesda, MD 20892 USA

The mechanisms by which estrogens and antiestrogens regulate the growth of human breast cancer have not been completely elucidated. Substantial amounts of information, often conflicting, have suggested on the one hand that estrogens exert no direct growth regulatory effects on breast cancer (BC)(1), while other work has suggested that estrogens directly regulate gene expression in human BC (2). In this presentation data will be reviewed supporting 4 hypotheses:

I. In human BC estrogens directly alter transcription of specific genes in BC and these gene products are involved in the growth response.

II. In hormone dependent human BC cells, estrogens increase and antiestrogens decrease the secretion of potent autocrine and paracrine growth factors. These growth factors are directly responsible for tumor growth and progression.

III. Hormone independence is conferred by the ability of BC cells to constituitively secrete a similar spectrum of autocrine and paracrine growth factors.

IV. The effects of antiestrogen and other growth inhibitors are induced by two mechanisms. First, by inhibition of stimulatory autocrine and paracrine growth factors and secondly, by induction of intracellular and extracellular factors with inhibitory activity.

In both defined and serum-containing media, estrogens and antiestrogens can be shown to alter the growth rate of human BC cells of various lineages (3-10). As part of this growth stimulation, numerous enzymes involved in DNA synthesis are appropriately regulated by estrogens and antiestrogens in proportion to their effects on growth (11-14). We have studied the regulation of thymidine kinase and dihydrofolate reductase in detail. Using a cDNA probe to the former, estrogens and antiestrogens alter messenger RNA concentrations for thymidine kinase and furthermore these effects occur at the level of gene transcription (15). We have also developed similar data for dihydrofolate reductase (16). Chambon and his colleagues have also demonstrated transcriptional regulation of another estrogen induced gene pS2 (17). Finally, we have recently isolated a collection of cDNA clones representing messenger RNA species which are induced within 6 hours of estradiol stimulation of human BC cells. Thus there is little doubt that estrogens can directly alter gene expression at the transcriptional level in human BC cells.

Notwithstanding the large number of estrogen regulated products in human BC cells, there exists the question as to which of these products are important in the regulation and progression of human BC. Preliminary experiments using conditioned media had suggested that factors might be present in such media which were autostimulatory (18). We therefore set about characterizing the growth factors produced by human BC cells their specific regulation by estrogens and antiestrogens. Many of our methods have been published elsewhere (19-21).

Human BC cells secrete material which cross reacts in sensitive radioimmunoassay with insulin-like growth factor-I(IGF-I). All BC cell lines tested - both hormone dependent and hormone independent - produce this activity. This material has molecular weight identical to authentic human IGF-I. Furthermore, using a cDNA probe to authentic human IGF-I, the human IGF-I messenger RNA is detected in these BC cells. All of the human BC cell lines that we have studied have IGF-I receptors on their surface and respond with growth stimulation to physiologic concentrations of IGF-I. Estradiol increases IGF-I secretion in hormone dependent human BC cells and secretion is inhibited by antiestrogen treatment. Thus, IGF-I is a hormone regulated growth factor which can function as autocrine growth regulator.

Human BC cell lines also secrete material of the epidermal growth factor (EGF)/transforming growth factor (TGFα) class. Three separate assay systems were developed. A soft agar cloning assay using non transformed NRK fibroblasts; a radioimmunoassay using antisera which reacts with TGFα but not EGF; and a radio receptor assay using A431 cells as a source of EGF receptor. Hormone dependent and hormone independent BC cells produce a major species of approximately 30,000 molecular weight and a smaller species. All 3 assays give coincident results with respect to molecular weight characterization. This activity is estrogen inducible in 3 estrogen responsive human BC cells and is secreted constituitively by hormone independent BC cell lines.

Human BC cell lines produce a growth factor belonging to the competency class. Using a bioassay in which quiescent fibroblasts are grown in platelet derived growth factor (PDGF) deficient serum, human BC cell lines that stimulate initiation of DNA synthesis. The human BC cell lines express RNA complementary to a c-sis probe. In addition, in collaboration with Harry Antoniades and colleagues at Harvard, it can be shown that this activity is immunoprecipitated by specific antiserum developed against PDGF. Its molecular weight, heat and reducing agent stability are characteristic for authentic PDGF. Thus, human BC cells secrete PDGF.

All the human BC cell lines that we have studied also secrete TGFβ. This has been demonstrated both by radioreceptor assay and (in collaboration with M. Sporn and his colleagues) a mRNA of appropriate size for the human TGFβ transcript. Its regulation is discussed later.

Finally, we have identified a high molecular weight epithelial cell stimulating activity which is currently under active investigation which is clearly separable from the above mentioned activities.

The role of these growth factor activities have been studied in a reconstituted nude mouse system. In ovariectomized nude mice, MCF-7 BC cells will not grow without estrogen supplementation (22). Animals were implanted with MCF-7 cells and then treated with either estradiol pellets or with implantation of Alza minipumps containing concentrated conditioned media from BC cells or growth factor preparations from which all estradiol had been removed. Using concentrated conditioned media, it is possible to induce formation of invasive adenocarcinomas though of a somewhat smaller size. Despite resupplementation with fresh conditioned media these tumors eventually regress as compared with estrogen treated cells in which continued tumor growth and progression is seen. These experiments suggest that secretion of some secreted factors are capable of functioning in an endocrine fashion to induce some tumor formation. Failure to achieve complete tumor formation may be due either to quantitative loss of specific growth factors, qualitative loss of required growth factors during the extraction and preparation of conditioned medium or the necessity for estradiol to induce other functions in the tumor (such as cell surface proteolysis) or specific effects on the host.

Hormone independent BC cells whose growth is not altered by estrogens and antiestrogens secrete similar growth factor activities. We provide further evidence for the hypothesis that hormone independence is due to the constituitive secretion of growth factor activities by experiments in which the v-ras^H gene was transfected into MCF-7 cells (23). These cells become hormone independent both _in vivo_ and _in vitro_. Furthermore, we have shown that these cells have upregulated secretion of growth factor activities suggesting that the mechanism by which they have become hormone independent is increased growth factor secretion (24).

Finally, in addition to providing evidence that antiestrogens may inhibit cell growth by lowering concentrations of TGF and IGF-I, we have also recently acquired some information that antiestrogens may exert part of their inhibitory effects through increased secretion of factors with some inihibitory activity. We have identified a 39,000 kDa glycoprotein which is strongly induced by estrogen deprivation. Most interestingly, we have recently shown that TGFβ is strongly induced by signals which slow the growth of cells. Antiestrogens, and glucocorticoids increase the secretion of TGFβ. Furthermore, several MCF-7 clones as well as estrogen independent breast cancer cell lines are inhibited by exogenous addition of TGFβ. A mutant MCF-7 cell line, LY2 (25), which is antiestrogen independent, fails to show TGFβ induction by antiestrogens. Inhibition of cell growth by TGFβ is proportional to the quantity of TGFβ receptor expressed on their surface. These experiments suggest that TGFβ is an important autocrine growth inhibitor; resistance to its activity may occur through loss of production of TGFβ or decreased TGFβ receptor.

Our work suggests that secreted stimulatory and inhibitory growth factor activities are an important component of the regulation of human breast cancer progression. Such mechanisms have obvious potential ramifications with respect to therapeutic interventions which are also actively under investigation.

REFERENCES

(1) Ikeda, T. and Sirbasku, D.(1984) J. Biol. Chem. 259, 4049-4064.
(2) Lippman, M.E., Bolan, G. and Huff, K. (1976) Cancer Res. 36, 4595-4601.
(3) Chalbos, D., Vignon, F. Keydar, I., et al (1982) J. Clin. Endocrinol. Metab. 55(2), 276-287.
(4) Darbre, P., Yates, J., Curtis, S. and King, R.J.B. (1983) Cancer Res. 43, 349-354.
(5) Noguchi, S., Kitamura, Y., Uchida, N., et al. (1984) Cancer Res. 44, 5644-5649.
(6) Katzenellenbogen, B., Norman, M.J., Eckert, R.L., et al (1983) Cancer Res. 44, 112-119.
(7) Leung, B.S., Qureshi, S. and Leung, J.S. (1982) Cancer Res. 42, 5060-5066.
(8) Natoli, C., Sica, G., Natoli, V. et al (1983) Breast Cancer Res. Treat. 3, 23-32.
(9) Page, M., Field, J., Everett, N. et al (1983) Cancer Res. 43, 1244-1250.
(10) Weichselbaum, R.W., Hellman, S., Piro, A. et al (1978) Cancer Res. 38, 2339-2342.
(11) Aitken, S.C. and Lippman, M.E. (in press) Cancer Res.
(12) Aitken, S.C. and Lippman, M.E.(1982) Cancer Res. 42, 1727-1735.
(13) Cowan, K.H., Goldsmith, M.E., Levine, R.M., Aitken, S.C., et al (1982) J. Biol. Chem. 257(24), 15079-15086.
(14) Bronzert, D.A., Monaco, M.E., Pinkus, L., Aitken, S. and Lippman, M.E. (1981) Cancer Res. 41, 604-610.
(15) Kasid, A., Davidson, N., Gelmann, E. and Lippman, M. (submitted) J. Biol. Chem.
(16) Levine, R.M., Rubalcaba, E., Lippman, M.E. and Cowan, K.H. (1985) Cancer Res. 45, 1644-1650.
(17) Jakowlew, S.B., Breathnack, R., Jeltsch, J., Masiaskowski, P. and Chambon, P. (1984) Nucleic Acid Res. 12, 2861-2874.
(18) Jakesz, R., Smith, C.A., Aitken, S. et al (1984) Cancer Res. 44, 619-625.
(19) Osborne, C.K., Hamilton, B., Titus, G. and Livingston, R.B. (1980) Cancer Res. 40, 2361-2366.
(20) Dickson, R.B., Huff, K.K., Spencer, E.M. and Lippman, M.E. (in press) Endocrinol.
(21) Bates, S. and Lippman, M.E. (1986) in Leukemia (Whittaker, J.D. and Delamore, I.W., eds.) Chapter 11, in press, Blackwell Scientific, Oxford, England.
(22) Soule, H.D. and McGrath, C.M. (1980) Cancer Lett. 10, 177-189.
(23) Kasid, A., Lippman, M.E., Papageorge, A.G., Lowry, D.R. and Gelmann, E.P. (1985) Science 228, 725-728.
(24) Dickson, R., McManaway, M. and Lippman, M.(submitted) Science.
(25) Bronzert, D.A., Green, G.L. and Lippman, M.E. (in press) Endocrinol.

LOCALIZATION OF THE GLUCOCORTICOID RECEPTOR IN STEROID-SENSITIVE AND STEROID-RESISTANT HUMAN LEUKEMIC CELL LINES.

T. ANTAKLY and E.B. THOMPSON Department of Anatomy, McGill University Montréal H3A 2B2, Canada and the Department of Human Biological Chemistry and Genetics, University of Texas Medical Branch, Galveston, Texas.

The preparation of antibodies to glucocorticoid receptor has added a new dimension to the study of this receptor.Using a sensitive and reproducible immunocytochemical procedure we localized the glucocorticoid receptor in both the cytoplasm and nucleus of traget cells (1-3). In these studies two different polyclonal and two different monoclonal antibodies gave similar results (3). These studies have established a basis for using immunocytochemistry as a tool to study glucocorticoid hormone action and glucocorticoid resistance at the cellular and subcellular level. In the case of normal glucocorticoid-resistant cells such as the cells of the intermediate lobe of the rat pituitary, the lack of response of these cells appears to be secondary to the absence of immunoreactive receptor (1,2) a comparison can be drawn between the pituitary cells and a well studied model system, the CEM leukemic cell lines where the degree of physiological response appears to be related to the number of glucocorticoid binding sites (4). Several mutants were selected following glucocorticoid treatment and chemical mutagen. These cell lines offer a unique system to correlate physiological response and receptor localization. We have investigated five C.E.M. cell lines: C7, C1, 4R4, 3R43, ICR-27 as well as a receptor-rich, IM9 lymphoblastic cell line (see ref. 4 for documentation on the cell lines).

The cells were grown in RPMI 1640 medium supplemented with 5% fetal bovine serum (charcoal-dextran absorbed). In most experiments, cells were used at mid-log phase. Fixation: In order to obtain reliable and reproducible immunocytochemical results, cells must be fixed to cross link the proteins and cell components *in situ*. However, results may vary depending upon the type of fixative used and subsequent procedures followed for sectioning the cells and enhancing the permeability of the cells to antibodies. In all these situations a compromise must be reached for a maximum preservation of the ultrastructure of the cells close to the native state and minimum denaturation of the antigenic sites. Therefore, in previous studies we have developed an immunocytochemical procedure for the intracellular and intranuclear localization of a variety of antigens in whole cells in culture (see 5 and references therein). In this study cells were fixed in paraformaldehyde, glutaraldehyde, picric acid-formaldehyde (Zamboni), Bouin, acetic acid-ethanol followed or not with brief permeabilization with Triton, saponin or ethanol. Subsequently, the cells were either smeared on glass slides in a Cytocentrifuge or handled as a cell suspension before incubation with a polyclonal or a monoclonal antibody to the receptor. The bound antibodies were revealed using a second antibody labelled with either peroxidase or fluorescein. Cells were observed at the light microscope level and in selected experiments at the electron microscope level. A total number of 60 experiments is reported herein. The overall staining intensity (at saturating antibody concentration), as evaluated visually by two observers is as follows:

cell line	IM9	C7	C1	4R4	3R43	1CR27
staining intensity	++++	++++	+++	++	+++	++

Although all fixative excepting ethanol-acetic acid gave consistent results, fixation in 4% paraformaldehyde gave most satisfactory results at the electron microscope level. The immunocytochemical reaction was found largely in the cell cytoplasm and to a lesser extent in the nucleus. Clearly, some nuclei were stained more intensely than others. Mitochondria were unstained. Rigorous immunocytochemical controls were performed to confirm the specificity of the immunocytochemical staining. These controls include preabsorption of the antibody with purified receptor and the use of non-immune serum.

These results confirm our earlier studies on normal cells (1-3) namely that the glucocorticoid receptor is found in both the cytoplasm and nucleus of target cells. We have never observed an exclusive nuclear localization of the glucocorticoid receptor either in these studies or in earlier ones. This observation was consistent under a variety of immunocytochemical staining protocols and using four different monoclonal and polyclonal antibodies (see 3). An unexpected finding was that the ICR-27 cell line, which is resistant to glucocorticoid action and contains no significant glucocorticoid binding sites (4), contains high level immunoreactive glucocorticoid receptor. These results suggest that a glucocorticoid receptor with altered binding site(s) exist in this cell line.

REFERENCES

1 - Antakly, T., Eisen H.J. (1982) J. Cell Biol. 95:437a.

2 - Antakly, T., Eisen H.J. (1984) Endocrinology 115:1984.

3 - Antakly, T. et al. (1985) Science 299:277.

4 - Thompson, E.B. et al. (1983) in Steroid Hormone receptors: structure and function (Eriksson, H. and Gustafsson, J.-A. eds.) pp. 171-194, Elsevier Science Public. Amsterdam.

5 - Antakly, T. (1980) J. Cell Biol. 86:377.

EFFECTS OF ESTROGEN ON APOLIPOPROTEIN AI SYNTHESIS IN THE HUMAN HEPATOCARCINOMA CELL LINE, HEPG2.

T.K. Archer, S.P. Tam and R.G. Deeley
Dept. of Biochemistry, Queen's University, Kingston, Ontario
Canada K7L 3N6

Recently we have examined the possibility of using a human hepatocarcinoma cell line, HepG2, to investigate the hormonal regulation of apolipoprotein synthesis in human liver (1,2). We have demonstrated that exposure of HepG2 cells to low initial concentrations of 17-β estradiol (20nM) results in the induction of both high- and low-affinity, nuclear estrogen-binding sites (1). This regimen of hormonal addition leads to a two fold increase in secreted apolipoprotein(apo) AI and a 2.5 fold increase in secreted apolipoprotein (apo) CII without affecting the steady state levels of the other major apolipoproteins. We were interested to determine if the hormone was acting at a pre- or post-translational stage and to examine the temporal correlation between the various effects of the hormone on these cells. To do this, we have synthesized a triacontanucleotide DNA probe, complementary to position -29 to +1 of human apoAI mRNA, for use in RNA blotting experiments and in a DNA excess, equilibrium, hybridization assay to determine absolute levels of apoAI mRNA in these cells. To correlate these results with the *in vivo* situation, we have carried out similar studies using human liver and tissue from non-human primates.

RESULTS AND DISCUSSION. Initial northern blotting experiments using the synthetic oligonucleotide detected a single mRNA species of 1100 nucleotides in total RNA isolated from HepG2 cells, in good agreement with similar studies using RNA isolated from human liver. The probe is complementary to a region of the mRNA which might be expected to be well conserved by virtue of its coding for part of the prepro region of apo AI which is involved in the secretion and processing of the mature protein. This was confirmed by using the oligonucleotide to determine the size and relative abundance of monkey apoAI mRNA by northern blotting experiments.

Previous experiments have documented the induction of estrogen receptors in HepG2 cells by 17-β estradiol. Examination of apoAI mRNA levels by DNA excess, equilibrium hybridizations demonstrated that levels were twice as high in cells treated with hormone as those in similar cells which did not receive estrogen. The levels of apoAI mRNA, calculated from a knowledge of its molecular weight and the specific activity of the probe, are 0.004% and 0.008% of the total RNA in control cells and cells treated with 20nM 17-β estradiol for 48h, respectively (Fig. 1A). There was no difference in the yield of total RNA from cells cultured in the presence or absence of the hormone and these percentages correspond to absolute levels of 425 molecules per cell for control cells and 850 molecules per cell for the estrogen treated cells. In order to establish if the response seen with 20nM estrogen was maximal, we used an extended range of estradiol concentrations (20M - 1000nM). The

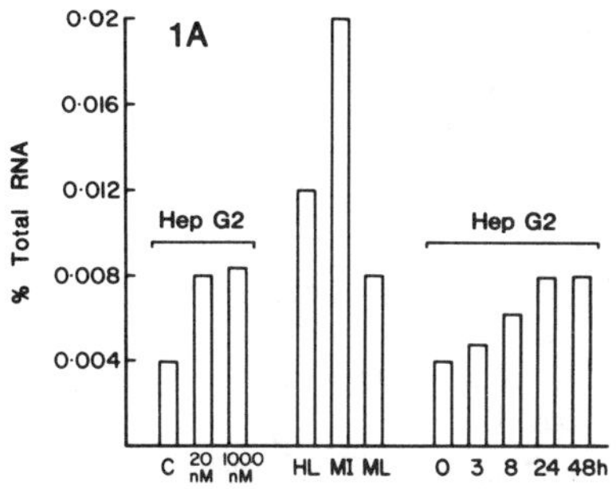

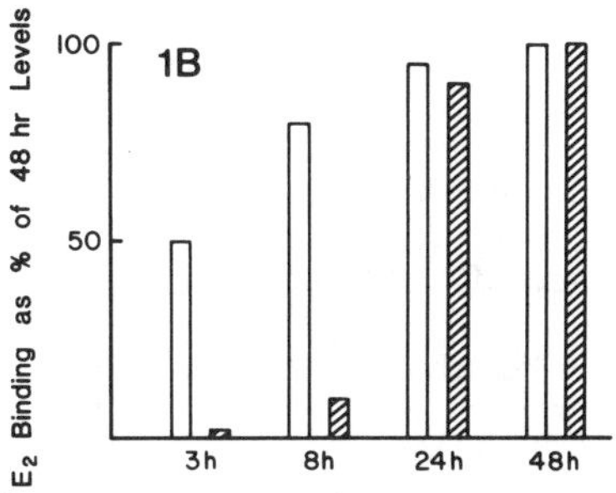

Fig.IA. ApoAI mRNA levels in HepG2 cells and primate tissues. C, control; 20nM, 17-β estradiol; 1000nM, 17-β estradiol; MI, monkey intestine; ML, monkey liver; 0h, 3h, 8h, 24h and 48h represent hours of treatment with hormone.
Fig.IB. Induction of high- and low-affinity estrogen binding sites in HepG2 cells. Open bars present high-affinity and hatched bars low-affinity binding sites. Times as in FigI.

results indicate that the two fold increase in apoAI mRNA levels is near maximal since a 50 fold increase in estrogen concentration (1000nM) led to only an additional 10% increase in mRNA levels (Fig. 1A). In order to compare the levels of apoAI mRNA seen in HepG2 cells with those observed _in vivo_, we determined the steady state levels in human liver as well as liver and intestinal epithelium of the cynomolgus monkey. In human liver, apoAI mRNA represents 0.012% of total RNA, which is 30% higher than the relative concentration in HepG2 cells treated with estrogen. ApoAI represents 0.008% of the total RNA in the monkey liver which is twice that in control HepG2 cells. In the intestine apoAI mRNA is 0.02% of the total RNA or 21/2 times the relative level in monkey liver (Fig. 1A).

We have extended our analysis of the influence of estrogen on apoAI mRNA synthesis by examining the temporal correlation of the induction of the estrogen receptor and the low-affinity binding component with the increase in apoAI mRNA levels. The receptor levels increase relatively rapidly to 50% and 80% of their maximal level within 3h and 8h of the initial exposure to estrogen, respectively. The low-affinity or type II receptor exhibits a lag of several hours reaching only 10% of the 48h level 8h after the addition of hormone (fig. 1B). The kinetics of apoAI mRNA induction are such that there is a 20% increase over control levels at 3h and a 55% increase at 8h after exposure to the hormone (Fig. IA). These results are consistent with a potential role for the estrogen receptor in the estrogen induced increase in apoAI mRNA.

REFERENCES

(1) Tam, S-P., Archer, T.K. and Deeley, R.G. (1985) J. Biol. Chem. 260, 1670-1675.
(2) Archer, T.K., Tam, S-P. and Deeley, R.G. (1985) J. Biol. Chem. 260, 1676-1681.

PARATHYROID HORMONE REGULATION OF THE RENAL PRODUCTION OF 1,25-DIHYDROXYVITAMIN D BY PHOSPHORYLATION AND DEPHOSPHORYLATION

H. James Armbrecht and Neal A. Siegel
Geriatric Center, VA Medical Center, St. Louis, MO 63125 and Depts. of Med. and Biochem., St. Louis Univ., St. Louis, MO 63104

Parathyroid hormone (PTH) markedly stimulates the renal conversion of 25-hydroxyvitamin D (25(OH)D) to 1,25-dihydroxyvitamin D ($1,25(OH)_2D$), the biologically active metabolite of vitamin D. This conversion takes place in the inner mitochondrial membrane by a hydroxylase system consisting of a cytochrome P450, a ferredoxin protein, and NADPH-dependent ferredoxin reductase. The specific mechanism by which PTH stimulates this system is largely unknown. It is known that PTH stimulates adenylate cyclase, increases intracellular cAMP levels, and stimulates cAMP-dependent protein kinase activity in the kidney (1). The purposes of this study were to determine if any components of the hydroxylase system undergo phosphorylation modification, if phosphorylation is modified by PTH, and if altered phosphorylation results in altered hydroxylase activity.

PHOSPHORYLATION OF THE P450 HYDROXYLASE SYSTEM

Slices of rat renal cortex were prelabeled with $[^{32}P]PO_4$ for 30 min. and then exposed to agonists for 5 min. The hydroxylase complex was isolated from solubilized mitochondria using a p-chloroamphetamine-sepharose affinity column (2). Solubilized mitochondria were loaded onto the affinity column, the column was washed exhaustively, and the P450 hydroxylase complex was eluted off with a higher concentration of detergent. The eluted column fractions contained both protein and large amounts of ^{32}P, which co-eluted. The eluted fractions were concentrated and found to contain cytochrome P450, which was detected spectrophotometrically. To determine which proteins were phosphorylated, the concentrated fractions were subjected to SDS-polyacrylamide slab gel electrophoresis. Silver-staining revealed multiple protein bands in the 10,000-70,000 mw region. However, autoradiography revealed only a single band of radioactivity in the 10,000-12,000 mw region. No radioactivity was seen in the 40,000-60,000 mw region which is characteristic of cytochrome P450's.

EFFECT OF PTH ON PHOSPHORYLATION

Exposure of renal slices to PTH (5 U/ml) before isolation of the P450 complex altered the protein phosphorylation pattern. PTH treatment consistantly decreased the amount of radioactivity associated with P450 complex by about 50%. Likewise, autoradiography revealed a decrease of about 50% in the amount of radioactivity in the 10,000-12,000 mw region of the gel. PTH treatment did not result in any new proteins being phosphorylated and did not alter the P450 content of mitochondria. Time course studies showed that the PTH-induced dephosphorylation was maximal at 5 min. Interestingly, treatment of renal slices with the calcium ionophore A23187 resulted in a significant increase in phosphorylation of the 10,000-12,000 mw band.

EFFECT OF PTH ON HYDROXYLATION

Parallel experiments were conducted to determine if PTH treatment altered the capacity of the isolated P450 complex to metabolize 25(OH)D. Hydroxylase activity was assayed by using tritiated 25(OH)D as a substrate and isolating the tritiated products by HPLC. Using this procedure, PTH treatment doubled $1,25(OH)_2D$ production by slices which were incubated under the same conditions that resulted in decreased protein phosphorylation.

DISCUSSION

This study shows that PTH treatment alters the phosphorylation state of a 10,000-12,000 mw protein associated with the 25(OH)D-1-hydroxylase activity isolated from renal mitochondria. Although the phosphorylated protein was not positively identifieid in this study, the renal ferredoxin has a molecular weight of 12,000 and is a likely candidate (3). We therefore propose the following sequence of events for PTH stimulation of renal $1,25(OH)_2D$ production. PTH binds to its receptor, stimulates adenylate cyclase activity, raises intracellular cAMP levels, and activates cAMP-dependent protein kinase. Protein kinase activates a protein phospatase, which then dephosphorylates the renal ferredoxin. The dephosphorylation of the ferredoxin results in increased hydroxylation of 25(OH)D by the P450 complex. Further work is needed to verify this hypothesis and to localize the protein kinase and phosphatase components. However, alterations in this phosphorylation/dephosphorylation scheme may explain the refractoriness to PTH seen in diabetes (4), aging (5), and other conditions.

REFERENCES

(1) Armbrecht, H.J., Wongsurawat, N., Zenser, T.V. and Davis, B.B. (1984) Amer. J. Physiol. 246, E102-E107.
(2) Warner, M. (1982) J. Biol. Chem. 257, 12995-13000.
(3) Pederson, J.I., Ghazarian, J.G., Orme-Johnson, N. and DeLuca, H.F. (1976) J. Biol. Chem. 251, 3933-3941.
(4) Wongsurawat, N. and Armbrecht, H.J. (1985) Acta Endocrinologica 109, 243-248.
(5) Armbrecht, H.J., Wongsurawat, N., Zenser, T.V. and Davis, B.B. (1982) Endocrinology 111, 1339-1344.

ACKNOWLEDGEMENTS

This work was supported by the Veterans Administration, USPHS Grant AM32158 (HJA), and USPHS Grant AG05366 (NAS).

MONOCLONAL ANTIBODY RECOGNITION OF ESTROGEN RECEPTOR ISOFORMS

A. Baldi, S.M. Hyder, N. Sato, D.M. Boyle and J.L. Wittliff
Hormone Receptor Laboratory, J.G. Brown Cancer Center, University of Louisville, Louisville, KY 40292 USA

Monoclonal antibodies (MAb) to estrogen receptors[1] (ER) allow a new means of recognition of these proteins in hormone sensitive breast tumors. We demonstrated that ER exhibits heterogeneity which may account for some receptor-positive patients not showing a response to hormone therapy[2]. It must be demonstrated that MAb recognizes all receptor isoforms in cytosols in a quantifiable fashion that correlates with established ligand binding procedures. We used HPLC to separate ER isoforms and then reacted these with the MAb. Procedures for HPLC fractionation, cytosol preparation, and estrogen receptor enzyme immunoassay (ER-EIA; Abbott Labs) are published elsewhere[3]. Studies documented here show that there was not an equivalent relationship between the ligand binding assay and the antibody-based assay.

ER-EIA was used to quantify ER in unfractionated cytosol or in samples fractionated by HPIEC and HPSEC. The EIA is purported to measure receptor content (mass)and is based on a sandwich technique which involves two different MAb sites on the ER. It should be noted that steroid binding sites associated with the immobilized MAb may be assayed by placing the bead in a gamma-counter and measuring bound radioactivity. The beads are then developed for the peroxidase assay as recommended. We also suggested various possibilites which may lead to discrepancies within the ligand-based and the antibody-based assay[3].

Table 1
Interaction of ER Isoforms With Monoclonal Antibody. Values shown are in fmol

	Radioactivity($^{125}IE_2$)		ER-EIA	
	Total Applied	Bead Bound	DES -	DES+
Isoform I (50 mM phosphate)	734	201 (27.3%)	667	998
Isoform II 115 mM phosphate)	1253	469 (37.4%)	1264	1768
Isoform III (200 mM phosphate)	469	181 (38.6%)	584	778

Table 1 demonstrates that the various ^{125}I-iodoestradiol ($^{125}IE_2$) labeled isoforms eluted from HPIEC only partially interact with MAb (25-40%). Unfractionated cytosol exhibited similar properties, i.e. ~30% binding to the MAb. The MAb is therefore unable to recognize all liganded receptor or the ligand $^{125}IE_2$ is blocking the immunodeterminant site of the receptor. In the presence of ^{3}H-estradiol, MAb binding is only slightly higher (~40%).

Fig. 1 Autoradiography of MAb-Immobilized autophosphorylated ER from MCF-7 cells separated by SDS-PAGE

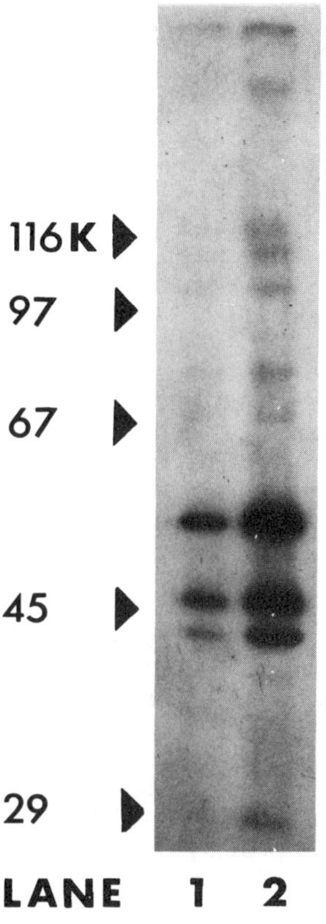

When radiolabeled receptor-MAb complex was compared with the total receptor mass detected by EIA, the [receptor] on the bead was 3-fold higher. The ER-EIA profile, however, was the same as that observed for elution of macromolecular bound radioactivity from the column. It appears the MAb also recognized other components present in ER positive tissues since ER negative tissues did not inhibit recognition of the immunodeterminant sites. Thus, immunodeterminant sites are distinguishable from steroid binding sites. Using ER-EIA, the ER concentration in samples containing DES and [^{125}I]E_2 was higher than that of samples containing only iodoestradiol suggesting that Iodine partially masks the ER-EIA measurement of the receptor. Other experiments were conducted toward understanding the stoichiometry between ligand-binding and MAb adsorption. Possibilities include multiple polypeptides being recognized or conformation-sensitive epitopes within a protein molecule. Steroid hormone receptors show subunit structure and are probably involved in regulatory phosphorylation reactions. Some of these demonstrate intrinsic protein kinase (autophosphorylating) activity. Immunoimmobilized proteins from cytosol from MCF-7 human breast cancer cells by this procedure are shown to contain autophosphorylating activitiesusing [Y-^{32}P]ATP as substrate[4]. The activity was dependent upon Mg^{2+} and inhibited by Ca^{2+}. As shown in Fig. 1, three major bands of radioactivity were detected at 57, 47, and 43 Kd. These are apparently not the result of proteolysis(lane 2). The presence of catalytically active ATP-binding proteins recognized by the bead could explain why ligand-binding does not equal mass.

Acknowledgements: This research was supported in part by USPHS Grant CA-42154 from the National Cancer Institute by Marie Overbey Memorial Award from the American Cancer Society and the Phi Beta Psi Sorority. S.M.H. is a postdoctoral research fellow from The Graduate School. N.S. is a visiting investigator form Iwate Medical University, Morioka, Japan, A.B. is a visiting professor from the Department of Biochemistry, University of Buenos Aires, Argentina.

References:

1. Greene, G.L., Nolan C., Engler, J.P. and Jensen E.J. (1980) Proc. Natl. Acad. Sci. U.S.A. 77, 5115.
2. Wittliff, J.L. (1984) Cancer 53, 630.
3. Sato, N., Hyder, S.M., Lee, C., Thais, A. and Wittliff, J.L. (1985) J. Chromatogr. (in press).
4. Baldi, A., Boyle, D. and Wittliff, J.L. Submitted.

TRANSFECTION STUDIES OF THE PROLACTIN GENE

E.A. Barron, A.J. Carrillo, and Z.D. Sharp
Dept. of Cellular and Structural Biology, University of Texas Health Science Center, San Antonio, Texas

The regulation of the rat prolactin gene in pituitary lactotrophs and in transformed pituitary tissue culture cells (GH_3) is known to be very complex. Numerous agents, such as estradiol (1), thyrotropin releasing hormone (2), vasoactive intestinal peptide (3), epidermal growth factor (4), dexamethasone (5), and dopamine (6), when applied to rat pituitary cells affect prolactin transcription. To investigate the regulation of this gene in more detail, we have constructed a prolactin minigene which can be easily manipulated and identified. This construction contains a) bacterial sequences which allow it to be amplified and selected in bacteria, b) prolactin 5' and 3' flanking sequences which presumably contain putative regulatory sequences, c) the first, second and last exons of the prolactin gene, and d) a sequence engineered into the first exon which allows this construct's transcipts to be recognized from the endogenous gene transcripts.

Minigene construction. To abbreviate the large prolactin gene (10 kb) and include as much flanking sequences as possible, a 10 kb Eco R1 fragment containing the first two prolactin exons and 7 kb 5' flanking sequence was ligated with a 2.5 kb Eco RI-PvuII fragment containing the last exon (exon 5) and 2.0 kb 3' flanking sequence. The resulting 12.5 kb prolactin minigene was then ligated to an Eco RI-PvuII fragment of pBR322 which included the plasmid's origin of replication and β-lactamase gene.

Addition of Identifier Sequence. Our plans are to manipulate the putative regulatory sequences of the minigene and transfect the new construct into cells which normally make prolactin. Furthermore, we intend to analyze the transcripts from both the endogenous prolactin gene and the minigene by primer extension. To do these experiments, an additional sequence was engineered into the first exon of the minigene. This identifier sequence is located 5' to the sequence which has been chosen for the primer. Since the primer will be able to hybridize with transcripts from both the endogenous gene and minigene, this additional sequence will lengthen the minigene transcript and thereby identify it.

We chose to use SalI linkers (8 bps) as our identifier sequence. These linkers were inserted into the first exon. The chosen site of insertion was an AvaII site at +34. Due to the frequency of AvaII sites throughout the prolactin minigene, a 0.9 kb HindIII- XbaI fragment containing the first exon was subcloned. This construct was digested with AvaII, the resulting 5' protruding ends were filled, and SalI linkers were attached by blunt end ligation. The former AvaII cut ends, changed to SalI ends, were then religated to form a new exon with an 8 bp addition at the AvaII site. This new HindIII-XbaI fragment was then returned to the correct position in the prolactin minigene.

Transfection and Expression. To date, we have transfected GH_3 cells with the prolactin minigene. Blot hybridization of total DNA isolated from nuclei of the transfected cells confirmed transfection of the minigene into the cells. Our next experiment planned is to isolate RNA from GH_3 cells shortly after they have been transfected with the minigene. The prolactin transcripts, including those off the endogenous gene and those off the minigene, will then be analyzed by primer extension.

Recently, 2.5 kb of 5' flanking region of the rat prolactin gene was sequenced revealing consensus promoter sequences, palindromes and alternating purine-pyrimidine tracts (7). These sequences may or may not have some cis-acting regulatory function. The construction of this minigene enables us to easily mutate (by deletion, insertion, or substitution) these sequences, analyze the resulting expression and determine their significance in the control of constitutive, stimulated, and depressed prolactin gene activity in GH_3 cells.

REFERENCES

(1) Maurer, R.A. (1982) J.of Biol. Chem. 257, 2133-2136.
(2) Murdoch, G.H., Franco, R., Evans, R.M., and Rosenfeld, M.G. (1983) J. of Biol. Chem. 258, 15329-15335.
(3) Carrillo, A.J., Pool, T.B., and Sharp, Z.D. (1985) Endocrinology 116, 202-206.
(4) Murdoch, G.H., Potter, E., Nicolaisin, A.K., Evans, R.M., Rosenfeld, M.G. (1982) Nature 300, 192-194.
(5) White, B.A., Bauerle, L.R., and Bancroft, F.C. (1981) J. of Biol. Chem. 256, 5942-5945.
(6) Maurer, R.A. (1981) Nature, 294, 94-97.
(7) Maurer, R.A. (1985) DNA 4, 1-9.

CLONING OF THE 90kDa HEAT-SHOCK PROTEIN INTERACTING WITH STEROID HORMONE RECEPTORS AND DIFFERENT VIRAL ONCOGENES

N. Binart[1], B. Chambraud[1], A. Zimiecki[2], D.M. Helfman[3], R., W.J.. Welsh[3], J.R. Feramisco[3], E.E. Baulieu[1] and M.G. Catelli[1].
1 INSERM U33, Lab Hormones, 94275 Bicêtre, France.
2 Ludwig Institute CH3010 Bern, Suisse.
3 Cold Spring Harbor Laboratory, New York, N.Y. USA.

Steroid hormone receptors found in the cytosol of target cells have ~ 8S sedimentation coefficient corresponding to an hetero-oligomeric structure of 250-300kDa. A monoclonal BF_4 antibody (1) raised against purified molybdate-stabilized 8S progesterone receptor is specific for an abundant and ubiquitous 90kDa soluble protein which does not bind steroids. This protein is a common component of all steroid hormone receptors in their 8S form (2), has been identified as the hsp90 (3) and interacts with oncogene products of several retrovirus (4).

(I) IDENTIFICATION

The 90kDa protein has been identified as an heat shock protein (Fig. 1a). In CEF infected by RSV, the 90kDa protein immunoprecipitated by L_2 polyclonal antibody presents the same V8 pattern digestion as the protein associated with $pp60^{v-src}$ and precipitated by TBR (tumor bearing rabbit) serum (Fig. 1b). The same hsp90 formed tight complex with the products of three members of the tyrosine protein kinase family of oncogenes (src, fes, fgr).

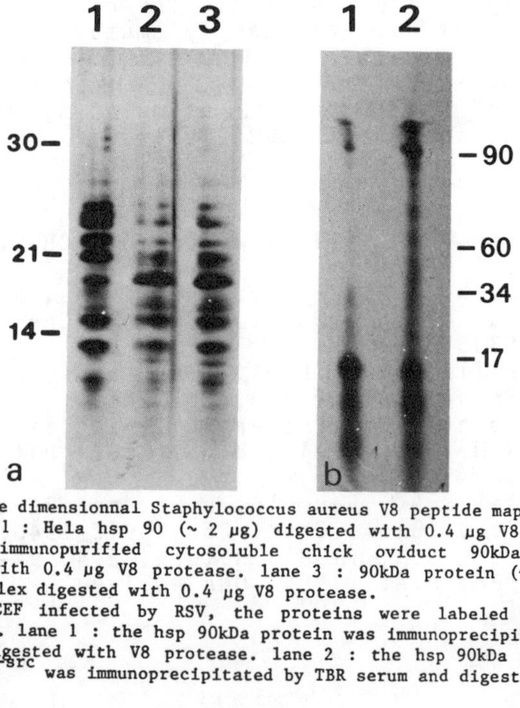

Fig. 1. One dimensionnal Staphylococcus aureus V8 peptide mapping.
1a : lane 1 : Hela hsp 90 (~ 2 µg) digested with 0.4 µg V8 protease. lane 2 : immunopurified cytosoluble chick oviduct 90kDa (~ 1 µg) digested with 0.4 µg V8 protease. lane 3 : 90kDa protein (~ 1 µg) of 8S-PR complex digested with 0.4 µg V8 protease.
1b : In CEF infected by RSV, the proteins were labeled with ^{35}S-methionine. lane 1 : the hsp 90kDa protein was immunoprecipitated with L_2, and digested with V8 protease. lane 2 : the hsp 90kDa associated with $pp60^{v-src}$ was immunoprecipitated by TBR serum and digested with V8 protease.

(II) CLONING

From a chicken smooth muscle cDNA expression library of 20,000 members (5) screened with monoclonal (BF_4) and polyclonal (L_2) antibodies, we characterized a p9.11 recombinant (1033 bp) (6). Northern blot analysis revealed a mRNA of 3kb isolated from various chicken tissues. Heat-shock treatment of CEF resulted in increased levels of 3kb transcripts. Southern blot analysis of genomic DNA showed that the cDNA hybridized to a single copy sequence. Comparison of p9.11 insert sequence data with yeast hsp90 and drosophila hsp83 DNA sequence (Fig. 2) demonstrated a high degree of homology 66.3 % and 82.6 % respectively, and indicates that we cloned the 5' portion of the coding sequence. The progesterone binding component (110kDa) of the chick progesterone receptor has been purified (7), cloning experiments are in progress and available results will be presented.

		ACC	AAG	GCT	TTC	ATG	GAA	GCA	CTG	CAG	GCA
Chicken	114	Thr	Lys	Ala	Phe	Met	Glu	Ala	Leu	Gln	Ala
Drosophila	103	Thr	Lys	Ala	Phe	Met	Glu	Ala	Leu	Gln	Ala
Yeast	101	Thr	Lys	Ala	Phe	Met	Glu	Ala	Leu	Ser	Ala
		GGG	GCT	GAT	ATT	TCC	ATG	ATT	GGT	CAG	TTT
C	124	Gly	Ala	Asp	Ile	Ser	Met	Ile	Gly	Gln	Phe
D	113	Gly	Ala	Asp	Ile	Ser	Met	Ile	Gly	Gln	Phe
Y	111	Gly	Ala	Asp	Val	Ser	Met	Ile	Gly	Gln	Phe
		GGT	GTT	GGT	TTC	TAC	TCT	GCT	TAC	CTT	GTT
C	134	Gly	Val	Gly	Phe	Tyr	Ser	Ala	Tyr	Leu	Val
D	123	Gly	Val	Gly	Phe	Tyr	Ser	Ala	Tyr	Leu	Val
Y	121	Gly	Val	Gly	Phe	Tyr	Ser	Leu	Phe	Leu	Val
		GCG	GAG	AAG	GTG	ACA	GTG	ATC	ACC	AAG	CAC
C	144	Ala	Glu	Lys	Val	Thr	Val	Ile	Thr	Lys	His
D	133	Ala	Asp	Lys	Val	Thr	Val	Thr	Ser	Lys	Asn
Y	131	Ala	Asp	Arg	Val	Gln	Val	Ile	Ser	Lys	Ser

Fig. 2. Chicken hsp 90 cDNA sequence. Comparison with yeast hsp 90 and drosophila hsp 83.

REFERENCES

1. Radanyi, C., Joab, I., Renoir, J.M., Richard-Foy, H. and Baulieu, E.E. (1983) Proc. Natl. Acad. Sci. USA, 80, 2854-2858.
2. Joab, I., Radanyi, C., Renoir, J.M., Buchou, T., Catelli, M.G., Binart, N., Mester, J. and Baulieu, E.E. (1984) Nature 308, 850-853.
3. Catelli, M.G., Binart, N., Jung-Testas, I., Renoir, J.M., Baulieu, E.E., Feramisco, J.R. and Welch, W.J. (1985) 4, in press.
4. Ziemiecki, A., Catelli, M.G., Joab, I. and Moncharmont, B. in preparation.
5. Helfman, D.M., Feramisco, J.R., Ricci, W.M. and Hughes, S.H. (1984) J. Biol. Chem. 259, 14136-14143.
6. Catelli, M.G., Binart, N., Feramisco, J.R. and Helfman, D.M. (1985) Nucleic Acids Res. 13, 6035-6047.
7. Renoir, J.M., Mester, J., Buchou, T., Catelli, M.G., Tuohimaa, P., Binart, N., Joab, I., Radanyi, C. and Baulieu, E.E. (1984) Biochem. J. 217, 685-692.

STUDIES OF NEURONAL TRANSDIFFERENTIATION IN CULTURED ADRENAL CHROMAFFIN CELLS

J.W. Brown[1], A. Carballeira[1], K.F.A. Soliman[2], and L.M. Fishman[1]
[1]V.A. Medical Center and Dept. of Medicine, University of Miami School of Medicine, Miami, FL; and [2]School of Pharmacy, Florida A & M University, Tallahassee, FL

INTRODUCTION: Normal adrenal chromaffin cells are exposed *in vivo* to high concentrations of glucocorticoid hormones from the adrenal cortex. When these influences are removed by *in vitro* culture techniques chromaffin tissue spontaneously transdifferentiates into neuronal complexes (1,2,3). Natural and synthetic glucocorticoid hormones can inhibit morphologic and biochemical aspects of this transition but steroid hormones without glucocorticoid activity are ineffective (4). In this report we show the induction of choline acetyltransferase during the transdifferentiation process and repression of this enzyme activity by dexamethasone (10^{-5}M). These alterations are inversely related to the occurrence of changes in epinephrine content and steroid 11 β-hydroxylase activity.

RESULTS: Table 1 shows the morphologic and biochemical alterations that occur in cultured bovine adrenal chromaffin cells derived from normal adult animals. With increasing times *in vitro* cells were found to develop neurite projections in a progressive manner. Changes were also seen in biochemical markers for cholinergic neurons as evidenced by a progressive increase in choline acetyltransferase activity. Two parameters of the endocrine function of these cells (i.e., epinephrine content and steroid 11 β-hydroxylase activity), however, declined under identical conditions.

Table 1. *In Vitro* Alterations in Markers of Neuronal and Endocrine Function

Function	Days in Culture			
	0	5	25	65
Neuronal Differentiation				
Neurite Projection (% of cells)	0	4	19	24
Synapse Formation (% of cells)	0	1	6	6
Choline Acetyltransferase (nmoles COASH* formed/minute/10^6 cells)	12.2	14.7	18.1	25.6
Endocrine Differentiation				
Epinephrine Content (μg/10^6 cells)	5.1	1.5	0.4	N.D.
Steroid 11 β-Hydroxylase (dpm/cell)**	N.D.	1.1	0.3	0.2

*COASH = CoA Sulfhydryl
**Cells were incubated for 72 hours in 1.0 ml of Medium 199 containing 1.0 μCi ^{3}H-DOC (41.8 Ci/mmol). 11 β-hydroxylase was measured by conversion of DOC (11-deoxycorticosterone) to corticosterone. N.D. means no data available.

Choline acetyltransferase activity was diminished with dexamethasone treatment (Table 2) but spontaneously increased in redifferentiating cultures in its absence (Table 1). We have also found that epinephrine content increases relative to control cultures in the presence of dexamethasone. Table 2 presents similar findings with another endocrine parameter, steroid 11 β-hydroxylase, whose presence in chromaffin tissue has been documented and discussed elsewhere (5).

Table 2. *In Vitro* Effects of Dexamethasone on Neuronal and Endocrine Function

Function	Control	Dexamethasone (10^{-5} M)
Neuronal Differentiation		
Neurite Projection (% of Cells)	34 ± 8	18 ± 6
Synapse Formation (% of Cells)	8 ± 3	4 ± 2
Choline Acetyltransferase (% of Control Activity)	100 ± 34	60 ± 4
Endocrine Differentiation		
Epinephrine Content (μg/10^6 cells)	0.41 ± 0.08	0.76 ± 0.01
Steroid 11-β Hydroxylase (% of Control Activity)	100 ± 2	154 ± 2

Data represent Mean ± Range or SE of 2 - 6 determinations. Bovine adrenal chromaffin cell cultures were grown in control medium or in medium containing dexamethasone (10^{-5}M) for 22-25 days before assay.

CONCLUSION: From these observations we conclude that glucocorticoid hormones can inhibit phenotypic aspects of neuronal transdifferentiation in cultured chromaffin tissue. These effects include the inhibition of neurite projection and resultant synapse formation and reduction in choline acetyltransferase activity. Dexamethasone also inhibits spontaneous *in vitro* declines in cellular catecholamine content and steroid hydroxylating capability. The molecular basis for steroid effects in these cells are yet to be determined. From findings in other systems (6) it is probable that complex transcriptional processes may be involved in these alterations.

REFERENCES: (1) Unsicker, K. (1977) Verh. Anat. Ges. 71, 1227-1229. (2) Unsicker, K., and Chamley, J.H. (1977) Cell Tiss. Res. 177, 247-268. (3) Unsicker, K., Griesser, G.H., Lindmar, R., Loffelholz, K., and Wolf, U. (1980) Neurosci. 5, 1445-1460. (4) Brown, J.W., Carballeira, A., and Fishman, L.M. (1984) Excerta Medica 652, 679. (5) Carballeira, A., and Fishman, L.M. (1980) Perspect. Biol. Med. 23, 573-579. (6) O'Malley, B.W., and Means, A.R. (1974) Science 183, 610-620.

ACKNOWLEDGMENTS: This project was supported by NIH Grant BRSG S07 RR-05363 and also by V.A. Merit Review 2839.01. We thank Dagoburto Trujillo and Linda Williams for technical assistance.

IDENTIFICATION OF A NUCLEAR SUBSTRATE OF THE CYCLIC AMP-DEPENDENT PROTEIN KINASE OF DICTYOSTELIUM DISCOIDEUM.

T. C. Chambers[+], J. Song[+], D. S. Campbell[+]. B. H. Leichtling[+] and H. V. Rickenberg[+*].

[+]Dept. of Molecular and Cellular Biology, National Jewish Center for Immunology and Respiratory Medicine, Denver, CO 80206 and *Dept. of Biochemistry, Biophysics and Genetics, University of Colorado Health Sciences Center.

We are investigating the control of transcription of genes regulated by cAMP during development of the cellular slime mold *Dictyostelium discoideum*. Specifically we consider the possibility that such control may be mediated by the phosphorylation of certain nuclear proteins by the cAMP-dependent protein kinase (cA-dPK). In this report we present evidence that a basic, nuclear non-histone protein of apparent M_r 38-kDa may be a substrate of the cA-dPK and we describe some of the properties of this phosphoprotein.

METHODS

D. discoideum nuclei, prepared as described (1), were isolated from vegetative amoebae, from multicellular aggregates at defined stages of development, and from prespore and prestalk cells. Three conditions of phosphorylation were studied. (I) *In vitro*: Nuclear extracts were incubated for 2 min at 23°C with γ^{32}P-ATP in the presence or absence of purified bovine or *D. discoideum* catalytic subunit. (II) *In situ*: As (I), except with intact nuclei. (III) *In vivo*: 1 mCi $^{32}P_i$ per 10^8 cells added 2 h prior to the preparation of nuclei. Phosphoproteins were analysed as described in the figure legend (see Ref. (2)).

RESULTS

Previous studies showed that *D. discoideum* cA-dPK is translocated from the cytoplasm to the nucleus in a developmentally regulated manner; maximum nuclear levels of both catalytic and regulatory subunits are found at the tipped aggregate and later stages of development (1). When nuclear extracts were incubated under phosphorylation condition I, the level of phosphorylation of a very basic phosphoprotein of apparent M_r 38-kDa (pp38) was markedly increased in the presence of added homologous or heterologous catalytic subunit (Fig. 1, B and C). Under conditions II and III (Fig. 1, A and D respectively), the level of phosphorylation of pp38 paralleled the level of activity of nuclear cA-dPK, i.e. *in situ* and *in vivo*, pp38 is most highly phosphorylated from the tipped aggregate to the early culmination stages of development. We find that pp38 does not copurify with the histones; e.g. it is distinct from histone H1 of *D. discoideum* which is not a substrate for cA-dPK (data not shown). Phosphoprotein pp38 occurs at very low abundance and is present in nuclei from vegetative amoebae and from multicellular aggregates at all stages of development, and is found in nuclei from both prespore and prestalk cells.

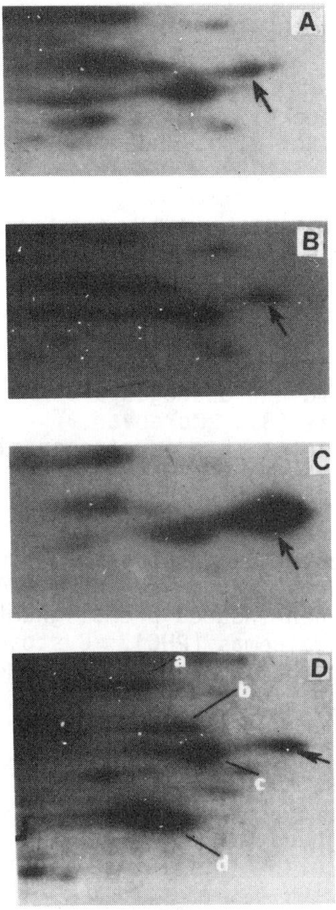

Fig. 1. 2D Gel Electrophoresis of pp38 (arrows). Nuclear phosphoproteins were separated by basic non-equilibrium pH gradient electrophoresis (left to right) and 12% acrylamide SDS gel electrophoresis (top to bottom). The basic portion spanning M_r 40-30 kDa of each autoradiograph is shown. (A) Nuclei from tipped aggregates phosphorylated *in situ*. (B) Nuclei from tipped aggregates phosphorylated *in vitro*, no added catalytic subunit. (C) As (B), with added bovine catalytic subunit. (D) *In vivo*, nuclei from early culminating $^{32}P_i$-labeled cells.

pp38 appears to be the major nuclear substrate for cA-dPK. In addition, we have found several presumptive nuclear substrates of the cA-dPK which occur predominantly in either prestalk or in prespore cells, respectively.

CONCLUSION

We have identified in *D. discoideum* a nuclear substrate of the cA-dPK. It is a very basic, non-histone protein of apparent M_r 38-kDa and seems to have properties distinct from nuclear substrates of the cA-dPKs identified in other cells (e.g. (3)). We have yet to compare phosphopeptide maps of pp38 phosphorylated *in vivo* and *in vitro*; therefore our studies do not rule out rigorously the possibility that pp38 is phosphorylated by a cyclic nucleotide-independent protein kinase which in turn is activated by cA-dPK.

REFERENCES

(1) Woffendin, C., Chambers, T. C., Schaller, K. L., Leichtling, B. H. and Rickenberg, H. V. (1985) Developmental Biology, in press.

(2) Morrissey, J. H., Devine, K. M. and Loomis, W. F. (1984) Developmental Biology, 103, 414-424.

(3) Waterman, M., Murdoch, G. H., Evans, R. M. and Rosenfeld, M. G. (1985) Science, 229, 267-269.

DECREASE IN GLUCOCORTICOID RECEPTORS DURING CHEMICAL-INDUCED HEPATOCARCINOGENEIS IN RAT

John Y. H. Chan, Nguyen T. Van, and F. F. Becker
Departments of Pathology and Hematology, UTSCC M. D. Anderson Hospital and Tumor Institute, Houston, Texas 77030

Experimental findings have indicated that steroid hormones and their receptors play a pivotal role in modifying the development of several cancers including the hepatocarcinomas. Adrenalectomy has been reported to decrease or completely block carcinogenesis while administration of deoxycorticosterone acetate protected against hepatomas (1). Gonadal steroids were shown to modify hepatic neoplasia (2) whereas antiglucocorticoid and antiandrogen are potential promoters for liver carcinogenesis (3). Moreover, glucocorticoid inhibited the promotion phase of skin carcinogenesis (4) and cellular transformation *in vitro* (5).

To determine if glucocorticoid receptors (GR) are altered during chemical hepatocarcinogenesis, we measure the specific binding of $[^3H]$ dexamethasone (DEX) to cytosolic receptor and that of receptor-hormone complex to nuclei isolated from normal rat liver (NRL), 24 hour regenerating rat liver (RRL), carcinogen-induced premalignant nodules (NN) and primary hepatocellular carcinomas (PHC). Cystosolic GR was measured by incubating cytosol with $[^3H]$ DEX in the presence and absence of 100-fold excess of unlabeled steroid at 2°C overnight. The unbound steroids were removed by charcoal-dextran, and the bound $[^3H]$ DEX was counted by liquid scintillation (6,7). Nuclear binding assay was performed by binding rat liver cytosol with $[^3H]$ DEX and then further incubated with isolated nuclei. After extensively washing with buffer, nuclear bound steroids were extracted with ethanol, and counted by liquid scintillation (6).

In 24-hr regenerating liver, cytosolic GR was reduced to 46% of normal liver controls while those of the nodules and PHC were reduced to 50% and 35%, respectively (Table I). Scatchard plot analysis indicates that the reduction is due to decreases in receptor number rather than to reduced affinity (Table II). When the nuclear binding of steroid receptor complex was compared, nuclei from nodules and PHC retained 50% and 43%, respectively, of the control GR level, while that of the 24-hr regenerating liver was unaltered (Table III).

The decreased cytosolic GR during liver carcinogenesis is in accord with previous report on reduced GR during chemical-induced skin carcinogenesis (7). Reduced GR nuclear binding has also been reported during acute carcinogen treatment in rat liver (8). These alterations may have some bearing on the reported alteration of hormone-induced enzyme regulatory mechanism in certain hepatomas (9), and in their escape from growth regulation during the neoplastic developmental process.

Table I - [^{3}H] Dexamethasone (DEX) binding to cytosol during hepatocarcinogenesis.

	fmole/mg Protein			
	Total	Nonspecific	Specific	%
NRL	360±20	40±5	320	100
Reg. L	182±16	36±7	146	46
Nodule	201±32	39±9	162	50
PHC	148±18	36±7	112	35

Table II - Effect of increasing [^{3}H] DEX on cytosolic receptor during hepatocarcinogenesis.

(fmole)	[^{3}H] DEX Bound (fmole/mg Protein)		
[^{3}H] DEX	NRL	Reg. L	Nodule
484	186	80	94
968	242	107	127
1452	292	116	141
Kd (nM)	1.97	1.9	2.1

Table III - Nuclear binding of steroid-receptor complex during hepatocarcinogenesis.

	Nuclei Bound [^{3}H] DEX (fmole/mg DNA)	%
NRL	545±80	100
Reg. L	505±74	93
Nodule	272±63	50
PHC	237±70	43

REFERENCES

1. Reuber, M.D. (1965) J. Nat. Cancer Inst. 34, 587-594.
2. Yeager, J.D., Jr. (1984) in Mechanism of Tumor Promotion (Slaga, T.J., ed.) CRC Press Vol 1, pp. 56-70.
3. Schulte Hermannn R., Ohde, G., Schuppler, J. and Timmermonn-Trosiener, T. (1981) Cancer Res. 41, 2556-2562.
4. Slaga, T.J. (1984) in Mechanism of Tumor Promotion (Slaga, T.J., ed.) CRC Press, Vol. 2, pp. 1-16.
5. Kennedy, A.R. (1984) in Mechanism of Tumor Promotion (Slaga, T.J., ed.) CRC Press, Vol. 3, pp. 13-56.
6. Higgins, S. Rousseau, G.G., Baxter, J.D. and Tomkins, G.M., (1973) J. Biol. Chem. 248, 5866-5872.
7. Davidson, K and Slaga, T.J. (1983) Cancer Res. 43, 3847-3851.
8. Kensler, T.W., Busby, W.F., Davidson, N.R. and Hogen F.N. (1976) Cancer Res. 36, 4647-4651.
9. Shapot, V.S. (1980) Biochemical Aspect of Tumor Growth (Shapot, V.S.,ed.) MIR Publishers Moscow, pp. 100-114.

Supported by NIH grant CA20657

REGULATED EXPRESSION FROM THE PRO-OPIOMELANOCORTIN PROMOTER PRESENT ON BOVINE PAPILLOMA VIRUS EPISOMAL DNA

J. Charron, and J. Drouin, Laboratoire de biologie moléculaire des eucaryotes, Institut de recherches cliniques de Montréal, 110 ouest, Avenue des Pins, Montréal, Canada H2W 1R7.

Regulation of eucaryotic gene expression by steroid hormones has provided the most detailed insight into the mechanism of transcriptional regulation. The gene encoding pro-opiomelanocortin (POMC) offers an interesting model system to study inhibition of transcription by steroid hormones. Indeed, glucocorticoids specifically inhibit transcription of the POMC gene in the anterior but not in the intermediate pituitary (1,2). This action was shown to take place at the transcriptional level and to effectively modify POMC mRNA levels in vivo (3,4). On the other hand, pituitary POMC gene transcription is stimulated by corticoliberin (CRH) and cyclic AMP. POMC is the precursor to a variety of hormones: ACTH, β-endorphin and the melanotropins. We have used the bovine papilloma virus (BPV) vector to study the control of POMC transcription. BPV replicates autonomously as an episome in rodent cells in culture and, thus, offers the possibility to characterize regulatory mechanisms in a well defined chromosomal environment (5).

BPV transformed cells

In order to study POMC regulatory mechanisms, we designed a hybrid transcription unit constituted of a rat POMC promoter fragment (from -709 to +63 bp) linked to SV40 T antigen coding sequences (POMC-Tag). We used four POMC-Tag/BPV plasmids containing POMC-Tag and BPV sequences (69% or 100%) in the two possible relative orientations. All four constructs were transfected in mouse C127 cells as supercoiled plasmids or deleted of the pBR327 sequences. Supercoiled plasmid DNAs produced fewer transformed foci, and none of these contained only unrearranged episomal BPV DNA. The four BPV constructs lacking pBR327 sequences produced similar numbers of transformed foci. Individual foci were cloned, propagated and their DNA was analysed by Southern blot. Overall, we find that constructs containing the 69% rather than the 100% BPV fragment more frequently yield transformed cell lines containing only unrearranged episomes and no chromosomal integration. The analysis of a number of representative clones is shown in Fig. 1a and three clones chosen for full investigation are further analysed in Fig. 1b.

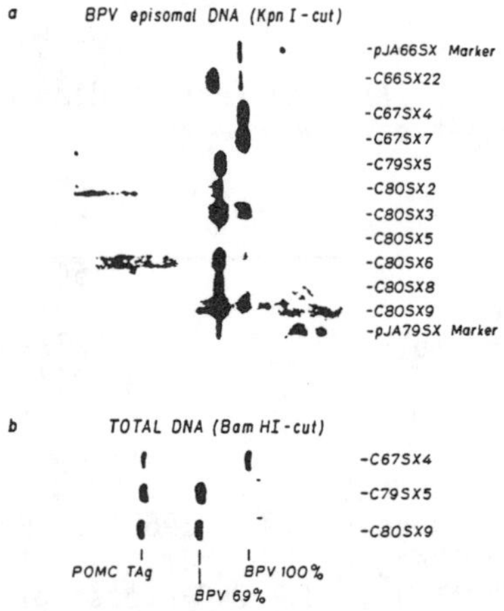

Fig. 1. Southern blot analysis of episomal (a) or total DNA (b) extracted from BPV-transformed cell lines.

Transcription and regulation

POMC-Tag, BPV and cellular actin transcripts were detected by Northern blotting of total cytoplasmic RNA; all cell lines contain the two expected POMC-Tag mRNAs encoding large and small T antigen. Incubation of these cells overnight in media containing 10^{-7}M dexamethasone (DEX) decreases POMC-Tag cytoplasmic mRNA levels 2 to 3-fold in various cell lines and experiments; this treatment did not alter BPV or cellular actin mRNA levels.

The precise 5' end of the POMC-Tag transcripts detected by Northern blot was determined by RNAase and nuclease S1 mapping (Fig. 2). In all cell lines, the probe protects the 87 nt only a fragment expected of transcripts initiating at the same site as in rat pituitary (6). The amount of protected fragment is also decreased about 3-fold by DEX treatment.

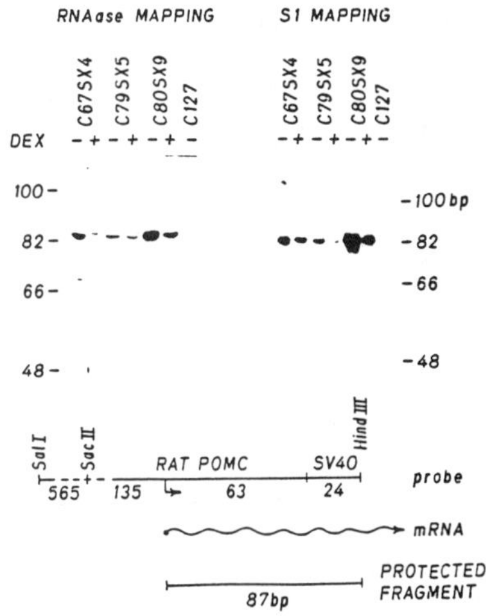

Fig. 2. Analysis of the 5'-end of POMC-Tag transcripts by RNAase and Nuclease S1 mapping.

In conclusion, transcription from the POMC promoter present on BPV episomes initiates at the correct site and is inhibited by glucocorticoids in the same way as in the anterior pituitary and as in AtT-20 cells electroporated with genes under control of the POMC promoter (7). It would therefore appear that inhibition of POMC transcription is not dependent on the activity of the POMC tissue-specific enhancer sequence (8) since this sequence element should not be active in C127 cells.

This work is supported by MRC and NCI of Canada.

REFERENCES

(1) Birnberg, N.C. et al. (1983) PNAS USA **80**, 6982-6986.
(2) Gagner, J.P. and Drouin, J. (1985) Mol. Cell. Endoc. **40**, 25-32.
(3) Bruhn, T.O. et al. (1984) Neuroendocrinology **39**, 170-175.
(4) Hollt, V. and Haarmann, I. (1984) Biochem. Biophys. R. C. **124**, 407-415.
(5) Sarver, N. et al. (1981) Mol. Cell. Biol. **1**, 486-496.
(6) Drouin, J. et al. (1985) FEBS Letters, in press.
(7) Drouin, J. et al. (1985) Short report submitted to this meeting.
(8) Jeannotte, L. et al. (1985) Short report submitted to this meeting.

ALTERNATIVE 3' ENDS OF HISTONE MRNA

Nunta Chodcoy*, Jane Levine**, Art Skoultchi** and William F. Marzluff*, *Dept. of Chemistry, Florida State Univ., Tallahassee, Fla. and **Dept. of Cell Biology, Albert Einstein School of Medicine, Bronx, N.Y.

Histone mRNA levels are stringently regulated in mouse cells both by controlling the transcription of histone genes and the halflife of histone mRNA (1,2). To investigate the sequences involved in histone gene expression a chimeric histone gene was constructed from two mouse histone genes and reintroduced by cotransfection with the thymidine kinase gene into mouse L cells. The chimeric genes were expressed and correctly regulated (3). However in addition to the expected histone transcript there was a longer transcript (RNA X) which was polyadenylated and was not regulated at the level of mRNA degradation (3). We have investigated the formation of RNA X by constructing other genes with altered 3' ends.

Three different histone genes containing this 3' end were introduced into mouse L cells; two chimeric genes and the native gene (Fig. 1). All three of these genes produced RNA X which was derived solely from the transfected gene. Thus part of the basis for formation of RNA X is the chromosomal location of the transfected gene far from the normal histone cluster.

Since RNA X appeared to be formed as a result of the failure of normal histone 3' end formation, we constructed deletions of the normal hairpin loop at the 3' end of histone mRNA (Fig. 1). When these genes were introduced into mouse L cells they were expressed but the major product was a new RNA species, RNA Y, which had a 3' end 155 bases 3' of the normal histone 3' end (Fig. 2). There was also a small amount of RNA X produced, similar in proportion to the amount produced in cells transfected with the intact gene. RNA Y is also polyadenylated and insensitive to DNA synthesis inhibitors. The ends of both RNA X and RNA Y were determined by S1 nuclease mapping. There is a consensus polyadenylation signal 35 bases before the end of RNA X and no polyadenylation signal near the 3' end of RNA Y (Fig. 3). This suggests that RNA Y represents a product of transcription termination or the product of a processing event which may be the normal precursor to histone mRNA 3' end formation.

To distinguish between these possibilities nuclear transcription experiments were done. There was equimolar transcription of the complete 3' flanking region and the H3.1-221 gene. This result suggests that RNA Y is formed by a cleavage reaction which may normally precede histone 3' end formation. We cannot competely rule out the possibility that RNA Y is formed by transcription termination *in vivo* which is not reproduced in isolated nuclei. The cleavage to form RNA Y is "leaky" in the transfected cells and then RNA X is formed by the normal polyadenylation mechanism.

References:
1. Sittman, D.B., Graves, R.A. and Marzluff., W.F. (1983) Proc. Nat. Acad. Sci. 80 1849-53.
2. Graves, R.A. and Marzluff, W.F. (1984) Mol. Cell. Biol. 4 351-57.
3. Alterman, R.A., Sprecher, C.S. Graves, R.A. Marzluff, W.F. and Skoultchi, A.I. (1985) Mol. Cell. Biol. 5 2316-24.

Supported by NIH grant GM 27789.

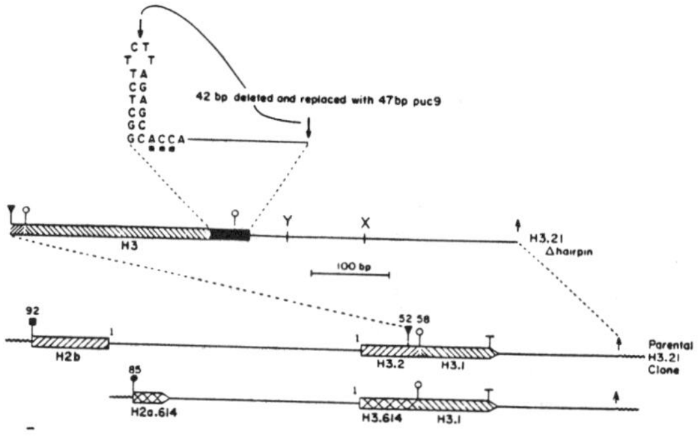

Fig. 1. The 3 constructions used are indicated.

P

X

Y

H3.1

H3

1 2 3 4

Fig.2 The products of the gene with the 3' end deletion were determined by S1 nuclease mapping. The band H3.1 is from the endogenous H3.1 gene, while X and Y are derived from the transfected gene. Lane 1: end-labeled probe; Lane 2: total RNA; Lane 3: Poly A^- RNA; Lane 4: Poly A^+ RNA.

```
                                                      H3.1
                                                        *
   TTTCTGT TAATCCACAC AACCACTTTA AAGGCTCTTC TTAGAGCCAC CCATCTTCCA
AAAAAAAGAA CTGTGCGCTT TTTCCAACTT GTGGGTATTA ATCAGTTTCA TTTGTGAAAG
TGCTAGGTCT CCTTTCATCA CACCGATCTA TTATAAGCAA GCAATATTTT GGTAAGTGAT

                              Y
                              **
ATCTTTACCC TTTTTCATGG AAATTGTACT CTTAGTTAGC AAAGCATAAA GATTGGAAAA
CTTTGCATGG TTACAGTAAT TTGGGCATTT ACCGAATTTA AAAAATAAAA TTATTAGTTG

                                  X
                          *       **
CAGATGTTTA CTTTGGAATT GTGAACTTTC TAAGGACAGA ACCACTAATA TTGTAACTCA
```

Fig. 3. The sequence of the 3' flanking region of the H3.1 gene is shown. The * mark the position of the 3 3' end sequences observed. The dyad at the normal histone 3' end and the polyadenylation signal are underlined.

DNA SEQUENCE ELEMENT RESPONSIBLE FOR INHIBITION OF PRO-OPIOMELANOCORTIN GENE TRANSCRIPTION BY GLUCOCORTICOIDS

J. Drouin, J.P. Gagner, L. Jeannotte, and R.K. Plante, Institut de recherches cliniques de Montréal, 110 ouest, Avenue des Pins, Montréal, Canada H2W 1R7.
Ö. Wrange, Karolinska Institute, Stockholm, Sweden.

The gene encoding pro-opiomelanocortin (POMC) offers an interesting model system to study negative control of transcription in eucaryotes. Indeed, glucocorticoids specifically inhibit transcription of the POMC gene and consequently decrease POMC mRNA levels in the anterior pituitary but not in the intermediate lobe of the pituitary where the single-copy POMC gene is also expressed.

We have isolated and characterized the rat POMC (rPOMC) gene (1,2). Glucocorticoid treatment decreases anterior pituitary POMC transcription rate about 10-fold in <u>in vivo</u> experiments and about 3-fold in cells in primary culture (3). This effect is specific to the anterior pituitary: glucocorticoids do not affect POMC gene transcription in the intermediate pituitary. In contrast, CRH treatment increases POMC transcription rate and this action appears to be mediated by cyclic AMP. Both glucocorticoid inhibition and CRH stimulation of POMC transcription are rapid and do not require <u>de novo</u> protein synthesis (4).

<u>POMC glucocorticoid-sensitive element (GSE)</u>

We have studied transcription from the rat POMC promoter linked to coding sequences for neomycin resistance. The POMCneo fusion gene was tested for glucocorticoid sensitivity after electroporation into AtT-20 and L cells. The POMC promoter is more active in AtT-20 than L cells because of tissue-specific enhancer sequences that are active in these cells (5). Pools of G418-resistant cells were used to test glucocorticoid sensitivity. Dexamethasone (DEX, 10^{-7}M) treatment decreases POMCneo transcripts and endogenous cellular POMC mRNA about 3-fold in AtT-20 cells electroporated with pPOMCneo plasmids containing 4500 or 709 bp upstream of the site of initiation of transcription. Sequences up to $^{-}709$ bp are therefore sufficient for full glucocorticoid sensitivity. RNAase mapping analysis demonstrated that these POMCneo transcripts have the same 5'-end as pituitary POMC mRNA (Fig. 1). L cells electroporated with the same plasmids contain POMCneo transcripts that are heterogenous in size and 5'-ends; however, some transcripts including those that correspond to the expected size (Northern and 5'-end) are decreased about 3-fold in DEX-treated cells. Insertion of a Moloney sarcoma virus (MSV) enhancer fragment upstream of the POMCneo unit stimulates constitutive expression in L cells, increases the specificity of transcription initiation and confers glucocorticoid inducibility (about 3-fold). In conclusion, it appears that, in these conditions, the MSV glucocorticoid-responsive element (GRE) overrides the POMC GSE. More experiments are needed to understand the interaction between these stimulatory and inhibitory elements.

Glucocorticoid receptor binding sites

The presence of glucocorticoid receptor (GR) binding sites on POMC DNA was tested directly using purified rat liver GR and end-labelled POMC DNA fragments. GR binding sites were defined by DNAaseI and exonucleaseIII footprinting (6,7); the interaction between GR and binding sites on POMC DNA was further probed by DMS protection (8). Five GR binding sites were identified; two in 5'-flanking sequences, one in exon 1 and two in intron A.

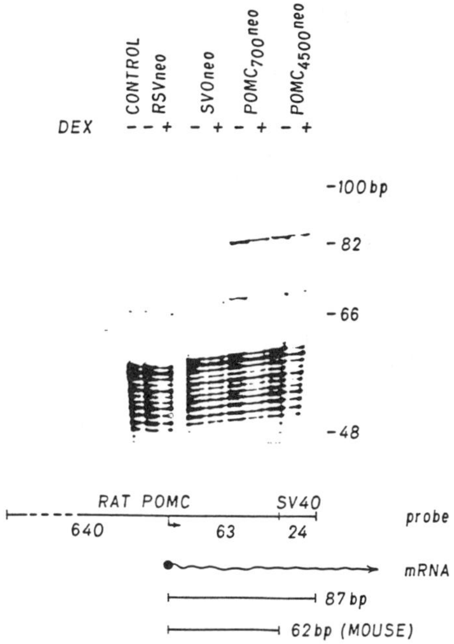

Figure 1. RNAase mapping assay of transcripts isolated from pools of AtT-20 cells treated or not overnight with 10^{-7}M DEX. The electroporated plasmids are indicated at the top and the structure of the SP6 probe is illustrated at bottom.

Both GR binding sites in 5'-flanking POMC DNA need not be present for glucocorticoid sensitivity; one of them confers the full activity. The intron A sites were not present in our test plasmids and the one half of the exon 1 site included in the plasmids doesn't have binding activity. The GR binding sites present in POMC are somewhat homologous to concensus sequences derived from the analysis of GR binding sites in up-regulated genes (6-8); however they diverge more from the concensus than sites in up-regulated genes. This divergence and a different DMS protection pattern suggest that GR interaction with POMC sequences may be different, although localization of these sites in 5'-flanking DNA may contribute to GR-mediated inhibitory activity.

This work is supported by MRC and NCI of Canada

REFERENCES

(1) Drouin, J. and Goodman, H.M. (1980) Nature **288**, 610-613.
(2) Drouin, J. et al. (1985) FEBS Letters, in press.
(3) Gagner, J.P. and Drouin, J. (1985) Mol. Cell. Endoc. **40**, 25-32.
(4) Gagner, J.P. and Drouin, J. (1985) Submitted.
(5) Jeannotte, L., Plante, R.K. and Drouin, J. (1985) Short Report submitted to this meeting.
(6) Payvar, R. et al. (1983) Cell **35**, 381-392.
(7) Scheidereit, C. et al. (1983) Nature **304**, 749-752.
(8) Scheidereit, C. and Beato, M. (1984) PNAS USA **81**, 3029-3033.

Monoclonal Antibodies to Human Leukemic Cell Glucocorticoid Receptor. B. Gametchu & E. Brad Thompson, Dept. of HBC&G, University of Texas Medical Branch, Galveston, TX 77550.

Until recently, methods for studying glucocorticoid receptors (GR) have depended on the ability of receptor protein to bind radiolabeled ligand. Difficulties with these studies include: there are two forms of the receptor (the active, steroid binding form and the inactive, non-binding form (1)); the steroid binding site can be cleaved from the receptor leaving an uncharacterized non-ligand binding domain which is necessary for biological activity (2). Immunochemical methods may solve these difficulties. Polyclonal antibodies have been raised against the human (3) and the rat (4) GR, and recently we (5) and others (6) have produced monoclonal antibodies to the rat GR. However, none of these monoclonals cross-react with the human GR. We describe here preparation of the first monoclonal antibodies to the human leukemic cell GR. [^{3}H] dexamethasone 21-mesylate-affinity labeled GR from the IM9 line of acute lymphoblastic leukemia cells was partially purified (7) and used to immunize Balb/C mice. Splenic lymphocytes from one animal were hybridized with myeloma cells and plated in 200 wells. After growth in selection medium, the supernatant media were assayed for antibodies (5). Fourteen of these wells contained anti-receptor antibodies. Fig. 1 illustrates results of the Western blot (W.B.) and autoradiography of the receptor using supernatant media from different uncloned hybrids (A-D). Affinity labelled human GR was analysed by denaturing gels and blotted onto nitrocellulose paper. The paper was reacted separately with each of the supernatant media (5). Autoradiography of the paper showed that the receptor preparation contained three radiolabeled protein bands of M_r 97kDa, 52kDa, and 36kDa (Fig. 1 A_1-E_1). The 97kDa and 36kDa protein bands were not seen when unlabeled steroid was included during the labelling period (competable). Therefore, these proteins are holoreceptor and a meroreceptor-like cleavage product, respectively. The 52kDa protein was not competable with excess unlabeled steroid. The W.B. results (Fig. 1, A-D) show that all the supernatants, except B, contained anti-holoreceptor antibodies. In addition, the supernatant media also contained

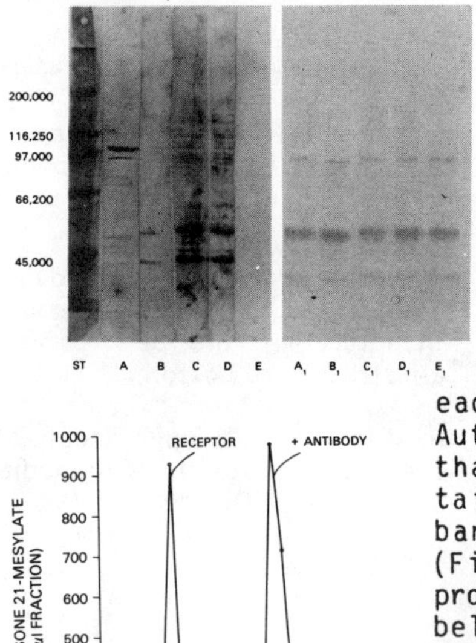

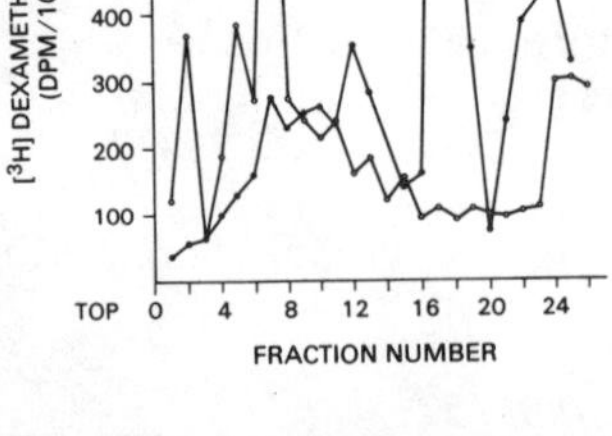

Top-Fig.1, Bottom-Fig.2

various antibodies that reacted with several additional proteins. The use of antibody free medium resulted in no binding (lane E). Supernate A was further analyzed by sucrose density gradient (SDG) (Fig.2). After incubation with the antibody containing medium, the receptor peak was shifted from 4S to two positions further down the gradient, indicating that the receptor-antibody complexes were formed (●). Incubation of supernatant media with labeled steroid alone did not produce a sedimenting peak, showing that the antibody did not interact with this steroid. Hybrids from well A were cloned and tested by W.B. and autoradiography for monoclonal antibodies to the GR. Figure 3 shows the results from one such clone, lane 3 contains protein standards, lane 2 W.B., lane 1 autoradiograph. The supernatant media contained antibody that reacted with only a 97kDa protein band, lane 2. This protein: 1) contained bound affinity ligand, (lane 1); 2) was competable with excess cold steroid, thus it is holoreceptor. Hence the monoclonal antibody was specific to the GR. Further confirmation of the specificity of this monoclonal antibody was obtained by SDG analysis (Fig. 4). Incubation of labeled receptor with the monoclonal antibody resulted in a shift of the receptor peak from 4S to a higher sedimentation value, suggesting the formation of antigen-antibody complex. In sum, we have produced the first monoclonal antibodies to the human leukemic cell GR. This reagent is a novel, inexhaustible tool for studies of GR in glucocorticoid sensitive cancers as well as for differentiating species-specific GR properties.

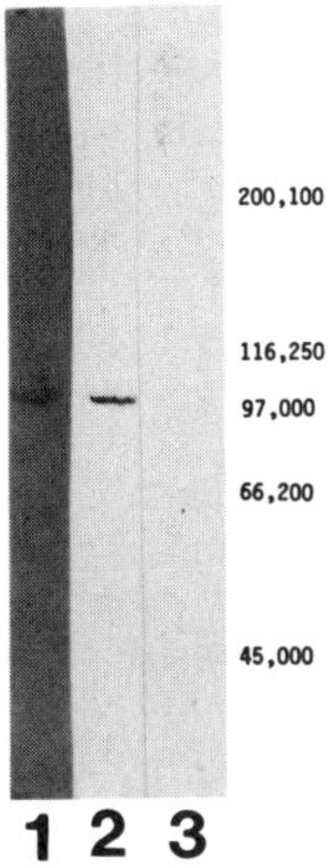

Figure 3.

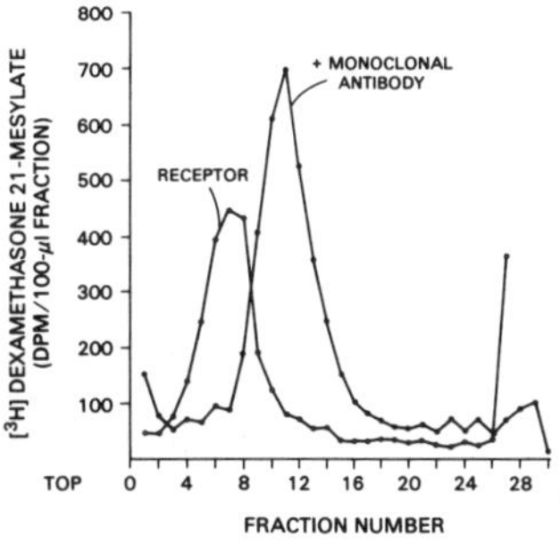

Figure 4 at left.

Acknowledgement: This research was supported in part by a grant from the Walls Medical Foundation.

References:

1) Housley, P.R., Dahmer, M.K. & Pratt, W.B. (1982). J.Biol. Chem. 257, 8615-8618.

2) McBlain,W. A.& Shymala,G.(1980). J. Biol. Chem. 255, 3884-3891.

3) Harmon,J.M., Eisen, H. J., Simons, S. S., Langley, C. L., Thompson, E. B. (1984). Cancer Research 44, 4540-4547.

4) Eisen,H.J.(1980).Proc. Natl. Acad. Sci. USA 77, 3893-3897.

5) Gametchu,B.& Harrison,R.W. (1984). Endocrin. 174, 274-279.

6) Okret,S.,*et al.*, (1984). Proc. Natl. Acad. Sci. USA 81, 1609-1613.

7) Eisen,H.J.& Glinsmann, W.H.(1978). Biochem. J. 171, 177-181.

THE HORMONE-REGULATED rDNA TRANSCRIPTION FACTOR (TFIC) DETERMINES THE EXTENT OF REINITIATION OF TRANSCRIPTION *IN VITRO*.

P. K. Gokal, A. H. Cavanaugh, P. B. Mahajan, and E. A. Thompson.
Department of Biology, University of South Carolina, Columbia, S.C. 29208.

INTRODUCTION: Cell free extracts (S100s) made from control P1798 cells can transcribe the cloned ribosomal RNA promoter *in vitro*. In extracts made from dexamethasone treated cells (S100F extracts), this ability is reduced to 5-10% that of control S100s (1). Transcription by S100F can be restored by the addition of TFIC, a phosphocellulose fraction of control S100 containing the RNA polymerase I transcription factor C (2).

In the present study, the role of TFIC in ribosomal RNA transcription has been examined. For this purpose S100F pellets were made, which can carry out only one round of transcription. When TFIC is added to these, the ability to transcribe is increased and the kinetics resemble transcription by control S100 extracts. Therefore, we propose that TFIC is responsible for carrying out multiple rounds of transcription.

MATERIALS AND METHODS: Procedures to make S100 and S100F extracts have been previously described (1). Pellets were made as described (3). Briefly, S100 or S100F extracts were preincubated with the template in transcription cocktail, then centrifuged at 12,000g and resuspended in transcription cocktail. Standard transcription protocols have been previously described (1). All reactions were preincubated at 30° for 5' with 0.5 mM ATP and 0.5 mM CTP. This allows initiation to occur since ATP and CTP are the first two nucleotides (respectively) in the transcription of ribosomal RNA. The time points refer to the time between the addition of NTPs + ^{32}P-UTP and termination by addition of SDS/tRNA. RNA was extracted by ammonium acetate/ethanol precipitation and run on polyacrylamide-urea gels. Gels were dried before autoradiography. Autoradiograms were scanned with a Beckman DU-8 spectrophotometer and the number of mol of product was calculated by the formula, $^{32}P(dpm) = [5.21 \times 10^{4} \text{ (peak area)} + 247] \times \text{(exposure time in min)}^{-1}$

RESULTS: Figure 1 shows transcription of rDNA in control S100 extract. At 30°C, there is a linear increase of transcription with time. At 10°C the level of transcription is reduced and reaches a plateau by 20-30 seconds. This implies that at 10°C reinitiation does not occur. Transcription at 10°C is due to a single round of transcription from initiation complexes that were formed during preincubation at 30°C in the presence of ATP and CTP. This is consistent with other data from our laboratory (4). Assuming that at 10°C one transcript was formed per initiation complex, one may estimate that 5μl of this extract was capable of forming approximately 4×10^{-16} mol of initiation complex.

Transcription of S100F pellet in the presence and absence of forming presumptive initiation complexes: With 5μl of this particular extract, approximately 1 x 10^{-16} mol of complex was formed. However, the transcription reaction was complete within 30 seconds and reinitiation did not occur at 30°C. Substantial reinitiation was observed when pellets were reconstituted with partially purified TFIC (Figure 2). The kinetics of transcription under these circumstances resembled those observed in unfractionated S100 extracts from control cells.

CONCLUSIONS: Extracts from hormone-treated cells (S100F) are depleted of transcription factor TFIC. Formation of initiation complexes is reduced in such extracts. Moreover, the extent of reinitiation is greatly reduced. The data suggest that TFIC plays a role in determining the extent of reinitiation and may function in a stoichiometric manner to determine the number of transcripts formed.

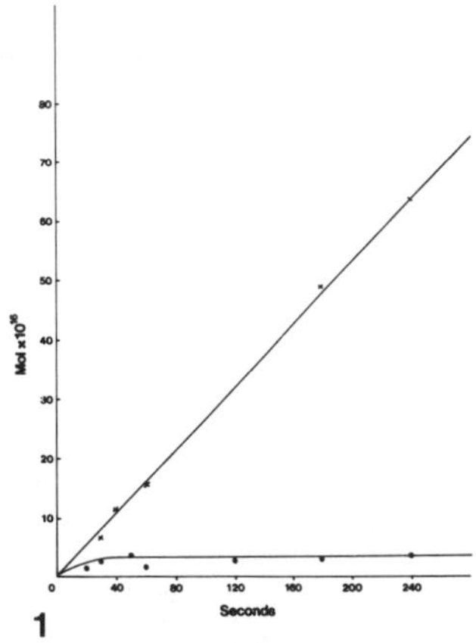

1

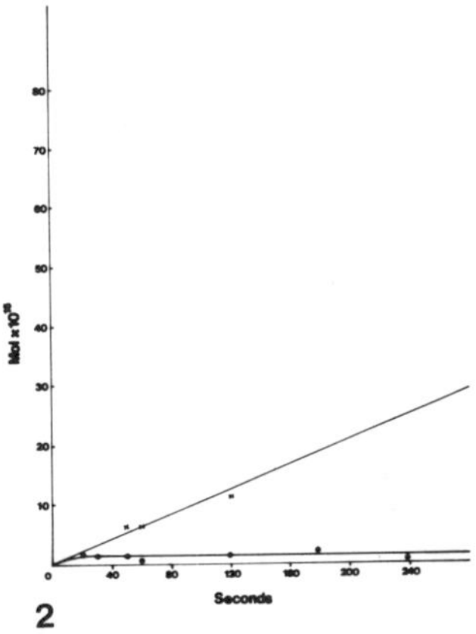

2

FIGURE 1: Transcription of S100 extract made from control cells at 10°C• and 30°C.×
FIGURE 2: Transcription of pellets made from S100F extracts from dexamethasone treated cells. Pellets were made as described in the Materials and Methods section. In the + TFIC experiment, TFIC was added when the pellets were resuspended, prior to the 30°C pre-incubation with ATP and CTP. S100F pellet• S100F pellet + TFIC×

REFERENCES:
(1) Cavanaugh, A. H., Gokal, P. K., Lawther, R. P., and Thompson, E. A. (1984). Proc. Natl. Acad. Sci. (U.S.A.) 81, 718.
(2) Cavanaugh, A. H. and Thompson, E. A. (1985) Nucleic Acids Res 13, 3357-3369.
(3) Culotta, V. C., Wides, R. J. and Souner-Webb, Mol. Cell. Biol., in press.
(4) Cavanaugh, A. H. and Thompson, manuscript submitted.

ESTROGEN REGULATES THE DEGRADATION, NOT THE STABILITY OF APOLIPOPROTEIN II AND VITELLOGENIN II mRNAs IN CHICK LIVER

D. Gordon and D.L. Williams
Department of Pharmacology, SUNY at Stony Brook, Stony Brook, New York 11794

I. INTRODUCTION

In addition to effects on gene transcription, estrogens (E) are believed to have major effects on the stability of E-induced mRNAs (1). In the case of the chick liver model, Wiskocil, et. al. (2) have shown that after a single E injection, apolipoprotein II (apo II) and vitellogenin (VTG) mRNAs accumulate in vivo with kinetics that are indicative of 26 h and 22 h half-lives of decay (t1/2) respectively. When the animals are treated for 2 weeks with an E implant which is subsequently removed, these mRNAs degrade with a t1/2 of 2-3 h. The authors concluded that E stabilizes these mRNAs ~10 X. Similar findings have been reported for the VTG mRNA in Xenopus laevis liver (1). Little is known about how estrogens modulate mRNA stability.

II. METHODS

Estrogen was administered to male white leghorn chicks by subcutaneous implantation of pellets containing 100 mg of 17β-estradiol. For mRNA decay experiments the pellets were removed at the indicated times and the antiestrogen Tamoxifen citrate (Tam) was administered intramuscularly. Livers were removed and total RNA was prepared (3). Apo II mRNA was quantitated by an ultra-sensitive DNA excess solution hybridization assay using a single stranded probe (3). A similar assay using an intron probe (4) was used to measure absolute amounts of nuclear precursors. VTG II mRNA was measured by the dot-blot assay described by White, et. al. (5) using a nick translated probe for VTG II mRNA (6).

III. RESULTS AND DISCUSSION

Figure 1 is a typical mRNA accumulation experiment showing that apo II and VTG II mRNAs accumulate at very similar rates following E administration. Both mRNAs show a slow accumulation at early times after E followed by a period of rapid increase until a steady state is reached between 24 h and 48 h. The levels of the mRNAs do not change significantly between 48 h and 14 days (d) (Data not shown).

Using an approach to steady state analysis (7), these data yield a t1/2 for decay of these mRNAs of 12-15 h in the presence of E. It should be noted that the slow initial accumulation of mRNA is not predicted by this theoretical analysis. However, by altering the mRNA synthesis rate in a stepwise fashion in the first few hours after E administration, the data are consistent with t1/2s of 12-15 h.

Figure 2 shows the decay of apo II and VTG II mRNAs when birds were pretreated with E for 1 d before pellet removal and Tam administration. As is clear apo II and VTG II mRNAs decay with equivalent kinetics indicative of a first order process with a t1/2 of 10.5 h. To ensure that pellet removal and Tam administration effectively terminated apo II gene transcription, parallel hybridization measurements were made with an intron probe. The data show that the nuclear precursors of apo II mRNA de-

FIGURE 1. APPROACH TO STEADY STATE OF APO II AND VTG II mRNAS.

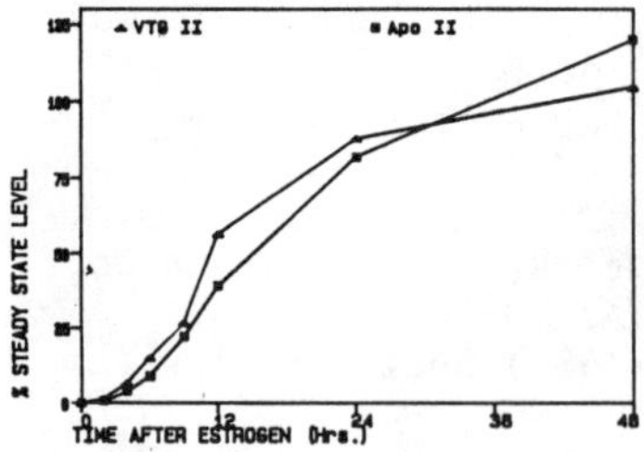

FIGURE 2. DECAY OF APO II AND VTG II mRNAS AND NUCLEAR PRECURSOR (INSET) AFTER 1 d OF E.

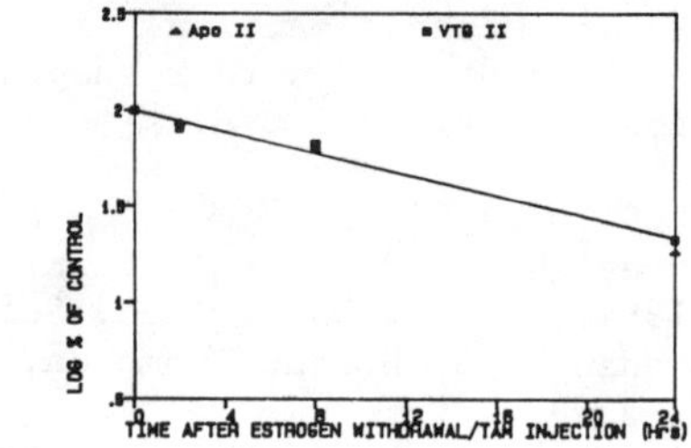

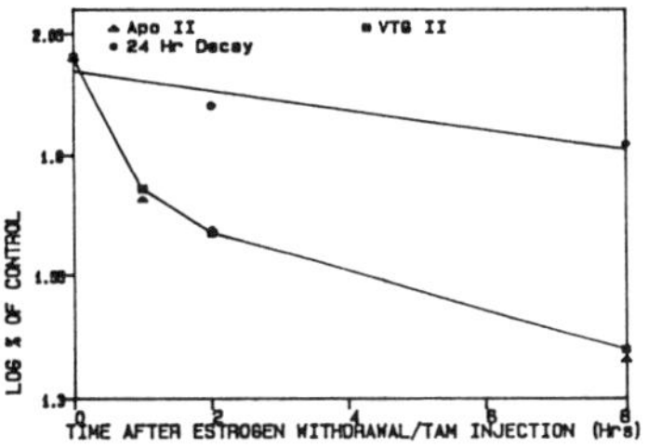

FIGURE 3. DECAY OF APO II AND VTG II mRNAS AFTER 1 d AND 14 d OF E.

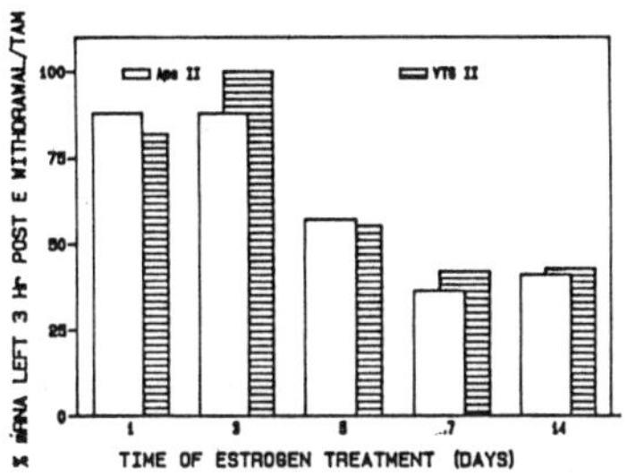

FIGURE 4. TIME COURSE OF SHIFT FROM SLOW DECAY MODE TO FAST DECAY MODE.

clined with a t1/2 of 11 min after Tam administration and were reduced by ~90 % within 30 min (Data not shown). Thus, the slow decay (t1/2=10.5 h) of mature apo II mRNA is not due to continued transcription after Tam treatment.

In contrast to the t1/2 for decay seen after 1 d of E treatment, Figure 3 shows that when animals were treated with E for 14 d, apo II and VTG II mRNAs decay much faster. In addition, the decay kinetics are not linear when examined in a log-linear plot whereas the decay kinetics seen after 1 d of E treatment showed first order kinetics. The results indicate that after 14 d of E treatment, apo II and VTG II mRNA decay is not only faster but also may occur via a different mechanism.

In order to determine when the shift from the slower decay mode to the faster decay mode occurs, birds were treated with E for various times before pellet removal and Tam administration. Apo II and VTG II mRNA content was measured at 3 h after Tam treatment, a time interval that readily distinguishes the slow and fast modes of decay. As shown in Figure 4, mRNA decay was unchanged at 1 and 3 d but increased thereafter until it was maximal by 7 d. No further change was seen between 7 d and 14 d of E treatment.

These data show that the degradation t1/2 for apo II mRNA is similar when estimated by the kinetics of approach to steady state (t1/2=12-15 h) or by directly measuring mRNA decay following the termination of hormone stimulation at 24 h. VTG II mRNA shows nearly the same t1/2 as apo II mRNA in these two situations. These results argue that E has no significant effect on the stability of these mRNAs during the 2 d necessary to attain the new steady state level of mRNA. Hence changes in mRNA stability are not playing a significant role in the extensive accumulation of apo II and VTG II mRNAs. However, termination of hormone stimulation after 14 days leads to the rapid decay (t1/2=1-2 h) of both apo II and VTG II mRNAs. Measurements of mRNA decay at intermediate times show a shift from the slow decay mode to the fast decay mode. These results suggest that E stimulation leads to the gradual accumulation of a cellular capacity to selectively degrade those mRNAs induced by the hormone. Since the steady state levels of apo II and VTG II mRNAs are unchanged between 2 d and 14 d, it seems likely that the new degradative capacity is not active until the hormone is withdrawn. The observation that the mRNA decay kinetics at 14 d of E treatment deviate substantially from the first order kinetics seen at 1 d of E treatment also argues that the new degradative activity is qualitatively different and not a simple up-regulation of a general cellular mechanism for degrading mRNA. In some manner hormone withdrawl selectively targets apo II and VTG II mRNAs for rapid degradation.

IV. REFERENCES

1. Schapiro, D.J. and Brock, M.L. (1984) in Biochemical Actions of Hormones (Litwak, G., ed.) Academic Press, N.Y.
2. Wiskocil, R., Bensky, P., Dower, W., Goldberger, R.F., Gordon, J.I. and Deeley, R.G. (1980) Proc. Natl. Acad. Sci. 77, 4474-4478.
3. Elbrecht, A., Lazier, C.B., Protter, A.A. and Williams, D.L. (1984) Science 225, 693-641.
4. Shelness, G.S. and Williams, D.L. (1984) J. Biol. Chem. 259, 9929-9935.
5. White, B.A. and Bancroft, F.C. (1982) J. Biol. Chem. 257, 8569-8572.
6. Protter, A.A., Wang, S.-Y., Shelness, G.S., Ostapchuk, P., and Williams, D.L. (1982) Nucl. Acids Res. 10, 4935.
7. Kafatos, F.C. (1972) in Gene Transcription in Reproductive Tissues (Diezfalusy, E., ed.) pp 319-345. Karolinska Institute, Stockholm.

SEQUENCE ORGANIZATION AND SPECIFIC PROTEIN/DNA INTERACTIONS IN REGIONS FLANKING THE ESTROGEN-DEPENDENT AVIAN VERY LOW DENSITY APOLIPOPROTEIN II GENE

R.J.G. Haché, R.N. Roy, M. Vasa and R.G. Deeley
Department of Biochemistry, Queen's University, Kingston, Ontario Canada K7L 3N6

The avian very low density apolipoprotein II (apoVLDL II) gene, expressed in the liver of the laying hen, codes for a small phospholipid binding protein (MW 9500) that is a major constituent of the yolk of the developing oocyte. Expression of the gene is entirely under the control of estrogen, with transcription being inducible in the hen, rooster and embryo beginning around day nine of embryogenesis (1). Prior to day nine the liver is not competent to respond. It has been our goal to distinguish between events that dictate the competence of the apoVLDL II gene to be transcribed and those that occur during gene activation. In this report we describe the DNA structure and the specific protein binding characteristics of the 5' flanking region of the apoVLDL II gene for non histone DNA binding protein(s) present in nuclear extracts. We have correlated these observations with changes that occur in the chromatin structure of this region, reflected by changes in methylation and DNAse I hypersensitivity patterns, as the gene becomes transcriptionally competent and following its subsequent activation.

RESULTS AND DISCUSSION. Our analysis of the 5' flanking region of the avian apoVLDL II gene has revealed structural features and specific protein binding sites that may be involved in the developmental programming of the gene and its hormonally induced expression. A summary of the data is presented in the figure.

Repetitive Sequences. Sequencing of the 5' flanking region of the apoVLDL II gene has revealed the presence of two intermediately repeated DNA sequences located between 2.4 to 3.6 kb upstream from the gene. One of these sequences has been identified as a member of the CR1 family of dispersed repetitive elements(2). The other is present at approximately 2-5% the frequency of CR1 element. Both of these repeats are also found in a similar region upstream from the avian serum albumin gene. The boundary between these two elements is reflected by a DNAse I hypersensitive site (site A in figure) that is present at all times during development, but is lost upon activation of the gene. The region in which this site is located is also sensitive to S1 nuclease in supercoiled DNA. In addition, a second stronger S1 site is observed 400 nucleotides 5' to the repeated elements.

Protein Binding. One of the mechanisms by which gene expression may be modulated is through the selective binding of non-histone proteins around the transcription unit. We have identified three sequences in the area extending from 1.4 to 2.3 kb upstream from the apoVLDL II gene that, as purified fragments, will specifically

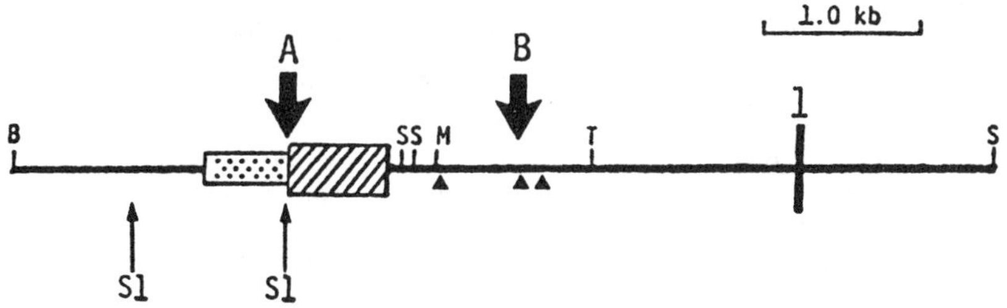

Figure 1: Schematic representation of the organization of the 5' flanking sequence of the avian apoVLDL II gene. Restriction enzyme sites; B=BamHI; M=Mspl/HpaII; S=Sacl; T=Taql. 1 illustrates the position of exon 1 of apoVLDL II. ▲ indicates the DNA binding sites of protein(s) in nuclear salt extracts. A and B are DNase I hypersensitive sites. S1 denotes S1 nuclease sites. CR1 element=hatched box, lower frequency repeat=stippled box.

retain (a) protein(s) found in a nuclear salt extract. These protein binding sites, shown in the figure, contain sequences corresponding to the viral enhancer core sequence GTGG$^{AAA}_{TTT}$G(3). Although these protein binding sites show some homology nuclear factor I and TGGCA binding protein recognition sequences(4,5), they differ significantly from both consensus sequences. Preliminary analysis of the chromatin structure in this region has revealed a DNAse I hypersensitive site (denoted "B" in the figure) present near the middle of the group of protein binding sites. This site is not present at day seven of embryogenesis, but is detectable at later stages in development. Its appearance is not estrogen dependent. In addition, affinity for the upstream binding site is decreased when the MspI/Hpa II site at -2 kb is methylated. Demethylation of this site has been shown to occur between day seven and nine of embryogenesis (6). The functional significance of these protein/DNA interactions is currently being investigated by gene transfer experiments.

ACKNOWLEDGEMENTS

This work was supported by a grant from the Medical Research Council of Canada to R.G.D. R.H. is the recipient of an Ontario Graduate Scholarship.

REFERENCES

(1) Elbrecht, A., Williams, D.L., Blue, M.L., and Lazier, C.B. (1981) Can. J. Biochem. 59, 606-613.
(2) Stumph, W.E., Hodgson, C.P., Tsai, M-J., and O'Malley, B.W. (1984) Proc. Natl. Acad. Sci. U.S.A. 81, 6667-6671.
(3) Khoury, G. and Gruss, P. (1983) Cell 33, 313-314.
(4) Nagata, K., Guggenheimer, R.A., Enomoto, T., Lichy, J.H., and Hurwitz, J. (1982) Proc. Natl. Acad. Sci. U.S.A. 79, 6438-6442.
(5) Nowock, J., Borgmeyer, U., Püschel, A.W., Rupp, R.A.W., and Sippel, A.E. (1985) Nucl. Acid. Res. 13, 2045-2061.
(6) Colgan, V., Elbrecht, A., Goldman, P., Lazier, C.B. (1982) J. Biol. Chem. 257, 14453-14460.

GENOMIC EFFECTS OF 1,25-DIHYDROXYVITAMIN D_3 UPON THE RACHITIC CHICKEN INTESTINE: INDEPENDENCE FROM SERUM CALCIUM STATUS

A. K. Hall and A. W. Norman, Department of Biochemistry, University of California, Riverside, CA 92521, USA

One of the most salient features of vitamin D deficiency is that of hypocalcemia which is a biological consequence of impaired intestinal calcium absorption (1). In a previous study (2) we have demonstrated that the D-replete (+D) chick intestine is less sensitive to $1,25(OH)_2D_3$ than its -D counterpart in terms of calbindin-D_{28K} (a 28,000 dalton vitamin D-dependent calcium binding protein, CaBP) and calbindin-mRNA accumulation. The present study was therefore designed primarily to examine whether or not this differential sensitivity was a reflection of the secondary effect of vitamin D deficiency, namely that of hypocalcemia *per se*.

METHODS

Animal Treatments. One-day-old White Leghorn cockerels were raised on a rachitogenic diet for 14 days prior to being maintained on a D-deficient diet containing either a high calcium (3%, w/w) or low calcium (0.4%, w/w) content for a further two weeks. After this time both groups of chicks received a range of doses of $1,25(OH)_2D_3$ (0 to 16 nmoles/animals) and were killed 48 hours later. Blood was collected whilst intestinal mucosa was scraped, pooled and frozen in liquid nitrogen.

Isolation of RNA and Measurement of Calbindin-mRNA. Total cellular RNA was extracted from intestinal mucosa by the guanidinium thiocyanate procedure. Nick-translated (^{32}P)-labelled cDNA (pCaBP-2, a 350 bp insert in pBR322) was hybridized to RNA (30 ug) immobilized on nitrocellulose paper filters which were used to expose X-ray film at -70C with intensifying screens. Exposed films were scanned with a densitometer.

Measurement of Calbindin. Samples of pooled intestinal mucosa were homogenized in 4 volumes of a buffer containing Tris-HCl, EDTA and DTT. The calbindin was then determined by an enzyme-linked immunosorbent assay (ELISA). Results are expressed as ug of CaBP per mg total protein.

RESULTS

As can be seen in Table 1, serum calcium was "normalized" by placing D-deficient chicks on the high calcium diet. Intestinal calbindin levels (Fig. 1) were stimulated by $1,25(OH)_2D_3$ in a dose-dependent manner in both HCa and LCa chicks; no difference in sensitivity of CaBP was seen. Stimulation of intestinal CaBP-mRNA (measured by dot-blot) was dependent upon the administered dose of steroid (Fig. 2). The response to low doses of steroid was essentially the same in HCa and LCa chicks. However, pharmacologic doses (16 nmoles) were less effective in the HCa group in stimulating CaBP-mRNA levels.

Table 1. Serum calcium (mg%) in high calcium (HCa) and low (LCa) chicks versus the dose of injected $1,25(OH)_2D_3$.

Dose of Hormone (nmoles)	Dietary Treatments LCa	HCa
	(mean ± 1 S.D.)	
0	4.42 ± 0.48	8.90 ± 0.91
0.065	4.59 ± 0.48	9.02 ± 0.53
0.325	4.47 ± 0.37	9.41 ± 0.23
0.65	5.10 ± 0.32	9.54 ± 0.80
3.25	6.42 ± 0.20	9.19 ± 0.41
6.50	6.46 ± 0.40	8.12 ± 1.04

FIGURE.1.

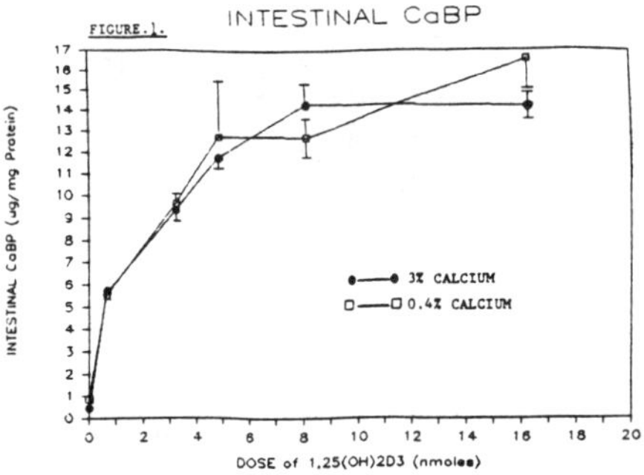

FIGURE.2.

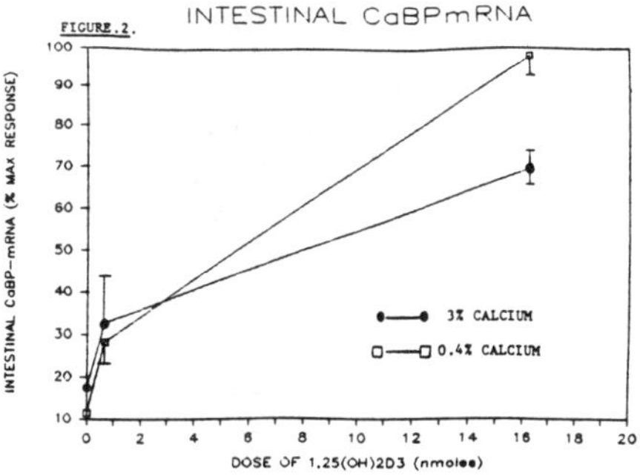

CONCLUSION

The recent synthesis and molecular cloning of cDNA to the mRNA encoding calbindin-D in our laboratory (3) has facilitated the precise measurement of the genomic effects of $1,25(OH)_2D_3$ in the intestinal epithelial cell. The present study has used these cDNA probes to demonstrate that $1,25(OH)_2D_3$ stimulation of CaBP gene expression is not influenced by ambient changes in serum calcium in the -D chick intestine. This finding therefore also implies that other calcium homeostatic hormones (such as parathyroid hormone and calcitonin) whose secretion is modulated by serum calcium, play insignificant roles in regulating the stimulation of intestinal CaBP and CaBP-mRNA by $1,25(OH)_2D_3$.

ACKNOWLEDGEMENTS

Supported in part by Grant AM-09012-021. A.K.H. is the recipient of a Fulbright Award.

REFERENCES

(1) Norman, A. W. (1979) Vitamin D: The Calcium Homeostatic Steroid Hormone, in Nutrition: Basic and applied Science (Darby, W. J., ed) Academic Press, NY.

(2) Hall, A. K. and Norman, A. W. (1985) in Vitamin D: Chemical, Biochemical and Clinical Update, pp. 353-354, Walter de Gruyter, Berlin.

(3) Hunziker, W., et al. (1983) Proc. Natl. Acad. Sci. 80, 4228-4234.

PREDICTING HORMONAL ACTIVITY FROM THE STEREOCHEMISTRY OF NUCLEIC ACIDS: A PROSPECTIVE STUDY WITH NOVEL ESTROGENIC STEROIDS

L.B. Hendry*†, T.G. Muldoon†, E.D. Bransome, Jr.*†, A.F. Lehner*†, M.S. Hutson§, N.K. Uberoi†, R.B. Myers†, A. Segaloff**, and V.B. Mahesh†
Departments of Medicine*, Endocrinology† and Pathology§, Medical College of Georgia, Augusta, Georgia 30912 and Alton Ochsner Medical Foundation**, New Orleans, Louisiana 70121

We have demonstrated with molecular models that naturally occurring small molecules are stereochemically complementary to double-stranded DNA (1-3). Complementarity is defined as the ability of a given molecule to: conform to the topography of the double helix when inserted into cavities between base pairs; form stereospecific linkages between each functional group and hydrogen bonding positions in the double helix. The mammalian steroid hormones fit between base pairs in the site 5'-dTdG-3'•5'-dCdA-3'; heteroatoms on the steroid skeleton are capable of forming at least two hydrogen bonds to phosphate groups thereby bridging double-stranded DNA. As indicated in the table below, different hydrogen bonding patterns reflect different hormonal activities.

POSITIONS ON THE STEROID NUCLEUS WHICH FORM H-BOND LINKAGES TO DNA

3	11β	17α	17β	18	20	21
ESTRADIOL						
OH••$^{-}$OP (3'-C)			OH••$^{-}$OP (3'-T)			
TESTOSTERONE						
C=O••HOP (3'-C)			OH••$^{-}$OP (3'-T)			
PROGESTERONE						
C=O••HOP (3'-C)					C=O••HOP (3'-T)	
CORTISOL						
C=O••HOP (3'-C)	OH••HOH••O=C (T at O_4)	OH••O (sugar O_4')			C=O••HOP (3'-T)	OH••$^{-}$OP (5'-T)
ALDOSTERONE						
C=O••HOP (3'-C)				C=O••HN (A)	C=O••HOP (3'-T)	OH••$^{-}$OP (5'-T)

For further details of steroid orientation cf. ref. (3)

Examination of the potential fit of a large number of steroids as well as other molecules into DNA revealed a close correlation between relative biological activity and degree of complementarity (4). These findings led to criteria for predicting structural characteristics of hormonal agonists i.e. the structure must fit between the same base pairs and in the manner of the natural hormone; degree of fit predicts degree of biological activity. Using a series of compounds related to estradiol, we report here the first *in vivo* and *in vitro* experimental test of such predictions (4).

Bioassays for estrogenicity were conducted by standard methods using ovariectomized Holzman female rats (4). Restoration of uterine weight and prevention of LH rise were used as endpoints in the assay. Good agreement was found for both methods; thus, a single value for relative estrogenic activity is reported below.

STEREOCHEMICAL FIT INTO DNA CORRELATED WITH ESTROGENIC POTENCY

COMPOUND	ABILITY TO HYDROGEN BOND TO DNA ††	TOPOGRAPHICAL COMPLEMENTARITY TO DNA	ESTROGENIC ACTIVITY PREDICTED	ESTROGENIC ACTIVITY FOUND
11β-ACETOXY ESTRADIOL	+ + +	+ +	+ + + + +	444
ESTRADIOL-17β	+ +	+	+ + +	100
11β-HYDROXY ESTRADIOL	+ + -	+	+ +	0.58
9β-ESTRADIOL	+ +	-	+	0.78
11α-HYDROXY ESTRADIOL	+ + -	-	0	<0.058

††Functional groups which can (+) and cannot (-) hydrogen bond.

To be considered an estrogenic agonist, the candidate molecule must fit into the double-stranded site 5'-dTdG-3'•5'-dCdA-3', and form two hydrogen bonds to phosphate oxygens on adjacent strands. The results (above) demonstrated a close correlation between fit into DNA and estrogenic activity of the compounds tested. A. 11α-hydroxy estradiol did not fit completely between base pairs and the 11α-hydroxy group would not hydrogen bond to DNA; this compound was virtually inactive. B. 9β-estradiol was a poor fit to the topography of the space between base pairs and possessed relatively poor activity. C. 11β-hydroxy estradiol was capable of fitting into DNA but would not hydrogen bond at the 11β-hydroxyl to DNA; poor activity was observed for this analog. D. 11β-acetoxy estradiol fit better into DNA than estradiol in that it filled more of the space between base pairs and an additional hydrogen bond could be formed; it was also more active than estradiol.

The close correlation between biological activity of these compounds and fit into DNA supports our contention that the biological activity of hormonal steroids and other natural products can be predicted from gene structure (2).

REFERENCES

(1) Hendry, L.B., Witham, F.H. and Chapman, O.L. (1977) Perspect. Biol. Med. 21, 120-130.
(2) Hendry, L.B., Bransome, E.D., Jr., Hutson, M.S. and Campbell, L.K. (1984) U.S. Patent 4,461,619.
(3) Bransome, E.D., Hendry, L.B., Muldoon, T.G., Mahesh, V.B., Hutson, M.S. and Campbell, L.K. (1985) J. theor. Biol. 112, 97-108.
(4) Uberoi, N.K., Hendry, L.B., Muldoon, T.G., Myers, R.B., Segaloff, A., Bransome, E.D. and Mahesh, V.B. (1986) Steroids, in press.

HIGH CAPACITY INTRACELLULAR STEROID BINDING PROTEINS

H. Homma and I. Listowsky
Dept. Biochemistry, A. Einstein Col. of Medicine, Bx., NY 10461

A subclass of glutathione-S-transferases (GST) are steroid binding proteins. Pure preparations of the Y_b-forms of the rat protein, adhere to corticosterone affinity matrices (1), bind steroids with high affinity (1), and have been identified as the major rat liver proteins to react with a glucocorticoid affinity label, dexamethasone 21-mesylate (DM) (2). Since these are relatively abundant proteins found in many cell types (3), they provide potential for high capacity binding of steroid hormones. In this report glucocorticoid binding to the multiple rat liver Y_b-transferases and temperature dependent transformations are analyzed.

<u>Binding</u>: Glucocorticords preferentially bind to the Y_b subclass of rat GST's and with much lesser affinity to Y_a,Y_c forms (ligandins). Figure 1 shows that all of the multiple Y_b-transferases resolved by chromatofocusing retain glucocorticoid binding capacity. All forms are also labeled by DM.

<u>Temperature dependence</u>: In view of observations that anionic GST's undergo temperature dependent redistribution to multiple forms (4), steroid binding was analyzed at 4° and 27°. Figure 2a shows that pure Y_b-proteins containing bound steroid are converted from forms that are retained by DEAE-Sephacel at 4° to forms that are no longer adsorbed by the anion exchange resin at 27°. The latter forms are retained by DNA-cellulose (Figure 2b). The temperature dependent transition characteristic of Y_b-type glutathione-S-transferases has been attributed to increased rates of dissociation of GSH from the protein at elevated temperatures (27°) resulting in generation of more basic forms (4). The loss of an anionic steroid binding component of cytosol at 27° seemingly reflects a shift of the anionic Y_b forms to more basic components. In this context it may be noted that "activation or transformation" of putative steroid receptors at elevated temperatures also converts these proteins to more basic forms that bind to DNA.

<u>Cell culture systems</u>: Normal rat hepatocytes in culture were incubated with DM, cytosolic proteins isolated, and Y_b identified as the predominant form covalently labeled by the reagent. Studies on hepatoma tissue culture cells (HTC) indicated that Y_b and Y_p forms predominate. Ligandins (Y_a,Y_c forms) are virtually nonexistant in these cells. A variant HTC cell line that is relatively resistant to effects of glucocorticoids, has increased amounts of Y_p, but DM preferentially labeled Y_b.

<u>Points to consider</u>: The Y_b-GST family of proteins, based on their abundance, their presence in cytosol as well as nuclei, and their high affinity binding of steroids, have the potential to function prominently in an intracellular steroid binding capacity. Indeed

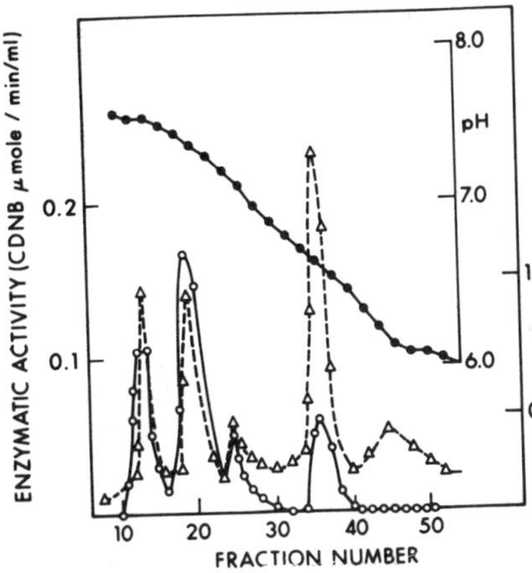

<u>Fig. 1. Corticosterone binding by the Y_b-GST family; chromatofocusing:</u> Y_b-GST (1.0 mg/ml) in 0.025 M Tris-acetate buffer pH 8.3 was incubated with 1.0 nM [^{3}H] corticosterone, passed through a dextran-charcoal plug, and applied to a 1.0 x 30 cm column of PBE-83 chromatofocusing gel. The column was eluted with polybuffers PB 96 (30%) and PB 74 (70%) (diluted 1:10) pH 5.6. Fractions of 3 ml each were collected and assayed for enzymatic activity (o) and radioactivity (Δ, dotted line).

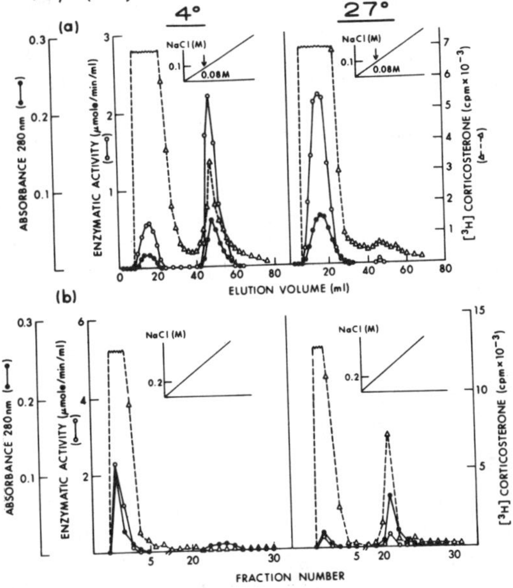

<u>Fig. 2. Temperature dependence:</u> Purified preparations of Y_b type GST (0.6 mg/ml) in 10 mM Tris-HCl buffer pH 8.0, were incubated with 2.0 nM [^{3}H] corticosterone for 30 min at 4° (left panels) and 27° (right panels). The protein solutions were then applied to DEAE-Sephacel columns (1.4 x 10 cm) ((a), upper panels) and DNA-cellulose columns (1.4 x 4 cm) ((b), lower panels).

these proteins have probably been ignored and categorized among "non-specific" binders because they are not ordinarily saturable in traditional laboratory binding studies. Preferential binding of glucocorticoids to these proteins in cells and cell extracts however, suggest that they could at least govern accessibility of steroids to their receptors, or perhaps have a more direct role in steroid metabolism or action.

REFERENCES

(1) Maruyama H. and Listowsky, I. (1984) J. Biol. Chem. <u>259</u>, 12449.
(2) Homma H. and Listowsky I. (1985) Proc. Natl. Acad. Sci. <u>82</u>, 7165.
(3) Mannervik, B. (1985) Adv. Enzymol. <u>57</u>, 357.
(4) Homma H. and Listowsky I. (1985) Biochem. Biophys. Res. Commun. <u>127</u>, 425.

HIGH-PERFORMANCE LIQUID CHROMATOGRAPHY PURIFICATION OF TOPOISOMERASE I FROM HUMAN BREAST CANCER CELLS

Salman M. Hyder, Alberto Baldi and James L. Wittliff
Hormone Receptor Laboratory, J.G. Brown Cancer Center, University of Louisville School of Medicine, Louisville, KY 40292, USA

DNA topoisomerases catalyze the removal of superhelical turns from supercoiled DNA by cleavage and rejoining. These enzymes participate in cellular processes including synthesis and possible control of RNA transcription, site specific recombination and segregation of daughter DNA molecules[1]. Recent studies with human breast cancer cells suggest that changes in the Topoisomerase I (TpI) activity may be one of the primary effects of estrogens and antiestrogens in the regulation of cell proliferation[2]. In this report we describe TpI purification utilizing HPLC in several protein separation modes. Whereas partial purification of TpI was obtained with every HPLC mode employed, only a combination of anion-exchange and size-e xclusion chromatography provided enhanced purification. HPLC in the cation-exchange mode provides the best first step purification of the TpI activity. This study[3] provides the first demonstration that HPLC may be used as a rapid, efficient method of purification for TpI, a labile regulatory enzyme.

Topoisomerase I Assay: Cellular pellets were resuspended in 1 µl per 10^3 cells in TKM buffer (10 mM Tris-HCl pH 7.5, 25 mM KCl, 5 mM $MgCl_2$, 1 mM DTT, 1 mM phenylmethyl-sulfonyl fluoride, PMSF). The procedure for cell lysis and TpI extraction has been described.[3]

TpI activity was determined by the decreased mobility of relaxed pBR322 DNA in a 1% agarose gel after treatment of the supercoiled form with various fractions obtained following HPLC. Assays contained 50 mM Tris-HCl pH 7.5, 0.2 M NaCl, 1 mM DTT, 30 µg/ml BSA, 1 mM EDTA and 0.1 µg of supercoiled pBR322. Reactions proceeded for 15 min at 37°C and were terminated by the addition of a solution composed of 5% SDS, 40% glycerol, and 0.005% bromophenol blue (all w/v). Samples were separated by electrophoresis on 1% agarose gels in TEA buffer (40mM Tris-acetate pH 8.0, 1 mM EDTA), and TpI activity was visualized by UV irradiation of the products. Plasmid bands were scanned on a Beckman DU 8B spectrophotometer. One unit is defined as the amount of protein which reduces the plasmid concentration by half.

HPLC purification of Topoisomerase I: Analytical details of our HPLC procedures are documented in a previous publication[4]. Partial purification (5-10 fold) of TpI was obtained following HPLC in the anion-exchange (HPIEC) or size-exclusion mode (HPSEC). However, separation on HPSEC was obtained only if the mobile phase (50 mM phosphate, 1.5 mM EDTA, 1 mM DTT and 10% v/v glycerol) contained 0.5% propanol. Still, the protein was eluted with a retention time greater than total column volume. This indicated that TpI exhibits hydrophobic properties which influence its separation on TSK 3000 SW size-exclusion columns. Enhanced purification of TpI was obtained when the HPIEC (SynChrom AX-1000) eluted protein was then separated by HPSEC (30-60 fold). Attempts to purify the HPIEC eluted protein using hydrophobic interaction chromatography (SynChrom propyl 500 column) were unsuccessful, again indicating the hydrophobic characteristic of TpI. Marked resolution of TpI activity was observed with HPIEC using a SynChrom CM-300 column (Table 1).

Table 1
Purification of DNA Topoisomerase I from Human Breast Cancer Cells (T47-D) on CM-300 Column

Fraction	Total Protein (μg)	Total Activity (units)	Specific Activity (units/μg)	Purification
Sample injected onto CM-300	1020.00	34,000	33.0	-
Flow through fraction	312.00	3,000	9.6	-
150-200 mM phosphate eluted peaks	6.75	2,250	333.0	10
250-350 mM phosphate eluted peaks	0.50*	2,000	4,000.00	121

Enzyme activity was noted in the void volume, at 150-200 mM and at 250-350 mM phosphate concentration. Silver stained polyacrylamide gels of TpI eluted from a CM-300 column showed considerable purity and a distinct protein band at 100-110 Kd in the 250-300 mM eluted peak.

Conclusion: We conclude that Topoisomerase I from human breast cancer cells is a highly charged molecule exhibiting binding to both anionic and cationic matrices. Further TpI appears to display strongly hydrophobic characteristics which are reflected in the separation of this protein on both size exclusion and hydrophobic columns.

To date, the most successful multi-step purification was obtained with a combination of HPIEC (SynChrom AX-1000) and HPSEC (TSK-3000 SW). However, the SynChrom CM-300 column provided the best resolution. Further analysis of the TpI activity separated first by the CM-300 column may provide the best path for subsequent purification by HPSEC. In contrast to the lengthy protocol (16-48 h) required for TpI purification by open column chromatography (giving approximately similar purities as those reported in this paper), we have demonstrated that the labile enzyme, TpI, can be purified approximately 100 fold within 4-8 h using HPLC methodologies.

Acknowledgments: This research was supported in part by USPHS Grant CA-19657, Phi Beta Psi Sorority and by CONICET of Argentina. S.M.H. is a postdoctoral research fellow of The Graduate School.

References:

(1) Wang, J.C. (1985) Ann. Rev. Biochem. 54, 665-697.
(2) Crespi, M.K., Baldi, A. and Wittliff, J.L. (1985) 13th Intl. Cong. Biochem., Amsterdam. Abs. p. 765.
(3) Hyder, S.M., Baldi, A., Crespi, M. and Wittliff, J.L. (1985) J. Chromatogr. (in press).
(4) Wittliff, J.L., Shahabi, N.A., Hyder, S.M., van der Walt, L.A., Myatt, L., Boyle, D.M. and He, Y.-J (1985) in Modern Methods in Protein Chemistry, (L'Italian, J.), ed., Plenum Press (in press).

TISSUE-SPECIFIC PROMOTER SEQUENCES IN THE PRO-OPIOMELANOCORTIN GENE

L. Jeannotte, R.K. Plante and J. Drouin, Laboratoire de biologie moléculaire des eucaryotes, Institut de recherches cliniques de Montréal, 110 ouest, Avenue des Pins, Montréal, Canada H2W 1R7.

Pro-opiomelanocortin (POMC), the precursor to ACTH, β-lipotropin, β-endorphin and the melanotropins, is expressed in specific cells of the anterior and intermediate lobes of the pituitary, in certain brain areas (1), in the testes (2), ovaries and placenta (3). We have isolated the single-copy rat POMC gene (4,5) and shown that regulation of POMC transcription is specific to each pituitary lobe (6), as is the processing of the precursor (7) and the control of peptide release (8). We have investigated the possibility that cis-acting sequence elements are necessary for tissue-specific expression of POMC in one or many POMC-expressing tissues. Tissue-specific promoter sequences were described in various cellular genes; these sequences activate transcription and some of them have properties of enhancer elements (9).

We have used a focus formation assay to assess POMC promoter utilization in various cell lines. The mouse pituitary tumor cell line, AtT-20, provides a good host to study the tissue-specificity of the POMC promoter as this cell line retains most characteristics of anterior pituitary corticotrophs. The fibroblastic mouse L cells were used as control. Electroporation was used to introduce recombinant plasmids into cells. POMC promoter activity was tested with plasmids containing POMC 5'-upstream sequences fused to neomycin resistance gene. Two POMC fragments containing upstream sequences and part of exon 1 were used. They have the same 3' end, but $pPOMC_{700}neo$ contains 709 bp upstream flanking sequences while $pPOMC_{4500}neo$ includes flanking sequences up to 4500 bp. Plasmids pRSVneo, pSV2neo and a promoter-less control plasmid (pPLneo) were also tested. Figure 1 illustrates graphically the efficiency with which the different plasmids produce G418-resistant colonies relative to pPLneo. The pPOMCneo plasmids are about 20 times more efficiently utilized in AtT-20 cells than in L cells. In the latter, the pPOMCneo plasmids are as inactive as the negative control pPLneo. Insertion of the MSV enhancer in $pPOMC_{700}neo$ appears to increase promoter utilization by about 10 fold in L cells, but only 2 fold in AtT-20 cells. In both cell types, this effect is orientation independent. Deletion mutants have been

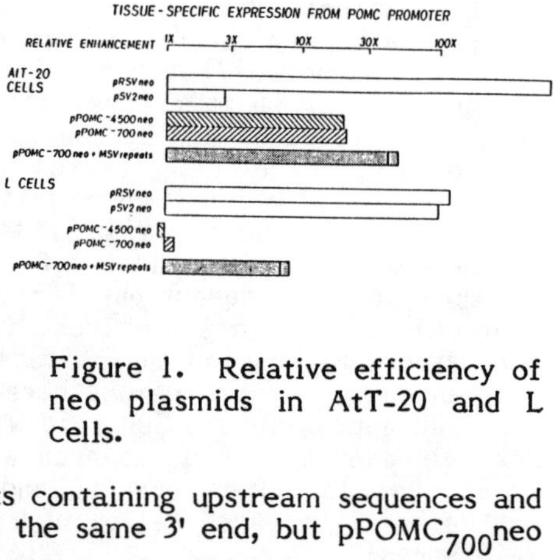

Figure 1. Relative efficiency of neo plasmids in AtT-20 and L cells.

constructed and as shown in Figure 2, no more than 478 bp upstream of the site of initiation are required for tissue-specific expression in AtT-20 cells.

In order to support the hypothesis that the colony numbers reflect promoter utilization rather than DNA integration, we analyzed genomic DNA extracted from pools of G418-resistant clones. Southern blots show that plasmid DNA copy number is similar in cells electroporated with the different plasmids. POMCneo transcripts were analyzed in the same pools. Transcription from the POMC promoter starts at the correct site as demonstrated by RNAase mapping. Thus, in AtT-20 cells, the exogenous POMC promoter is correctly transcribed; it is also regulated by glucocorticoids to the same extent as the endogenous cellular POMC gene (10).

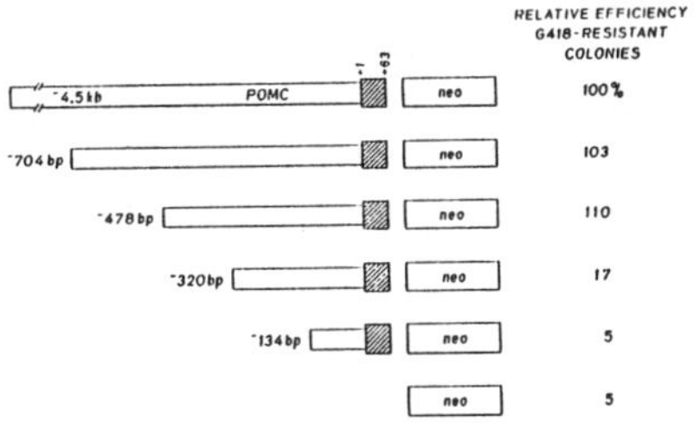

Figure 2. Relative efficiency of POMC gene fragments containing 5' deletions.

In order to determine if POMC 5'-flanking sequences possess enhancer properties, we have introduced POMC fragments upstream and downstream of an heterologous promoter. Insertion of a 575 bp POMC fragment on each side of the tk-neo gene activates transcription of this gene in AtT-20 cells. Thus, the rat POMC gene contains a tissue-specific enhancer element situated in upstream flanking sequences; this element does not overlap with sequences responsible for glucocorticoid inhibition of POMC transcription (10). It will be interesting to test whether the same POMC sequences are active in other POMC-expressing tissues.

This work is supported by MRC and NCI of Canada

REFERENCES

(1) Civelli, O. et al. (1982) J. Biol. Chem. **257**, 6783.
(2) Chen, C.-L. C. et al. (1984) Proc. Natl. Acad. Sci. USA **81**, 5672-5675.
(3) Chen, C.-L. and Chang, C.-C. (1985) Prog. 67th Annual Meeting Endocrine Society, 161.
(4) Drouin, J. and Goodman, H.M. (1980) Nature **288**, 610-613.
(5) Drouin, J. et al. (1985) FEBS Letters, in press.
(6) Gagner, J.P. and Drouin, J. (1985) Mol. Cell. Endoc. **40**, 25-32.
(7) Eipper, B. and Mains, R. (1982) Endocr. Rev. **1**, 1-27.
(8) Vale, W. et al. (1983) Endocrinology **113**, 1121-1131.
(9) Chambon, P. et al. (1984) Recent Prog. Horm. Res. **40**, 1-42.
(10) Drouin, J. et al. (1985) Short report submitted to this meeting.

ANDROGEN INDUCTION OF CDP mRNA, A HUMAN BREAST TUMOR MARKER

C.A. Kelton, J.E. Monahan
Cambridge Research Laboratory
195 Albany St.
Cambridge Ma. 02139

CDP or GCDFP-15 is a human breast Gross Cystic Disease Fluid Protein with a approximate monomer size of 15,000 daltons. CDP is a glycoprotein which is present in cystic disease fluid at a concentration of 1-10mg /ml. Human Breast Gross Cystic Disease is a premenopausal disease in women. It is the most common benign disease of the breast with an incidence of about seven percent in women. The disease has been considered to arise from excessive apocrine cystic secretions induced by a imbalance in the hormonal stimulus to the apocrine cells or in their response to these stimuli. CDP is present in normal plasma at less than 150 ng /ml. A number of studies have been performed to determine the value of CDP as a tumor marker for metastatic breast cancer (1,2). Clinically, plasma levels of CDP are elevated in approximately forty percent of patients with metastatic carcinomas. Plasma levels of CDP have been shown to correlate with the therapeutic response of metastatic breast carcinomas to hormonal therapy or palliative chemotherapy. In addition, an androgen stimulation of plasma CDP has been observed in patients with metastatic breast carcinoma (5). The CDP cDNA clones were obtained from the T47-D human breast tumor cell line. We have cloned and sequenced the complete coding region of the CDP mRNA and the 3' non-coding region to the poly A tail (7). The sequence reported completely agrees with the partial amino acid sequence for CDP reported by Haagensen (8).

(I) EFFECT OF DIHYDROTESTOSTERONE DOSE ON CDP mRNA INDUCTION.

Total RNA was isolated from replicate flasks containing T47-D cells grown for three days in DME media plus 10% DCC-stripped fetal calf serum. The dihydrotestosterone (DHT) in ethanol was added to the media to achieve a final concentration ranging from 1 pM to 100 nM. An equivalent amount of ethanol (0.1%) was added to the media of the control cells. Total RNA was extracted by the guanidinium isothiocyanate /cesium chloride method. Appropriate amounts (0.2-0.5 ugm) of total RNA were loaded onto a Gene Screen Plus membrane using a Schleicher & Schuell slot-blot apparatus. The filter was prehybridized and the RNA hybridized to a single-stranded, CDP specific DNA probe synthesized from a M13mp8 subclone of CDP (6). After washing, the amount of probe which had hybridized to the RNA was quantitated by liquid scintillation counting. The results of this analysis are shown in figure 1. The data is expressed as a

Fig. 1. DOSE RESPONSE of CDP mRNA induction

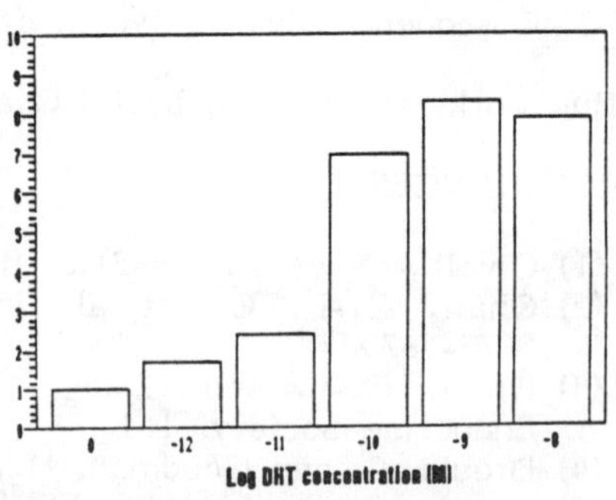

fold induction of CDP mRNA as compared to cells in flasks not treated with DHT. The induction of CDP mRNA was minimal at DHT concentrations at or below 10 pM. Maximal induction with DHT results in an approximately eight fold higher level of mRNA specific for CDP. Half maximal induction CDP occured at about 0.05 nM DHT. While there are a number of estrogen regulated markers in human breast cancer these results demonstrate for the first time the mRNA induction of a breast tumor marker with DHT. This induction occurs at a DHT concentration which suggests that the response is mediated by the androgen receptor. The androgen receptor in the MCF-7 human breast tumor cell line has a K_d of between 0.1 - 1.0 nM (13). Further work is in progress to define the steroid specificity for CDP mRNA induction.

(II) TIME COURSE OF CDP mRNA INDUCTION. Replicate flasks containing T47-D cells were grown as decribed above in the presence or absence of 10 nM DHT. This experiment was initiated at a cell density of approximately 10^6 cells per 100mm dish. Cells were harvested, RNA isolated, and filter hybridizations performed as described above. The results are shown in figure 2. The fold induction of CDP mRNA is relative to RNA extracted from cells harvested at time zero. During the course of this experiment there was no change in the level of CDP mRNA in the cells not treated with DHT. An induction of CDP mRNA levels is apparant after 24 hours and is maximally increased after 2-3 days of DHT treatment. Further work is in progress to identify the regulatory step(s) responsible for the induction of CDP mRNA.

Fig. 2. TIME COURSE of CDP mRNA induction

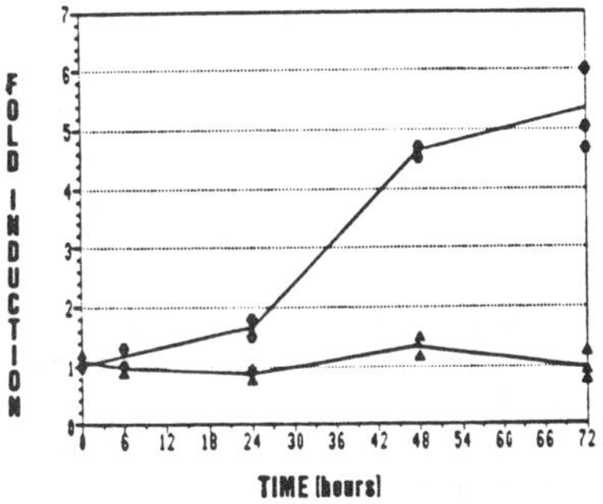

REFERENCES

(1) Haagensen, D.E., Jr., Mazoujian, G., Holder, W.D., Kister, S.J., Wells, S.A., Jr. Ann. Surg. 185:279-285 (1977).
(2) Silva, J.S., Leight, G.S., Jr., Haagensen, D.E., Jr., Tallos, P.B., Cox, D.E., Dilley, W.G., and Wells, S.A., Jr. Cancer 49(6):1236-1242 (1982)
(3) Dilley, W.G., Leight, G.S., Jr., Silva, J.S., Ammirata, S., Haagensen, D.E., Jr., and Wells, S.A., Jr. J. Natl. Cancer Inst. 70(1):69-74 (1983).
(4) Kelton, C.A., Monahan, J.E. Manuscript in preparation, 1985.
(5) Haagensen, D.E. Jr. U.S. Patent #4,452,904. June 5, 1984.
(6) Jeffreys, A.J., Wilson, V., and Thein, S.W. Nature 314:67-73 (1985).
(7) Lippman, M., Bolan, G., and Huff, K. Cancer Research 36: 4610-4618 (1976).

THE MOLECULAR ACTION OF 1,25-DIHYDROXYVITAMIN D_3 IN RAT INTESTINE: ISOLATION AND CHARACTERIZATION OF DIFFERENT VITAMIN D_3-RESPONSIVE cDNA-CLONES

L. Lamm, M. A. Kessler, H. Darwish, and H. F. DeLuca
Department of Biochemistry, University of Wisconsin-Madison, 420 Henry Mall, Madison, Wisconsin 53706

The mechanism of action of vitamin D through its active metabolite, 1,25-dihydroxyvitamin D_3 (1,25-$(OH)_2D_3$), follows the general model of steroid hormones in target tissues. This involves the binding of the hormone to a specific receptor and subsequent interaction with the nuclear genetic material resulting in gene transcription. Vitamin D exerts its effects on different organs and tissues, including intestine, kidney and bone. One of the primary effects of vitamin D is the stimulation of intestinal calcium transport and the induction of a cytosolic calcium-binding protein (CaBP). While it is well established that the mode of action of vitamin D involves the initiation of gene expression, very little is known about the nature and the number of the affected genes and the molecular mechanism of this stimulation. We have used the technique of differential hybridization to screen a rat intestinal mucosa cDNA library for 1,25-$(OH)_2D_3$-inducible sequences. This library consisting of 10^6 independent recombinants was constructed in the vector λgt10 using poly$(A)^+$RNA extracted from vitamin D-deficient rats 12 h subsequent to an intrajugular dose of 500 pmol of 1,25-$(OH)_2D_3$. Duplicate filters were hybridized to cDNA probes synthesized from poly$(A)^+$RNA prepared from the small intestines of either vitamin D-deficient or vitamin D-replete animals (Fig. 1). Of the 20,000 clones screened thus far, 20 clones representing 4 distinct sequences survived 3 rounds of screening. Sequence analysis and a computer search of the Genebank Data File (1) enabled us to identify 3 of the 4 clones as: 1) rat CaBP, 2) cytochrome c oxidase subunit I, and 3) cytochrome c oxidase subunit III. The fourth clone, a > 90% full length with mature message size of 1,000 bp, does not match any of the previously reported sequences. The message size and time course of induction were determined for these sequences by Northern blots as shown for CaBP (Fig. 2). This message undergoes a maximum induction of about 16-fold 12 h after an intrajugular dose of 1,25-$(OH)_2D_3$ as measured by densitometry (Fig. 3). In Figures 2 and 3, the far right-hand data point represents the levels of CaBP message in samples from rats on a diet sufficient in vitamin D but low in calcium. The time course of induction of 2 of the other mRNAs was similar to that of CaBP. However, cytochrome c oxidase subunit I had a unique biphasic response with maxima at 6 and 18 h, paralleling the time course of vitamin D-induced energy-dependent calcium transport (2). Using the CaBP cDNA-clone, an EcoRI rat genomic library constructed in λ Charon 4 vector was screened for the CaBP gene. A recombinant clone was isolated which contains the putative CaBP gene. These studies may enable us to elucidate the molecular basis for the physiological action of 1,25-$(OH)_2D_3$.

REFERENCES

(1) Devereux, J., Haeberli, P., and Smithies, O. (1984) Nucl. Acids Res. 12, 387-395.
(2) Halloran, B. P. and DeLuca, H. F. (1971) Arch. Biochem. Biophys. 146, 574-578.

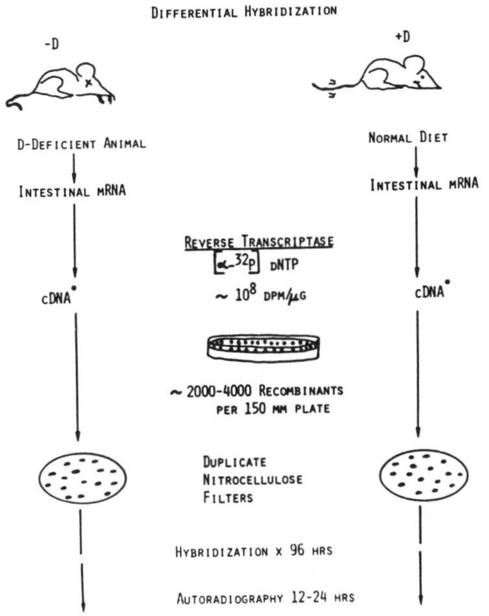

Fig. 1: Schematic description of the differential hybridization protocol.

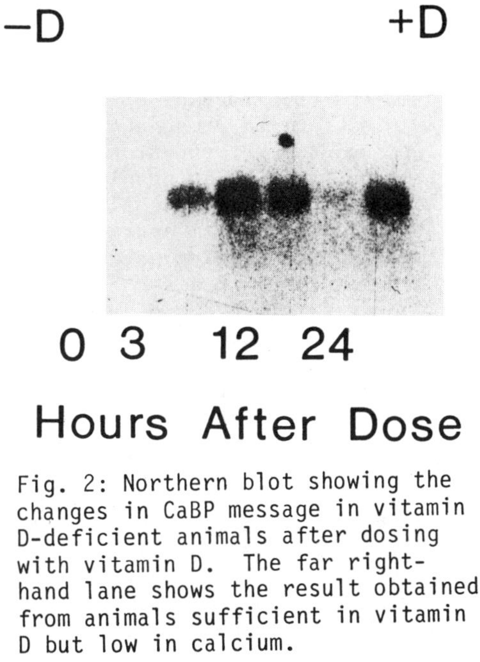

Fig. 2: Northern blot showing the changes in CaBP message in vitamin D-deficient animals after dosing with vitamin D. The far right-hand lane shows the result obtained from animals sufficient in vitamin D but low in calcium.

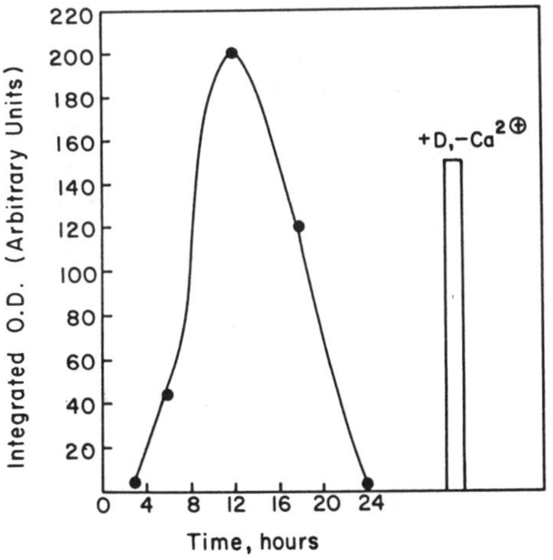

Fig. 3: Densitometerscanning of the Northern Blot as shown in Fig. 2.

THE PHYTOESTROGEN COUMESTROL APPEARS CAPABLE OF INSERTION BETWEEN BASE PAIRS IN DNA IN AGREEMENT WITH A STEREOCHEMICAL RATIONALE FOR HORMONE ACTION

A.F. Lehner*†, T.G. Muldoon†, V.B. Mahesh†, E.D. Bransome, Jr.*†, and L.B. Hendry*†
Departments of Endocrinology† and Medicine*, Medical College of Georgia, Augusta, Georgia 30912.

Gonadal steroid hormones and related agonists have been predicted by stereochemical reasoning to fit between base pairs in the partially unwound DNA sequence 5'-dTdG-3'·5'-dCdA-3' with topological congruence to the perimeters of the cavity defined by the bases and with hydrogen bonding of oxygen functions in the steroid 3 and 17β or 20 positions to phosphate residues in the DNA backbone (1,2). This finding does not appear to be merely coincidental as excellent structure-activity relationships have been demonstrable purely on the basis of stereochemical analysis. For example, the series of estrogens diethylstilbestrol, estradiol-3,17β, coumestrol, genistein, and daidzein have decreasing estrogenic potency in the order given even though phenolic A rings and hydroxyl groups are similarly spaced in each molecule; this order of biological activity correlates well with a corresponding decreasing fit into the 5'-dTdG-3'·5'-dCdA-3' sequence. We have therefore sought physicochemical support for our hypothesis that hormones fit into DNA by examining in vitro estrogen/DNA interactions. Here we report our initial findings with coumestrol, an estrogenic coumarone with readily exploitable spectral properties.

DNA TEMPERATURE OF DENATURATION (T_m). Coumestrol altered the T_m of polydeoxynucleotides with alternating pyrimidine-purine sequences in the order poly(dA-dT)·poly(dA-dT) >> poly(dT-dG)·poly(dC-dA) ≥ poly(dG-dC)·poly(dG-dC). However, these effects were small in comparison to those of the classical intercalating agents acridine, adriamycin or ethidium on these sequences.

ULTRAVIOLET/VISIBLE ABSORBANCE SPECTROSCOPY. Wavelength scans on acridine, adriamycin, ethidium or coumestrol in the presence of increasing concentrations of calf thymus DNA disclosed common features of bathochromic and hypochromic shifts of peaks corresponding to major $\pi \rightarrow \pi^*$ transitions at wavelengths above 300 nm.

FLUORESCENCE SPECTROSCOPY. There was significant quenching of the fluorescence of coumestrol on exposure to double-stranded calf thymus DNA in a manner similar to acridine and adriamycin (ethidium fluorescence was enhanced); however, in contrast to effects on the intercalators, single-stranded (denatured) DNA had no effect on coumestrol, suggesting specificity for double-strandedness (Fig. 1).

EFFECTS OF METAL CATIONS. Various monovalent and divalent metal cations were compared as modifiers of DNA effects on the intensity of coumestrol fluorescence. On an equimolar basis, the monovalent cations had less dramatic effects than divalent cations in reversing

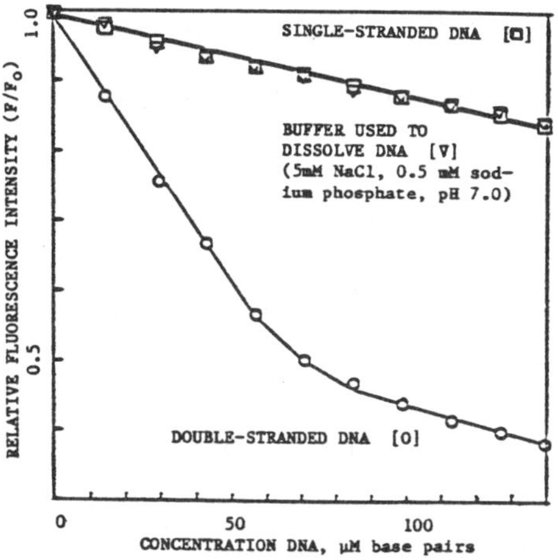

Fig. 1. Effects of increasing concentrations of calf thymus DNA (double- or single-stranded) or buffer alone on fluorescence of 10 μM coumestrol in 0.5 mM sodium phosphate, pH 7.0; λ_{em} = 365 nm, λ_{em} = 440 nm.

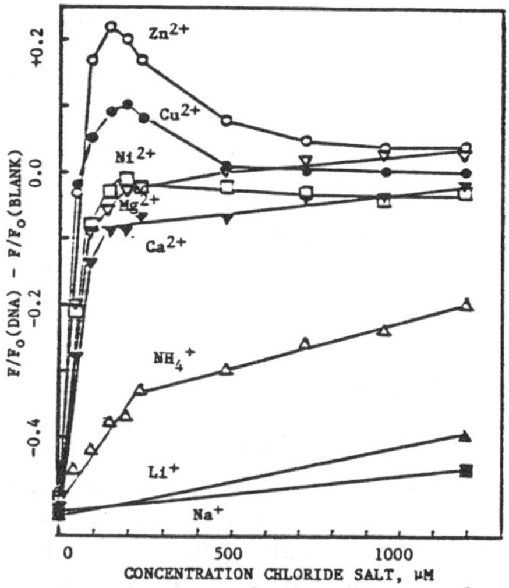

Fig. 2. Effects of various metal cations on quenching of 24 μM coumestrol fluorescence by 140 μM DNA (ion effects on coumestrol subtracted; F/F_0 = relative fluorescence; rest as in Fig. 1).

the effects of DNA; the cations also presented a range of effects (Fig. 2). The order of effectiveness $Zn^{2+}>Cu^{2+}>Ni^{2+}>Mg^{2+}>Ca^{2+}>>NH_4^+>>Li^+>Na^+$ correlates well with the capacity of these ions to unwind double-stranded DNA: $Cu^{2+}>Zn^{2+}>Ni^{2+}>Mg^{2+}>NH_4^+>Li^+>Na^+$ (3,4).

CONCLUSIONS. A model in which coumestrol is inserted between base pairs of partially uncoiled B DNA readily accommodates the requirements of the data: electron cloud distortion e.g. by stacking interactions, weak cross-linking of strands, preference for double-strandedness and sensitivity to helical unwinding. An insertional model is attractive not only because of its prediction on theoretical grounds (1,2) but also because coumestrol fulfills criteria considered essential for ideal intercalants (5). If the findings with coumestrol can be extrapolated to steroids, then it remains to be determined whether the mechanism of action of these hormones involves stereochemical insertion between base pairs in concert with the binding of receptor proteins to DNA.

REFERENCES

(1) Hendry L.B., Witham F.H., and Chapman O.L. (1977) Perspect. Biol. Med. 21, 120.
(2) Bransome E.D. Jr., Hendry L.B., Muldoon T.G., Mahesh V.B., Hutson M.S. and Campbell L.K. (1985) J. Theor. Biol. 112, 97.
(3) Eichhorn G.L. and Shin Y.A. (1968) J. Amer. Chem. Soc. 90, 7323.
(4) Anderson P. and Bauer W. (1978) Biochem. 17, 594.
(5) Miller K.J. and Newlin D.D. (1982) Biopolymers, 21, 633.

STRUCTURE OF THREE MOUSE HISTONE H2A AND H2B GENES INCLUDING ONE PSEUDOGENE ON CHROMOSOME 13

Ta-Jen Liu, Landie Liu and William F. Marzluff. Department of Chemistry, Florida State University, Tallahassee, Florida 32306.

We have previously described the isolation of three clusters of mouse histone genes containing several genes for each type of core histone protein (1). Two of these clusters, MM221 and MM291, are found on mouse chromosome 13 and contain multiple H2a and H2b histone genes (Fig. 1). The third cluster, MM614, is found on chromosome 3 and contains an H2a and H3 gene but we have not characterized any other genes on this cluster. The complete sequence of the H2b genes and H2a genes on chromsome 13 have been determined, including the entire 5' intragenic regions between the H2b and the neighboring H2a (MM291) or H3 (MM221) genes.

The H2b genes encode 3 different proteins (Table 1) differing from one another in a single amino acid in each case. None of these genes encodes the protein sequence reported for histone H2b, although the consensus of these 3 sequences is that expected for histone H2b. All three of these genes are expressed as judged by S1 nuclease mapping and are coordinately regulated with DNA synthesis (1). The three H2b genes are very similar in nucleotide sequence in the coding region, differing in only 10-15 base changes in addition to the change responsible for the amino acid change. This is partly due to the stringent pattern of codon usage in mouse histone genes (2) but reflects a strong evolutionary relationship between the coding regions of these closely linked genes. In contrast there is no detectable conservation in the 5' flanking regions of any of the H2b genes, except for the TATAA and CCAAT sequences found in all genes transcribed by RNA polymerase II. The 3' flanking regions each contain the expected dyad sequence characteristic of the 3' end of mouse histone genes. Other than this sequence there is no other homology in the 3' flanking regions of these genes.

The H2a genes show a similar phenomenon. None of the H2a genes code for the same protein (Table 2). The H2a.614 gene has the sequence expected for the H2a.2 protein, while the other H2a genes have the characteristic amino acids (but not the exact sequence) expected for the H2a.1 protein (3). The H2a.291A is a pseudogene derived from a presumably functional real gene. This pseudogene has two major defects. The first 12 amino acids (including the initiator ATG codon) are missing as is a TATAA box. The last 3 amino acids as well as the dyad sequence characteristic of the 3' end of histone genes is also missing. However, the protein is in frame from amino acid 12-125 and encodes the sequence expected for the H2a.1 protein in this region. The number of nucleotide changes between the different H2a genes in the coding region is very few, similar to the H2b genes. The gene on chromosome 3 (H2a.614) is more divergent from the genes on chromosome 13 than the genes on chromosome 13 (including the pseudogene) are from each other as expected. Since the pseudogene has two major, presumably independent, defects we postulate that gene conversion involving only the coding region has maintained the constancy of the nucleotide sequence in the histone coding regions and that the flanking regions have diverged greatly with little selective pressure. Gene conversion has maintained the sequence of the coding region of the non-expressed pseudogene and the elements necessary for expression 5' and 3' of the gene have been lost due to the lack of selective pressure.

References

1. Graves, R.A., Wellman, S.E., Chiu, I-M. and Marzluff, W.F. (1985) J. Mol. Biol. 183 179-94.
2. Sittman, D.B., Graves, R.A. and Marzluff, W.F. (1983) Nuc. Acids Res. 11 6679-91.
3. Franklin, S.G. and Zweidler, A. (1977) Nature 266 273-74.

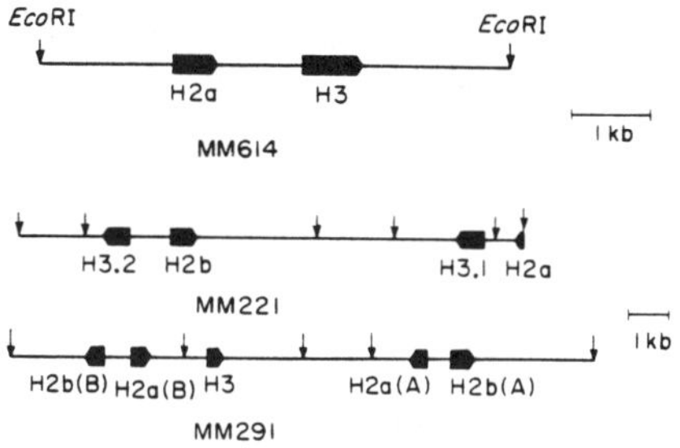

Figure 1. Restriction maps of the histone gene clusters. (a) The 3 recombinant phage MM291, MM221 and MM614 are shown. The location and orientation of the genes is shown. The arrows indicate the *Eco*RI sites. (b) A

TABLE 1. The position of amino acid changes in H2b genes

amino acid #	4	18	75
H2b-221	Ala	Leu	Gly
H2b291A	Ala	Val	Ser
H2b291B	Thr	Val	Gly

TABLE 2. The position of amino acid changes in H2a genes

amino acid #	16	40	51	99	126
H2a-221(92-129)	--	--	--	Arg	Pro
H2a-614	Ser	Ala	Met	Lys	Ala
H2a-291A	Thr	Ser	Leu	Arg	Ala
H2a-291B(12-125)	Thr	Ser	Leu	Arg	--

3,5,3'-L-TRIIODOTHYRONINE (L-T_3) BINDING TO RATS SUBCELLUAR FRACTIONS

A.Llopart-Román and L.K.Stitzer, Department of Physiology, Ponce School of Medicine, Ponce, Puerto Rico 00732

INTRODUCTION

Modulation of L-T_3 receptor at subcellular levels play an important role in understanding the mechanism of action of this hormone and its variable metabolic effects (1).

In previous studies we found that in vitro L-T_3 binding characteristics vary from thyroid hormone "responsive" to "non-responsive" tissues. We concluded from our binding data that the affinity to L-T_3 nuclear and mitochondrial receptors for the hormone was higher in "responsive" tissues while in "non-responsive" tissues the affinity was very low, although the number of active receptors was high. Here we present the results of an in vitro study of L-T_3 binding under the effect of acute hypo-and hyperthyroid conditions.

MATERIALS AND METHODS

Adult male albino rats were separated in three groups of 10 rats each: control or euthyroid, hypothyroid and hyperthyroid rats. The animals were treated with saline, the anti-thyroidal agent PTU and T_4, respectively.

The studied tissues were fractionated by differential centrifugation to obtain nuclear and mitochondrial fractions.

The fractions were incubated with $4x10^{-12}M$, ^{125} I-L-T_3 at 37°C for 30 min and a 1000 fold molar excess of non-labeled L-T_3 was added to determine non-specific binding. The mixture was centrifuged, decanted and the pellet redioactivity measured in a gamma counter.

RESULTS

Scatchard analysis (2) of the binding data in nuclear fractions resulted in the affinity constants (Ka's) and number of active L-T_3 receptors (B.C.'s) depicted in Table I.

Table I. Ka's and B.C.'s of Nuclear L-T_3 Receptors in Hypo-and Hyperthyroid Rats

A. Ka (10^9M^{-1})

Tissue	Euthyroid	Hypothyroid	Hyperthyroid
Liver (TR)	2.6 ± 0.2	0.51 ± 0.2*	0.4 ± 0.1 *
Kidney (TR)	5.1 ± 1.6	0.85 ± 0.1*	1.1 ± 0.09*
Brain Cortex (TNR)	0.55± 0.05	1.25 ± 0.5*	1.2 ± 0.1 *

B. B.C. ($10^{-12}M$)

Tissue	Euthyroid	Hypothyroid	Hyperthyroid
Liver (TR)	43.0 ± 1.0	130.0 ± 9.0*	175.0 ± 9.0 *
Kidney (TR)	10.0 ± 4.0	59.0 ± 5.0*	66.0 ± 1.0 *
Brain Cortex (TNR)	80.0 ± 8.5	44.0 ± 1.0*	68.0 ± 1.0 *

* Significantly different from euthyroid condition, $p < 0.01$
TR Thyroid hormone responsive tissue
TNR Thyroid hormone non-responsive tissue

The affinity constants (Ka's) and number of active L-T_3 receptors (B.C.'s) for the mitochondrial fractions are shown in Table II.

Table II. Ka's and B.C.'s of Mitochondrial L-T_3 Receptors in Hypo-and Hyperthyroid Rats.

A. Ka (10^9 M^{-1})

Tissue	Euthyroid	Hypothyroid	Hyperthyroid
Liver (TR)	5.0 ± 0.5	4.1 ± 0.4 N.S.	7.2 ± 0.05**
Kidney (TR)	4.3 ± 0.1	2.5 ± 0.01*	10.5 ± 0.01*
Brain Cortex (TNR)	2.5 ± 0.8	5.0 ± 0.5 *	3.0 ± 0.2 N.S.

B. B.C. (10^{-12}M)

Tissue	Euthyroid	Hypothyroid	Hyperthyroid
Liver (TR)	11.0 ± 0.9	18.0 ± 1.0 *	8.0 ± 0.2**
Kidney (TR)	28.1 ± 1.0	31.4 ± 0.02*	12.5 ± 0.5 *
Brain Cortex (TNR)	19.8 ± 0.5	8.5 ± 0.5 *	17.0 ± 0.1 *

* Significantly different from the euthyroid condition, $p < 0.01$
** Significantly different from the euthyroid condition, $p < 0.05$
N.S. Not significantly different from euthyroid condition, $p < 0.01$ or $p < 0.05$

DISCUSSION

These results reveal that different regulatory mechanisms exist for L-T_3 receptors in nuclei and mitochondria when the metabolic state of the animal is altered. It appears that both organelles under hypothyroid conditions recruite additional L-T_3 receptors. These "new" active receptors are considered " spare receptors" (3) and show low affinity for L-T_3. Nuclear and mitochondrial fractions of brain cortex showed an increase in affinity and a decrease in the number of active L-T_3 receptors. These results are not in accordance with those reported by Hamada and co-workers (4), although they agree that the severe hypothyroidism induced by thyroidectomy could account for their unexpected results. In our study we induced a less severe hypothyroid condition by using PTU (5).

The results under hyperthyroid conditions revealed that the nuclear fraction made similar adjustments in its L-T_3 receptors as those for hypothyroid conditions. Mitochondrial fraction on the other hand, lowered the number of active receptors for L-T_3 but increased their ability to bind the hormone. This mitochondrial modulation may help explain why several of its enzymatic systems respond differently to thyroid hormones (6). Further studies will be needed in order to determine if the adjustments of L-T_3 receptors under acutely induced metabolic changes correlate with long-term metabolic changes.

REFERENCES

(1) Samuels, H.H., et.al., 1977, J. Biol. Chem., 252:6052
(2) Scatchard, G., 1949, Ann. NY Acad. Scie., 51:660
(3) Baxter, J.D., et.al., 1979, N. Engl. J. Med., 301:1149
(4) Hamada, S., et.al., 1983, Endocrinology, 112:207
(5) Cooper, D.S., et.al., 1983, Endocrinology, 113:921
(6) Yoshimasa, Y., et.al., 1983, Biochem J., 210:331

EXPRESSION OF U1b GENES IN MOUSE CELL LINES

Susan M.Lobo, Naguib Moussa and William F.Marzluff.
Dept.of Chemistry, Florida State University.

The mouse genome contains two major classes of U1 genes encoding the U1a and U1b RNAs. These RNAs differ in nucleotide sequence at six key positions. Both U1a and U1b RNAs are expressed in mouse embryos and in adult tissues such as the spleen, testis and thymus, which contain undifferentiated stem cells. Only U1a is expressed in differentiated adult tissues (1).

We transfected a 7.0 kb DNA fragment containing two U1b genes as well as subclones derived from this fragment (Figure 1) into two mouse cell lines, L cells and C127 fibroblasts. Expression of the U1b DNA was assayed by hybridisation of *in vivo* labeled RNA to a single stranded DNA probe immobilised on nitrocellulose.

L cells normally express U1a and small amounts of U1b RNA whereas C127 cells express only U1a. U1b RNA was not detected in C127 cells by our assay.

Upon transfection, L cells efficiently transcribed U1b RNA from constructs A through F, which contain 400bp or more of DNA flanking the 5'end of the gene (2). Subclone G, containing 150 bp upstream of the gene, was not expressed. These observations are in keeping with the data of Skuzeski et. al.(3) who showed that a TATAA sequence between -211 and -203 were required for transcription of the human U1 gene in Xenopus oocytes. There is a similar TATAA sequence in the mouse U1b gene.

C127 cells expressed U1b RNA only when transfected with the 7.0kb fragment. All the other constructs shown in Figure 1 were not expressed. This indicates that C127 cells and L cells have different sequence requirements for the expression of U1b RNA. It may be that a trans-acting factor, encoded by the 7.0 kb fragment, but not by subclones B through G, is required for the transcription of the U1b class of U1 genes.

References:

(1)Lund,E.,Kahan,B.and Dahlberg,J.,Science 229,(1985) 1271-1274.
(2)Moussa,N.M.,Lobo,S.M.and Marzluff,W.F.,Gene,36 (1985) 311-319.
(3)Skuzeski,J.M.,Lund,E.,Murphy,J.T.,Steinberg,T.H.,Burgess,R.R.and Dahlberg,J.E.,J.Biol.Chem. 259 (1984) 8345-8352.

Supported by NIH grant GM 29832.

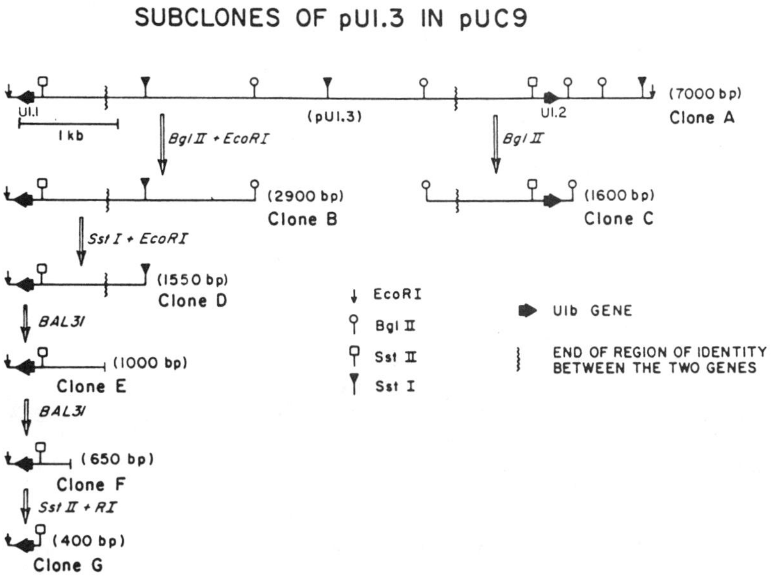

FIGURE 1.
Clone A was isolated from a mouse genomic library. It contains two U1b genes which are identical. The region of homology between the two extends to 650bp 5' of the genes. Constructs B through G were derived from A.

PROMOTER SEQUENCES INVOLVED IN THE DEVELOPMENTAL REGULATION OF THE DROSOPHILA MELANOGASTER HSP 23 GENE

R. Mestril, P. Schiller, J. Amin, H. Klapper, J. Ananthan and R. Voellmy. Dept. of Biochemistry, University of Miami School of Medicine, Miami Florida

The small heat shock protein genes (HSP 27, 26, 23 and 22 genes) of *Drosophila melanogaster* are specifically expressed in late third instar larvae and in prepupae, in the absence of external stress (1,2). At these developmental stages titers of the insect molting hormone ecdysterone (a steroid hormone) are high. The hormone activates the same set of genes in certain *Drosophila melanogaster* cell lines (2). In cultured cells as in the developing organism this induction occurs without the concomitant synthesis of other HSP genes (2).

We have constructed a hybrid gene by functionally linking a 1.75 kb *D. melanogaster* DNA segment containing 1.5 kb of 5' nontranscribed sequence, the 5' nontranslated region and the first 45 codons of the HSP 23 gene to a truncated *E.coli* beta-galactosidase gene. This hybrid gene and mutant derivatives of this gene with HSP 23 gene promoter segments of different lengths have been introduced into *D. melanogaster* S3 cells by DEAE-dextran mediated transfection. Addition of ecdysterone to transfected cultured cells leads to an at least 10 fold increase in the level of HSP 23 hybrid gene expression. This hormonal effect on HSP 23 gene expression is selective since the activities of analogous HSP 70 and HSP 84 hybrid gene constructs are not influenced by ecdysterone (3).

Analysis of mutants with internal deletions in the HSP 23 gene promoter segment has led to the identification of two promoter regions which are required for ecdysterone but not for heat-induced expression. Mutants in which either one or both of these promoter regions have been deleted (d217/186 and d239/197) are still heat but not ecdysterone-regulated (Fig.1). A mutant that lacks the sequences between these two regions (d 217/197) is both heat- and hormone-inducible (Fig.1). A mutant that lacks the heat shock regulatory sequences at -401 and -135 (d379/143/63) was found to be hormone but not heat shock regulated (Fig.1).

Inspection of the DNA sequence in the two regions involved in ecdysterone regulation of the HSP 23 gene, revealed the presence of an imperfect inverted repeat (Fig.2A). This sequence element is an isomer of the one found in the promoter of another *Drosophila* gene that is also under the control of ecdysterone, the Sgs 4 gene (Fig.2B). A naturally occuring deletion in this region of the Sgs 4 gene affects its expression (4). Another *Drosophila* developmental gene that has recently been cloned and sequenced also exhibits a related repeat in the 5' nontranscribed region between -257 and -287 (5). The functional importance of the latter sequence has not been investigated. Similar inverted repeats also appear to be present in the promoter regions of the other small HSP genes (Fig.2B). We propose that the inverted repeat between -239 to -186 in the HSP 23 gene promoter is a recognition site for an ecdysterone-receptor complex.

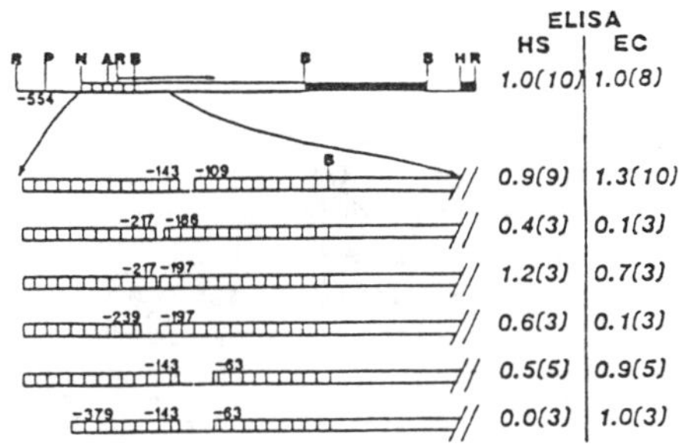

Figure 1.

The HSP23 - beta-galactosidase hybrid gene and derivatives with internal promoter deletions. 5' nontranscribed, leader and coding region of HSP 23 gene, E.coli beta galactosidase coding region, 3' trailer of HSP 70 gene. Expression of HSP23 hybrid genes was measured by an ELISA method, using antibodies specific against E.coli beta galactosidase (3). Activities are relative to that of the hybrid HSP 23 gene which contains 554 bp of the HSP 23 promoter. The number of independent experiments are given between parenthesis.

A) -270

TCCACCAAGC CTTTTCATTC CCACTCCCCT AGGAGATTGC TCATTTTCCA
TAGCGATACT CTCACTTTCA ATGGCAGATA ATGCGTAATT
-180

B) HSP 23: -228 ATTTTCCAT-19-ATGGCAGAT -192
Sgs 4: -354 AAATGGAAA-3-TACCTTTCT -344
74F: -284 AATTTGCAT-13-ATGGAAACT -254
HSP 27: -155 TATTTGCAT-11-AGGGAAAAC -133
HSP 26: -261 TCATGGCAT-4-TGGGAAAGG -240
HSP 22: -304 GTATGGAAA-2-GACCTTCCC -284

Figure 2.

A) DNA sequence of a segment of the HSP23 promoter containing elements involved in the ecdysterone regulation.
B) Inverted repeats found in the promoters of HSP 23, Sgs 4 (4), 74F (5) and other HSP genes.

REFERENCES

(1) Sirotkin, K.and Davidson, N. (1982) Dev. Biol. 89: 196-210.
(2) Ireland, R.and Berger, E.(1982) PNAS 79: 855-859.
(3) Lawson, R., Mestril, R.,Luo, Y.and Voellmy, R. (1985) Dev. Biol. 110: 321-330.
(4) McGinnis, W.,Shermoen, A.,Heemskerk, J.and Beckendorf, S.(1983) PNAS 80: 1063-1067.
(5) Moritz, Th., Edstroem, J.and Pongs, O.(1984) EMBO J. 3: 289-295.

INVESTIGATION OF GLUCOCORTICOID RECEPTOR REGULATION OF AUTOCRINE GROWTH IN A SMOOTH MUSCLE TUMOR CELL LINE

J.S. Norris[1,2], L.E. Cornett[2], S.E. Harris[3], A. Nag[5], P. Rossby[2], A. Srivastava[4], S.L. Macleod[1] and R.G. Smith[5,6].
Departments of Medicine[1] and Physiology[2], University of Arkansas for Medical Sciences, Little Rock 72205; W. Alton Jones Cell Science Center[3], Lake Placid, NY 12946; University of Indiana Medical School, Indianapolis[4]; Departments of Urology[5] and Cell Biology[6], Baylor College of Medicine, Houston, TX 77030.

Introduction: DDT_1 MF-2 cells (CRL 1701) are a smooth muscle tumor derived cell line of Syrian hamster origin. Growth of DDT_1 MF-2 cells is stimulated by androgens and inhibited by glucocorticoids (1). We have previously determined that glucocorticoid inhibition of growth was due to transcriptional and/or posttranscriptional regulation of expression of the c-sis proto-oncogene (codes for platelet derived growth factor, PDGF) (2,3). DDT_1 MF-2 cells blocked in G_0/G_1 by glucocorticoids are stimulated to re-enter the cell cycle in a dose dependent manner by exogenously applied PDGF but not by epidermal growth factor, insulin or tumor growth factor ß (TGFß) (2). No regulation of sis gene expression or cell growth is observed in a variant of the DDT_1 MF-2 cell line termed DDT_1 MF-2 GR which lacks glucocorticoid receptor (4). These data, in conjunction with Northern and Southern blotting data (4), suggest that growth of DDT_1 MF-2 cells is regulated by the production of a PDGF-like molecule which is secreted into the media, binds to DDT_1 MF-2 growth factor receptor (implied) and stimulates growth of the cells, i.e., autocrine regulation of growth.

Methods: To further our understanding of the mechanisms of hormonal regulation of sis gene expression as a functional aspect of autocrine growth, we constructed the following expression vector. Plasmid pSM-1 (kindly provided by S.F. Josephs and F. Wong-Staal), a transforming plasmid containing human c-sis cDNA, was restricted at the unique Hind III site and the mouse mammary tumor virus LTR from plasmid pSVMgpt (kindly provided by G. Ringold) was inserted. A plasmid demonstrated by restriction mapping to have a MMTV LTR oriented as in pSVMgpt was designated pSMTV.

Plasmids were introduced by cotransfection with pSV2 neo and selected by 800 µg/ml Geneticin (Gibco). Twenty-nine colonies were identified and cloned. The first 6 clones analyzed by restriction mapping were determined to contain pSMTV inserted into genomic DNA.

Cell growth studies are carried out as previously described (4) using an initial 10,000 cell inoculum. The cells are treated with appropriate vehicle or hormone (testosterone, T; triamcinolone acetonide, TA) and media is changed every two days. Cells are harvested and counted on day 8.

Results of cell growth experiment: If the mechanism of growth regulation by glucocorticoids was as simple as the shutoff of hamster c-sis gene expression , i.e., reduced production of PDGF, then the transfected cells (if the inserted pSMTV construct is glucocorticoid upregulated) would produce PDGF (now human PDGF) and the cells would continue to grow. To test this hypothesis, growth assays were carried out. Our results for the first two clones assayed are presented as Table I. From these data it is clear that glucocorticoids are continuing to downregulate cell growth. However, it is also clear that the growth rates of control transfected cells are higher than in the wild type DDT_1 MF-2 which perhaps is a result of increased constitive production of PDGF from the introduced plasmid.

TABLE I. Hormonal Regulation of Cell Growth

Treatment	Cell Number x 10^6		
	Clone 1	Clone 5	Wild Type
Control	1.96	2.07	0.54
T (1x10^{-8}M)	2.38	2.31	1.42
TA (1x10^{-8}M)	0.72	0.29	0.50
T + TA (1x10^{-8}M)	0.61	0.22	0.32

Results of Northern Blotting: We have also initiated studies examining expression of pSMTV in the transfected cells. Preliminary Northern blotting experiments indicate glucocorticoids are inducing accumulation of sis transcripts. Mapping the transcripts with S1 nuclease is in progress to verify their pSMTV origin.

Conclusions: It would be premature to make definitive conclusions about these results although it is clear that glucocorticoids are upregulating inserted plasmid vectors (not shown) while continuing to inhibit growth of the transfected cells. However, until we can determine that transfected cells are translating the human c-sis cDNA into a biologically active PDGF and that exogenously applied PDGF continues to overcome glucocorticoid induced cell cycle block in the transfectants, further conclusions cannot be made.

References

(1) Syms AJ, Norris JS, Smith RG. Biochem Biophys Res Commun 116:1020-1025, 1983.
(2) Syms AJ, Norris JS, Smith RG. Biochem Biophys Res Commun 122:68-74, 1984.
(3) Norris JS, Cornett LE, Hardin JW, Kohler PO, MacLeod SL, Srivastava A, Syms AJ, Smith RG. Biochem Biophys Res Commun 122:124-128, 1984.
(4) Syms AJ, Nag A, Norris JS, Smith RG. (Submitted)

Supported by NIH grants CA36264, GM30669 and NSF ISP8011447.

ISOLATION OF TRANSLATABLE MESSENGER RIBONUCLEIC ACID FOR ESTROGEN INDUCED UTERINE CREATINE KINASE FROM IMMATURE RAT UTERUS

Ana C. Pastini and J. D. Manjula Devi
Wadsworth Center for Laboratories and Research, New York State Department of Health, Empire State Plaza, Albany, NY 12201, USA

One of the earliest responses of the immature rat uterus to the administration of 17-β-estradiol is the enhanced synthesis of a protein termed "induced protein" (1). Reiss and Kaye (2) using mixed preparations of estrogen-stimulated immature rat uterine and brain cytosols found that the induced protein was indistinguishable from the BB isoenzyme of creatine kinase (CK-BB). Earlier studies from this laboratory reported the purification of the induced protein solely from the target uterine cytosol and its identification as creatine kinase (EIP-CK) (3). Although the amino acid composition closely corresponded to that of rat brain creatine kinase, there were differences in elution from hydroxyapatite, stability, molecular weight (as determined by SDS-PAGE) and in isoelectric points. while purified brain creatine kinase eluted from the hydroxyapatite ultrogel column at a high phosphate concentration, CK-EIP was discharged at low phosphate concentrations. Isoelectric focussing of the two enzymes showed that CK-EIP was more acidic than CK-BB. Double diffusion precipitation tests indicated that rat CK-BB was less antigenic than CK-EIP and showed partial identity with CK-EIP when tested with rabbit anti-CK-EIP IgG (4). Titration with a monoclonal antibody mAb 28, raised against CK-EIP showed significant differences between CK-BB, indicating nonidentity between the two proteins (5). Microheterogeneity of the muscle and brain isoenzymes of creatine kinase are reported in literature. Thus, CK-EIP may be a variant of the BB type isoenzymes which is under the control of estrogens. The aim of the present study was to obtain identifiable CK-EIP mRNA from which a cDNA probe could be synthesized and used for the eventual isolation of the native CK-EIP gene.

Unless otherwise stated, total uterine RNA was isolated from 18-21 day old female Wistar rats by the guanidinium/$CsCl_2$ or the phenol-cresol method and repeatedly precipitated with ethanol several times. After heat denaturation total RNA was applied to an oligo dT cellulose column and poly A+ RNA was eluted by standard procedures (6). In vitro translation of the mRNAs was carried out using the rabbit reticulocyte assay system containing either the ^{3}H-leucine or ^{35}S-methionine. The products were separated on SDS-PAGE and either analyzed by slicing the gel into 2 mm segments and measuring radioactivity or visualized by autoradiography. Fig. 1 shows the ^{3}H-labeled translation products of poly A+ RNA from uteri of adult (3 month old) and immature rats (18-21 days old). Immature rats were injected intraperitoneally either with estrogen (5 ug/rat) or with 1% ethanol in saline and uteri removed after one hour. Poly A+ RNA from adult and estrogen treated immature rats supported the synthesis of a protein (43-45 kDa) which closely corresponded to the molecular weight of CK-EIP. This protein band was not present in the translation products of poly A+ RNA from control immature rat uteri. Since the CK-EIP mRNA is a nonabundant species, partial pur

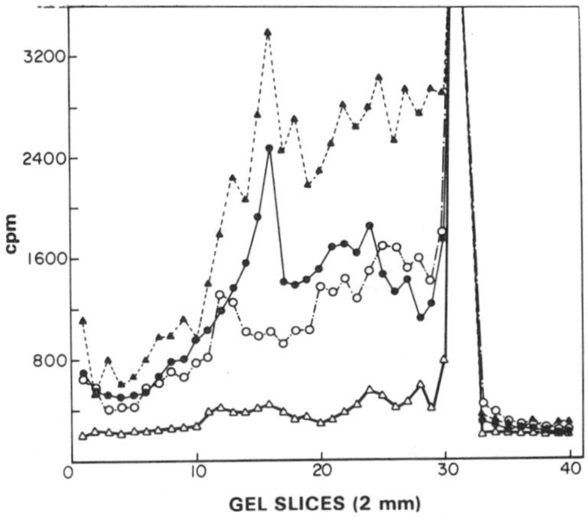

top bottom

Fig. 1. SDS-10% PAGE analysis of translation products of poly A+ RNAs from uteri of adult and immature rats. ▲—▲, uteri of adult (3 months) rats, ●—●, uteri of immature rats dissected out one hour after intraperitoneal injection of 5 ug of 17β-estradiol in 0.3 ml normal saline containing 1% ethanol, o—o, uteri of immature rats injected with 0.3 ml of normal saline with 1% ethanol, Δ—Δ, without any added poly A+ RNA. Segments (2 mm) were sliced, digested in H_2O_2 and assayed for radioactivity.

ification of the poly A+ RNA from estrogen treated immature rat uteri centrifugation through 4-20% sucrose density gradient containing 70% formamide was attempted. An enrichment of poly A+ RNA which translated to a product migrating on SDS-PAGE closely corresponding to CK-EIP was achieved. This protein band cross reacted with rabbit anti CK-EIP, anti rat CK-BB, IgGs and mAb 28 (IgM) antibodies on western blots as visualized by autoradiography after complexing with ^{125}I-labeled protein A either directly in the case of IgGs or after reacting with IgG of goat anti rat IgM.

ACKNOWLEDGEMENTS

The authors thank Drs. S. A. Kumar and H. W. Dickerman for their participation in this project. Supoprted by NIH grants HD 18406 and AM 23075. Ana C. Pastini is a doctoral student of the University of Buenos Aires, Argentina.

REFERENCES

1. Katzenellenbogen, B.S. (1980) Ann. Rev. Physiol., 42, 17-35.
2. Reiss, N.A. and Kaye, A.M. (1981) J. Biol. Chem. 256, 5741-5749.
3. Kumar, S.A., O'Connor, D.L., Seeger, J.L., Beach, T.A. and Dickerman, H.W. (1983) Biochem. Biophys. Res. Comm., 111, 156-165.
4. Kumar, S.A., Macario, A.J.L., Dickerman, H.W. and Pastini, A.C. (1985) 13th Intl. Cong. Biochem. Amsterdam. Abs. #Th. 218.
5. Kumar, S.A. and Macario, A.J.L. (1985) Hybridoma, 4, 297-309.
6. Maniatis, T., Fritsch, E.F. and Sambrook, J. (1982) Molecular cloning A laboratory manual. pp. 196-198, Cold Spring Harbor Laboratory.

CLONING OF THE ESTRADIOL INDUCIBLE GLUCOSE-6-PHOSPHATE DEHYDROGENASE GENE OF THE RAT.

K. Yen Pham, C.H. Faust and K.L.Barker
Department of Biochemistry, Texas Tech University Health Sciences Center, Lubbock, TX 79430 U.S.A.

Glucose-6-phosphate dehydrogenase (G6PD) is the first enzyme in hexose monophosphate shunt that is responsible for converting glucose-6-phosphate to 6-phosphogluconate. This metabolic pathway is important, because it provides NADPH and ribose necessary for nucleic acid and lipid synthesis, which increase tremendously during tissue growth. In many tissues, specific hormones regulate this pathway by modification of G6PD activity. For example, insulin regulates G6PD in the liver and estradiol does the same in the uterus. Specifically, the study of estradiol action in the rat uterus in our laboratory has proved that G6PD activity (1) increases as a result of many events. These include: [1] an increase of translatable G6PD mRNA (2); [2] a decrease in ribosome transit time on G6PD mRNA (3); [3] a decrease of G6PD N-terminus processing time (3); [4] an increase of G6PD protein synthesis rate (3,4); and [5] a decrease of G6PD protein degradation rate (5). Another aspect which needs to be studied is how estradiol increases G6PD gene expression. Namely, is the expression of the G6PD gene controlled at the level of transcription or translation, or does its control involve both? This requires that we measure the amount of uterine G6PD mRNA and study its structure. It is also of interest to know the structure of the G6PD gene and elements of this gene which may affect its transcription and regulation of mRNA production. As a first step toward these goals, we have isolated several cDNA clones and genomic DNA clones encoding G6PD. Eventually, we will use the G6PD cDNA probe characterized above to quantitate G6PD mRNA and also to study its turn-over in the uterus in different hormonal states.

G6PD is encoded by an mRNA of a low abundance class, and needed a very sensitive approach to isolate its cDNA clone. Therefore, we chose the gt 11 lambda bacteriophage expression vector. This vector contains a portion of the the beta galactosidase gene and its flanking sequences, including a ribosome binding site and the operator and promoter regions. This promoter can be induced by IPTG, with the subsequent expression of the cloned genes downstream. The phage will lyse the host bacteria and the released contents will bind to a nitrocellulose filter, and the expressed product will be detected by its monospecific antibody. This system allows us to screen a very large number of cDNA clones and to detect positive ones with higher sensitivity and greater efficiency than with plasmid vector systems.

Using this approach developed by Young and Davis, 1983 (6), we screened approximately 3 million plaques from a cDNA lambda gt11 library, which was constructed by Schwarzbauer et al, 1983 (7) from total rat liver mRNA. We detected G6PD expression with an affinity-purified rabbit monospecific anti-G6PD antibody and a second antibody conjugated with horseradish peroxidase. We found 9 immuno-positive clones with cDNA inserts ranging from 500 to 900 base pairs. Each insert was subcloned into the plasmid vector, pUC8, and characterized by restriction enzyme mapping, positive selection translation assays, Southern and Northern blot analyses. We found from Southern blot analysis that 8 cDNA clones were homologous to each other differing only in length, while one was not homologous to these 8. Positive selection translation assays of one clone from the group of 8 and the other unique clone suggested that the group of eight represented part of the total length of G6PD cDNA. This was confirmed by immunoprecipitation and competition with authentic purified G6PD against the cell-free synthesized products from the positive selection translation assays. When using this assay, we reproducibily observed several other specific protein bands besides G6PD. Negative controls, including the vector and the vector with an irrelevant insert, showed no protein bands with this assay. Northern blot analysis showed at least two hybdridzing mRNA populations -- one approximately 5 kilobases and the other approximately 2.3 kilobases. The restriction map of these 8 cDNA clones indicates that all have Pst I, Hind III and Bst EII sites, and none has any Bgl II, Cla I, Hpa I or Kpn I sites.

Using the G6PD cDNA characterized above, we screened one million plaques from a rat liver genomic DNA library constructed in the Eco RI site of the vector Charon 4A. We found 9 different independent G6PD clones. The Eco RI digestions of these individual clones indicate that their genomic DNA insert lengths range from 11-19 kilobase pairs; these digestions produced from two to seven Eco RI fragments per cloned insert. Seven of the nine genomic DNA clones each contain a single Eco RI band of 3 to 4 kilobase pairs hybridizing strongly to the cDNA probe, while all clones have other Eco RI bands hybridizing with less intensity.

CONCLUSIONS: We have idenified and characterized a G6PD cDNA clone and used this as a probe to isolate the genomic cognate sequences. We will use these cloned DNAs to: (1) study the structure of the rat G6PD gene; (2) study the effects of estradiol on the production and turnover of G6PD mRNA in the rat uterus; and (3) study the structure of the rat G6PD mRNA.

REFERENCES:

1. Moulton, B.C. and Barker, K.L. (1971) Endocrinology 89, 1131-1136.
2. Barker, K.L., Adams, D.J. & Donohue, T.M., Jr. (1981) in "Cellular and Molecular Aspects of Implantation" (S.R. Glasser and D.W. Bullock, eds.) p. 227-246. Plenum Publishing Co., N.Y.
3. Donohue, T.M., Jr. and Barker, K.L. (1983) Biochim. Biophys. Acta 739, 148-157.
4. Smith, E.R. and Barker, K.L. (1974)J. Biol. Chem. 249, 6541-6547.
5. Smith, E.R. and Barker, K.L. (1977) J. Biol. Chem. 252, 3709-3714.
6. Young, R.A. and Davis, R.W. (1983) Science 222, 778-782.
7. Schwarzbauer, J.E., Tamkun, J.W., Lemischka, I.R. and Hynes, R.O. Cell 35, 421-431.

STUDIES ON THE OESTROGEN REGULATION OF CELL-CYCLE REGULATED PROTEINS IN THE MOUSE UTERINE LUMINAL EPITHELIUM

Pollard, J.W., Cheng, S.V.Y., MacDonald, B.S. and Cullingford, T.E., MRC Group in Human Genetic Diseases, Dept. Biochemistry, King's College London, Campden Hill, London, W8 7AH, UK.

Oestrogens are trophic hormones in the rodent uterus. In the ovariectomized adult mouse, oestradiol-17β (E_2) produces a rapid proliferative response only in the luminal and glandular epithelium, tissues which constitute about 5% of the uterine cellular mass. Thus a single injection of 50 ng of E_2 induces luminal epithelial cells, after a lag, to enter DNA synthesis which reaches a peak at 12-15 hrs when essentially all the cells are engaged in DNA replication (1). By 15 hrs the cells enter into mitosis and the cell number doubles. Three daily injections of 1 mg progesterone (P) however, completely inhibits this E_2 induced proliferative response(1). Since the luminal epithelium can be removed with great purity from the underlying tissues we have chosen to use these endocrine regimes to study E_2 induced proteins and the correlation of their expression with cell proliferation.

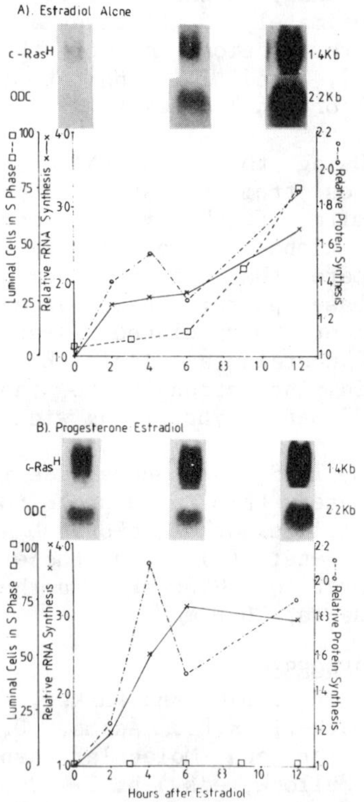

FIG 1. A composite figure of protein, rRNA and DNA synthetic rates in the mouse uterine luminal epithelium compared to the mRNA levels for the c-ras proto-oncogene and ornithine decarboxylase (ODC). Two weeks after ovariectomy adult Schneider mice were primed with 100 ng of E_2 and sacrificed one week later. Prior to sacrifice mice were either given a single injection of 50 ng E_2 (A) or 50 ng E_2 and 1 mg P after 3 daily injections of 1 mg P (B). Control animals were not given the E_2 on the day of sacrifice. At appropriate times thereafter the uteri were dissected out, slit longitudinally and processed in one of the following ways. Five uterine horns were incubated for 1 hr in media containing either a mix of ^{3}H-labelled amino acids to measure the protein synthetic rate (o--o), or ^{3}H-methyl-methionine to measure rRNA synthesis (x-x). Following removal of the luminal epithelium the resultant homogenates were processed to obtain the relevant synthetic rates/mg DNA as described in detail elsewhere (2) and displayed as a factorial stimulation over the control rate (A and B). The number of cells in S-phase was taken from Martin and Finn (1). For the determination of mRNA levels, total RNA was isolated (3) and 50μg per treatment group subjected to a Northern blot analysis. The blots shown are areas corresponding to the 1.4kb c-ras and 2.2kb ODC mRNA detected by probing with ^{32}P-nick translated pBS-9 plasmid (4) homologous to v-ras^H and pOD-48 (5) to most of the coding sequence of ODC. The autoradiograms show the mRNA levels 0, 6 and 12 hours after E_2.

In the luminal epithelium E_2 stimulated both protein and rRNA synthesis which commenced within 2 hrs of injection (Fig 1) and remained elevated until 12 hrs. This increase in synthetic rates also caused an accumulation of protein and rRNA per cell (2). This growth response, despite the complete inhibition of DNA synthesis, was not inhibited by progesterone pretreatment. In fact 12 hr after E_2 injection the rates of rRNA and protein synthesis were indistinguishable between those animals given progesterone and those that were not (Fig 1).

E_2 also increased the mRNA level for the c-ras proto-oncogene and ODC in the luminal epithelium (Fig 1). By 12 hr the c-ras level was 8 times and ODC 28 times the control level. Progesterone pretreatment however, again had no significant effect on the level of stimulation of these mRNAs at the 12 hr time point (Fig 1). Therefore, expression of these mRNAs appears to be closely correlated with the growth response of these cells,although temporally dissociated from the increase in protein and rRNA synthetic rates, rather than the proliferative state. This view is strengthened since progesterone alone causes a stimulation of both mRNAs and yet completely inhibited the basal level of proliferation (Fig. 1), although it does induce a small amount of cell growth (2). The correlation between cell growth and an increase in ODC mRNA and enzyme activity (6) is expected (6) however,the stimulation by E_2 of the ras proto-oncogene independently of the proliferative state of the cell is of particular interest since mutant forms of ras are associated with neoplastically transforming retroviruses and with certain carcinomas _in vivo_ (7). Furthermore, microinjection of the ras protein has been shown to initiate DNA synthesis in fibroblasts in culture (8). Experiments using single injections of P have shown that it exerts its inhibitory effect on the E_2 induced DNA synthesis within the first few hours of injection but this is clearly prior to the increase in ras mRNA level. P is known to re-model the pattern of synthesis of nuclear non-histone proteins (NHP, 9), and to specifically inhibit the synthesis of one NHP of Mw 32,000 daltons (10), which is similar to cyclin, a molecule thought to be involved in the regulation of cell proliferation. Studies are in progress to determine how E_2 stimulates the expression of these mRNAs and on the action of P in inhibiting cell proliferation in the luminal epithelium.

This work was supported by a grant from the Cancer Research Campaign.

1 Martin, L. and Finn, C.A. (1971) in Basic Actions of Sex Steroids on Target Organs, pp 172-188, Karger, Basel (Hubinont, P.O., Leroy, F. and Galand, P. eds)

2 Cheng, S.V.Y., MacDonald, B.S., Clark, B.F. and Pollard, J.W. (1985) Exp. Cell. Res. _160_, 459-470

3 Chirgwin, J.M., Przylyla, R.J., MacDonald, R.J. and Rutter, W.J. (1979) Biochemistry _18_, 5294-5298

4 Ellis, R.W., De Feo, D., Maryak, J.M., Young, H.A., Shih, T.Y., Chang, E.H., Lowy, D.R. an Scolnick, E.M. (1980) J. Virol. _36_, 408-42

5 McConolgue, L., Gupta, M., Wu, L. and Coffino, P. (1984) Proc. Nat. Acad. Sci. USA _81_, 540-544

6 Cheng, S.V.Y., MacDonald, B.S., Lary, S. and Pollard, J.W. (1985) Biochem. Soc. Trans. _13_, 350-351

7 Parada, L.F., Tabin, C.J., Shih, C. and Weinberg, R.A. (1982) Nature _297_, 474-478

8 Stacey, D.W. and Kung, H-F (1984) Nature _310_, 508-511

9 Pollard, J.W. and Martin, L. (1976) Mol. Cell. Endocrin. _6_, 223-229

10 Pollard, J.W. and Martin, L. (1975) Mol. Cell. Endocrin. _2_, 183-191

THYROGLOBULIN mRNA IS REGULATED BY INSULIN AND IGF-I AS WELL AS BY THYROTROPIN IN THE FTRL-5 THYROID CELL LINE

P. Santisteban, L.D. Kohn, and R. Di Lauro
LBM, NIADDK; and *LB, NCI, NIH, Bethesda, Maryland 20892

INTRODUCTION: Thyroglobulin (Tg), the major protein synthesized by the thyroid gland, is the macromolecular precursor of the thyroid hormones, T_3 and T_4 (1). Thyrotropin, TSH, is presumed to be the prime regulator of thyroid hormone formation and has been shown to increase Tg synthesis 2 fold both in vivo (2,3) and in a functioning rat thyroid cell line (FRTL-5) (4,5). The FRTL-5 cell line does not, however, depend on TSH alone for its growth and survival; insulin, for example, is also a growth requirement. In evaluating the relevance of insulin to FRTL-5 cell growth and function, we found that insulin also controled the synthesis of Tg by modulating the level of Tg mRNA. Thus, in the absence of insulin the concentration of Tg mRNA in the FRTL-5 cell line decreases 3 fold and returns to normal levels upon readdition of insulin to the culture medium. IGF-I apparently replaces insulin completely. Since the effect of insulin or IGF_1 on Tg synthesis occurs in the absence of TSH, we can conclude that regulation of Tg mRNA levels is controlled by multiple hormones, not only by TSH. Since the effect of insulin or IGF_1 occurs in the absence of cell growth, we can conclude that the insulin effect on Tg biosynthesis is not secondary to its growth regulation.

MATERIALS AND METHODS: Growth of the FRTL-5 cell line, extraction of total RNA and hybridization to a cloned rat thyroglobulin cDNA probe were performed as described (4, 5).

RESULTS AND DISCUSSION: FRTL-5 cells were grown in 5% serum and a mixture of six hormones, including insulin and TSH. When cells approached confluence, the serum concentration of the medium was decreased to 0.2% and insulin and TSH were removed. After 48 hours, insulin (10 μg/ml), IGF_1 (1 μg/ml) and/or TSH (1×10^{-8} M) were added as appropriate to the culture media for 36 hours (maximum time of induction of Tg synthesis according previous results). At this point the media was removed and the cells washed twice with PBS, scraped and the RNA isolated (5). Different concentrations of RNA from the cells subjected to various hormonal treatments, were spotted onto nitrocellulose paper. Hybridization was performed with a rat Tg cDNA clone (6) labelled by nick translation (7) to a specific activity of 10^8 cpm/μg. The induction of Tg mRNA was determined by autoradiography. Table 1 illustrates the induction of Tg mRNA under different conditions. Insulin, or IGF_1 in absence of TSH increased the level of Tg mRNA about 3.5-4 fold. Without insulin, a high dose of TSH (10^{-8} M) increased the level of Tg mRNA ~2 fold, concentrations of TSH below 1×10^{-9} M, i.e. those already maximal in their ability to increase cAMP levels in FRTL-5 cells (8), only minimally to increased Tg mRNA levels. The effect of insulin and IGF-I was not additive when each was added at a saturating level. Since the maximal effect of insulin was elicited at a concentration of 1 μg/ml and the maximal effect of IGF-I elicited at a concentration of 30 ng/ml, it is possible that the action of insulin in the induction of mRNA levels of Tg may mediated be via the IGF-I recpetor.

Insulin and IGF-I in the absence of TSH and at concentration eliciting maximal changes in Tg RNA had no affect on cell growth as measured by cell number. The present data thus indicate that regulation of Tg biosynthesis is not mediated by TSH alone but that IGF-I or insulin have an important and heretofore undescovered role. Measurements of Tg protein confirm this conclusion. Current experiments concern the mechanism by which insulin or IGF-I regulate mRNA, i.e. whether by inducing mRNA synthesis or by decreasing degradation.

Table I. Effect of TSH, insulin and IGF_1 on the Tg mRNA levels in FRTL-5 thyroid cells.

	Tg mRNA levels (Arbitrary units)
4H (no insulin, no IGF-I, no TSH)1	1
4H + TSH ($1x10^{-10}$ M)	1.2 ± 0.2
4H + TSH ($1x10^{-9}$ M)	1.5 ± 0.1
4H + TSH ($1x10^{-8}$ M)	2.1 ± 0.1
4H + Insulin (10 μg/ml)	3.25 ± 0.25
4H + IGF_1 (1 ng/ml)	3.85 ± 0.50
4H + Insulin + IGF_1	4.00 ± 0.24
4H + Insulin + TSH ($1x10^{8}$ M)	4.5 ± 0.20
4H + IGF_1 + TSH ($1x10^{-8}$ M)	5.2 ± 0.40

REFERENCES:

1. Salvatore, G., Stambury, J.B., and Rall, J.E.: In The Thyroid Gland, ed. by M. De Visscher, pp. 483-487. Raven Press, New York (1980).
2. Van Heuverswyn, B., Streydio, C., Brocas, H., Refetoff, S., Dumont, J., and Vassart G.: Proc. Natl. Acad. Sci. USA 81, 5941-5945 (1984).
3. Van Heuverswyn, B., Leriche, A., Van Sande, J., Dumont, J.E. and Vassart, G.: FEBS Letters 188, 192-196 (1985).
4. Ambesi-Impiombato, F.S., Picone, R., and Tramontano, D.: Cold Spring Harbor Conference Cell Proliferation 9, 483-492 (1982).
5. Avvedimento, V.E., Tramontano, D., Ursini, J.J., Monticelli, A., and di Lauro, R.: Biochem. Biophys. Res. Comm. 122, 472-477 (1984).
6. Di Lauro, R., Obici, S., Acquaviva, A.M., and Alvino, C.: Gene 19, 117-125 (1982).
7. Rigby, P.W., Dieckmann, M., Rhodes, C., and Berg, P.: J. Mol. Biol. 113, 237-251 (1977).
8. Valente, W.A., Vitti, P., Kohn, L.D., Brand, M.L., Rotella, C.M., Toccafondi, R., Tramontano, D., Aloj, S.M., and Ambesi-Impiomabato, F.S.: Endocrinology 112, 71-79 (1983).

POST-TRANSCRIPTIONAL REGULATION OF ALBUMIN GENE EXPRESSION BY ESTROGEN IN *XENOPUS* LIVER

D. R. Schoenberg, M. B. Martin and A. T. Riegel
Department of Pharmacology, Uniformed Services University of the Health Sciences, 4301 Jones Bridge Rd., Bethesda, MD 20814-4799

INTRODUCTION. Estrogen administration to male *Xenopus laevis* causes the *de novo* induction of the genes for the yolk precursor protein vitellogenin (vit) in a true primary response that is independent of protein synthesis (1). It was known for several years that vitellogenesis is also associated with the decreased synthesis of serum proteins present in the non-estrogenized animal (2). The purpose of our research was to identify the mechanisms responsible for the inhibition of serum albumin (alb) gene expression by estrogen.

MATERIALS AND METHODS. Changes in alb and vit mRNA were assayed by a quantitative cRNA excess hybridization assay (3). Transcription was assayed by a nuclear "run-on" assay in which isolated liver nuclei were incubated in a cocktail containing radioactive nucleotide triphosphates. The resultant RNA transcripts were isolated and hybridized to an excess of each cDNA immobilized on nitrocellulose filters (3). Quantitative changes in transcription were determined by scanning densitometry of autoradiograms.

RESULTS AND DISCUSSION. Steady-state levels of alb mRNA remained unchanged for 10 hr following estrogen administration; however, by 12 hr alb mRNA dropped to 30% of its control value. Albumin mRNA remained suppressed for 9 days, after which it returned to the control steady-state level (Fig. 1). During this interval, vit mRNA was induced to reach a maximal level by 4 days and subsequently declined to almost control values. The differential changes in alb and vit mRNAs are temporally uncoupled; alb mRNA is suppressed prior to the maximal induction of vit, and remains suppressed past the peak of vit mRNA.

Antiestrogens were utilized to investigate the role of the estrogen receptor in the suppression of alb mRNA. By themselves, the antiestrogens tamoxifen and 4-hydroxytamoxifen had little effect on the steady-state levels of alb mRNA. However, pretreatment with antiestrogen effectively prevented the suppression of alb mRNA by estradiol. Similarly, the drugs prevented the induction of vit mRNA by estrogen. Therefore, it appears that the inhibition of alb gene expression by estrogen requires the interaction of the estrogen receptor.

Two-to-three hr after estrogen administration there was a transient 80-90% decrease in alb transcription (Fig. 1). This returned to almost control levels by 4-6 hr and remained elevated throughout the following 12 days. Vit transcription also became apparent at 3 hr, reached a maximum 4 days after hormone, and subsequently dropped to barely detectable levels by day 12. The brief drop in alb transcription could not account for the sustained suppression of alb mRNA.

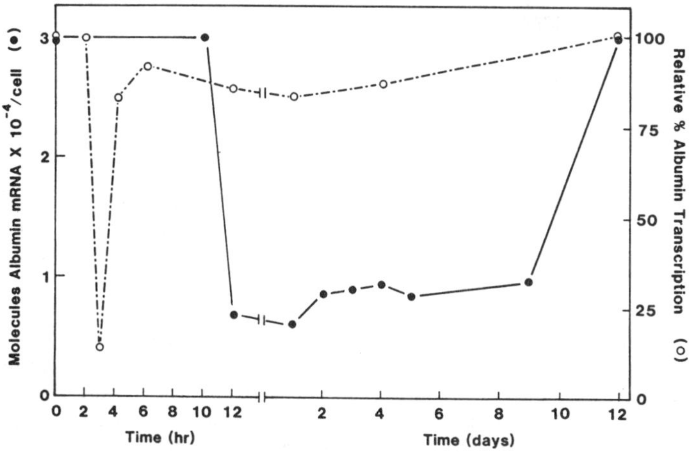

Fig. 1. Relationship between estrogen-induced changes in albumin mRNA and albumin gene transcription. Male Xenopus were injected at time 0 with 1 mg of estradiol and total liver RNA and liver nuclei were isolated at the indicated times. Albumin transcription is shown as the percent change in the albumin/globin ratio from scanning densitometry of autoradiograms.

These data indicate that alb gene expression is regulated predominately by the post-transcriptional destabilization of alb mRNA.

In addition to the transcriptional induction of vit, estrogen stabilizes vit mRNA (4) and induces the cellular protein synthetic apparatus. Therefore, the cell must have a mechanism to selectively target alb mRNA for destruction. We have recently examined the 2',5'-oligoadenylate synthetase/RNase L system in Xenopus and were unable to detect hormone-induced changes in the activities of these enzymes. The selectivity and mechanism of the post-transcriptional regulation of alb mRNA is the subject of present and future research in this laboratory.

ACKNOWLEDGMENTS. Supported by grants from the NIH and the Damon Runyon-Walter Winchell Cancer Fund.

REFERENCES

1) Hayward, M.A., Brock, M.L. and Shapiro, D.J. (1982) Nucl. Acids Res. 10, 8273-8284.
2) Follet, B.K. and Redshaw, M.R. (1974) in Physiology of Amphibia, B. Lofts, ed., 219-308, Academic Press, NY.
3) Martin, M.B., Riegel, A.T. and Schoenberg, D.R. (1986) J. Biol. Chem., in press.
4) Brock, M.L. and Shapiro, D.J. (1983) Cell 207-214.

CERVICOVAGINAL (CV) TUMOR LINE LW6214: A POTENTIAL MODEL FOR STUDYING THE ETIOLOGICAL EVENTS LEADING TO ADENO-SQUAMOUS CARCINOMA.

L.A. Scrocchi and L.A. Jones
Experimental Gynecology Laboratory, U.T. M.D. Anderson Hospital and Tumor Institute, Houston, Texas 77030.

INTRODUCTION:

Neonatal estrogen exposure of female BALB/cCRL mice has been shown to induce CV lesions after a long latency period (1). Tumor LW6214 is an adeno-squamous cell carcinoma from the CV region of a mouse neonatally treated with estrogen, which has been stable for more than ten years (2). Recently, an in vitro cell-line was derived from this solid tumor. Several cell culture experiments resulted in an optimal growth medium containing no hormones, a concentration of heat denatured FCS of 3.5%, and a calcium level reduced by Chelex treatment from 1.2mM to trace amounts (0.02mM). Several experiments have been performed with this medium in an attempt to characterize the behavior of these cells.

MATERIALS AND METHODS:

(1) Cellular Growth Studies: Effects of Estrogen or EGF on cell proliferation was determined by adding either estrogen or EGF to culture flasks in specific concentrations (See Figs. 2,3). Cell growth was determined by calculating number of cells per flask using a Hemocytometer.

(2) Two Dimensional Gel Electrophoresis: Samples were loaded onto isotube gels containing 3.0% polyacrylamide, urea, and ampholytes (pH 5-8, pH 3.5-9.5), and subjected to one dimensional separation on the basis of charge. Isotube gels were each loaded onto a 10%-20% linear gradient acrylamide Dalt slab gel, and loaded into a Dalt gel tank. Second dimensional separation occured through an electrical field as the proteins migrated through the slab gel on the basis of their molecular weight. Gels were stained using Silver Stain techniques described by Guevara et. al. (3).

RESULTS AND DISCUSSION:

Data from whole cell receptor assays indicate estrogen receptor (ER) levels similar to ER levels in the solid tumor LW6214 (4). However, like the solid tumor, the addition of estradiol to medium resulted in no increase in cell number when compared to medium without estradiol present (Fig. 2). In addition, no increase in cell growth was observed in response to the addition of EGF (0 - 200 ng/ml) to medium (Fig. 3). It is possible that these cells may produce a growth factor which controls their proliferation. Comparison of 2-D gel patterns between normal vaginal epithelia and LW6214 cells suggest numerous differences indicated by arrows (Figs. 4,5).

REFERENCES:

1. Jones L.A., Bern H.A. Cancer Research 39: 2560-2567, 1979.
2. Jones L.A., Pacillas-Verjan R. Cancer Research 39: 2591-2594, 1979.
3. Guevara J., Johnson D.A., Ramagli L.S., Martin B.A., Capetillo S., Rodriguez L.V. Electrophoresis 3: 197, 1982.

4. Jones L.A., Scrocchi L.A., Bern H.A., Siiteri P.K. (Unpublished data).

Figure 2

CELL LINE 6214
MEDIA SUPPLEMENTED WITH E_2 + 2% FBS

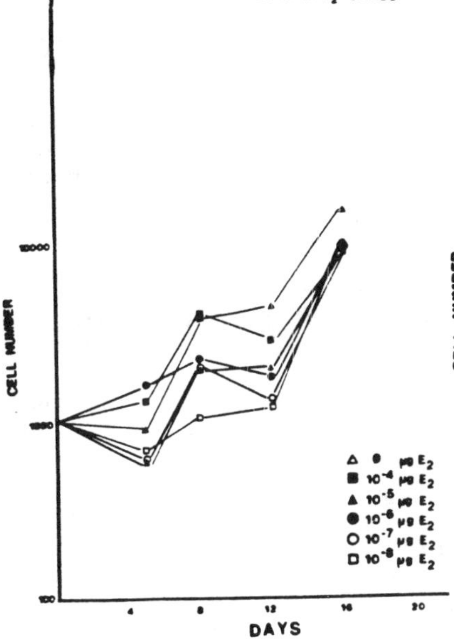

Figure 3

CELL LINE 6214
MEDIA SUPPLEMENTED WITH EGF

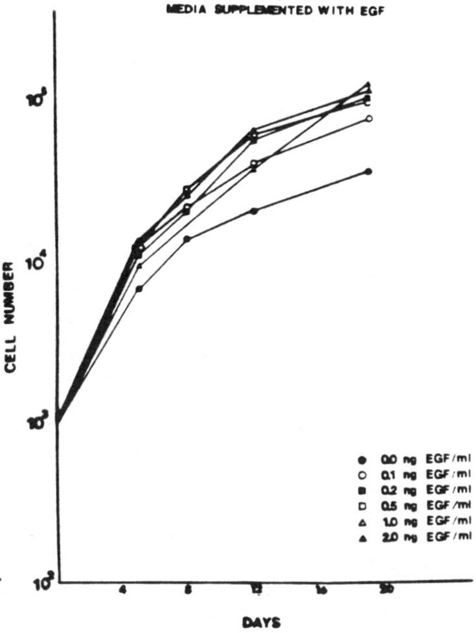

Figure 4
NORMAL MURINE VAGINAL EPITHELIAL CELLS

Figure 5
MURINE TUMOR CELL-LINE LW 6214

GLUCOCORTICOID REGULATION OF RAT INTESTINAL EXTRACELLULAR MATRIX AND EPITHELIAL CELL DIFFERENTIATION

K.M. Sterling, Jr.[1,2], M.J. Walsh[1], B. Martin[1], and N.S. LeLeiko[1]
Department of Pediatrics[1] and Biochemistry[2], Mount Sinai School of Medicine, New York, New York 10029

INTRODUCTION: The functional properties of suckling rat intestinal epithelium differs significantly from that of the adult (1). In rats, the adult pattern of intestinal epithelial cell function appears at the time of weaning (1). Adrenal corticosteroid hormones are widely accepted as regulators of rat small intestinal development which occurs at the time of weaning (1). Administration of exogenous glucocorticoids during the first two postnatal weeks induces precocious maturation of intestinal enzymes and other developmental changes (1).

The importance of the mesenchyme in the development of the small intestine has been demonstrated by the observation that villus formation, structural differentiation of villus epithelial cells and restriction of cell proliferation to the crypts results from the invagination of the mesenchyme (2). This implies changes in the structure of the extracellular matrix and concomitant alterations in the synthesis and accumulation of its components.

Steroid hormones have significant effects on extracellularmatrix protein synthesis (3) which suggests that glucocorticoids may mediate their effect on intestinal epithelial cell differentiation through the extracellular matrix.

RESULTS: Twelve day old rats previously treated with dexamethasone(0.8mg/kg) for 3 days had maltase, sucrase and lactase enzyme activities of the small intestine indicative of adult specific epithelial cell function (data not shown).

Table I

Radioimmunodot Assay of Small Intestinal Extracellular Matrix Proteins

Twelve Day Old Rats

CPM (^{3}H)-Protein A Bound to First Antibody per Milligram Protein x 10^{-4}

Antigen	Control	Dexamethasone
Type I procollagen	1.30 ± 0.28	0.59 ± 0.13
Type III collagen	1.27 ± 0.07	0.62 ± 0.03*
Type IV procollagen	1.55 ± 0.30	3.13 ± 0.26*
Fibronectin	2.49 ± 0.26	4.24 ± 0.46*
Laminin	1.21 ± 0.07	2.18 ± 0.05*

Legend: Rats were treated as described in the text. Twelve day old rat small intestine was homogenized in Tris-buffered saline (pH 7.5) and equal amounts of homogenate protein were applied to nitrocellulose using a Schleicher and Schuell minifold apparatus. Remaining binding sites were blocked with TBS plus 1% BSA and washed with TBS. First antibody was added in TBS plus 1% BSA and washed with TBS. Protein a, N-(propionyl-^{3}H)propionylated, 73 ci/mmole (Amersham) in TBS plus 1% BSA was then added, followed by washing with TBS. The samples were then analyzed by scintillation counting. In parallel experiments, second antibody (Goat-anti-rabbit IgG-linked to horseradish peroxidase, BioRad) was added in place of Protein A. After washing, the amount of specific antigen was determined by development of color with hydrogen peroxide and 4-chloro-1-napthol. This enzyme linked immunodot assay indicated a decrease in type I and III collagen content and an increase in procollagen type IV, fibronectin, and laminin content in glucocorticoid-treated 12 day old rat small intestine (data not shown). The values represent the mean plus or minus the standard error of the mean from 2 to 4 animals. An asterisk indicates significantly different values from control at $p \_ 0.05$ as determined by Student's nonpaired t-test.

Newly synthesized collagenase digestable protein was significantly less (data not shown) in the small intestine of dexamethasone treated rats, as was the accumulation of type I and III collagen (Table I). Type IV collagen, fibronectin and laminin accumulation was significantly increased in the small intestine of glucocorticoid treated rats (Table I). Type I and III procollagen steady state mRNA levels were significantly decreased while type IV procollagen, fibronectin and laminin steady state

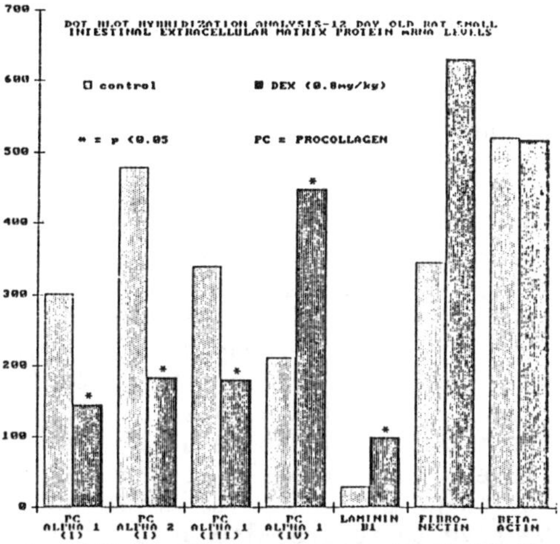

Legend Fig. 1: Rats were treated as described in the text. Total RNA was isolated by the method of Chirgwin, et al. (5). Nitrocellulose bound RNA was hybridized to ^{32}P-labeled DNA as described by Thomas (6). The ordinate indicates CPM ^{32}P-labeled DNA hybridized per microgram RNA. Asterisks indicate significantly different from control at p 0.05 as determined by Student's nonpaired t-test.

mRNA levels were significantly increased in the small intestine of dexamethasone treated rats (figure 1).

DISCUSSION: Glucocorticoid induced precocoius maturation of suckling rat intestinal epithelium was accompanied by a glucocorticoid mediated differential regulation of extracellular matrix proteins. Apparently significant is the observation that the interstitial collagens are decreased and basement membrane collagen is increased. It was previously shown that mammary epithelial cells will not differentiate when cultured on type I, II, or III (interstitial) collagen in the absence of _de novo_ collagen synthesis (4). Mammary epithelial cells synthesize type IV collagen and require it for growth and viability both _in vivo_ and _in vitro_ (4). The results of this investigation suggest that type IV collagen synthesis is related to intestinal epithelial cell differentiation as is the synthesis of fibronectin and laminin. Furthermore, the glucocorticoid induced precocious maturation of rat intestinal epithelium may be mediated, at least in part, through a differential effect on the synthesis of extracellular matrix components at the level of mRNA.

ACKNOWLEDGMENTS: We wish to thank Drs. J. Kelly, K. Burke, G. Martin, R. Hynes and S. Palm for their generous gift of antibodies to type I, III and IV collagen, fibronectin, and laminin, respectively. We also wish to thank Drs. D. Rowe, R. Hynes, B. deCrombrugghe, M. Kirkinen and D. Cleveland for cloned DNAs to type I, III and IV procollagen, fibronectin, laminin and beta actin.

REFERENCES:

(1) Martin, G.R. and Henning, S.J. (1984) Am. J. Physiol. 246:G695-G699.
(2) Smith, M.W. (1985) Ann. Rev. Physiol. 47:247-260.
(3) Cutroneo, K.R., Sterling, K.M. and Shull, S. (1985) in The Biology of the Extracellular Matrix. eds. Mecham, R.P. and Toole, B. Academic Press, New York, in press.
(4) Wicha, M.S., Liota, L.A., Lewko, W.M. and Kidwell, W.R. (1981) Cancer Letters 12:9-21.
(5) Chirgwin, J.M., Przybyla, A.E., MacDonald, R.J. and Rutter, W.J. (1979) Biochemistry 18:5294-5299.
(6) Thomas, P. (1980) Proc. Natl. Acad. Sci. USA 77:5201-5205.

TRANSCRIPTIONAL REGULATION OF THE CALBINDIN-D_{28K} GENE BY 1,25-DIHYDROXYVITAMIN D_3 IN CHICK INTESTINE.

G. Theofan, A.P. Nguyen, and A.W. Norman
Department of Biochemistry, University of California,
Riverside, CA 92521 USA

Using cDNA probes specific for chick intestinal calbindin-$D_{28}K$ (CaBP), we have previously demonstrated the accumulation of CaBP-mRNA in the intestine of vitamin D-deficient chicks following administration of 1,25-dihydroxyvitamin D_3 (1,25$(OH)_2D_3$), the most biologically active metabolite of vitamin D_3 (1). In this report we present data from in vitro nuclear transcription assays supporting a role for 1,25$(OH)_2D_3$ in the transcriptional regulation of the chick intestinal CaBP gene. We have also previously observed an inhibition of CaBP-mRNA levels following cycloheximide treatment in vitamin D-replete chicks (2). We have therefore also used nuclear transcription assays to examine the effects of cycloheximide on transcription of the CaBP gene in vitamin D-replete chick intestine.

METHODS. Chicks were raised from day of hatch on either a vitamin D-deficient (-D) or a vitamin D-replete (+D) diet for 3 weeks. Nuclei were prepared from duodenal mucosa of -D chicks at various times following a dose of 100 IU (6.5 nmoles) of 1,25$(OH)_2D_3$, and from +D chicks with and without cycloheximide pretreatment (600ug/chick, 1 hr prior to sacrifice). Nuclei were isolated from 0.5g of mucosa by homogenization (Potter-Elvehjem) followed by centrifugation. In vitro transcription with the nuclei and isolation of RNA for hybridization were carried out essentially as described by McKnight and Palmiter (3). Labelled transcripts were hybridized to nitrocellulose filters to which was attached either pBR322 alone or pBR322 containing a 1700bp insert of cDNA to CaBP-mRNA (1). Filters were then hybridized, washed, and ^{32}P determined by scintillation counting (3).

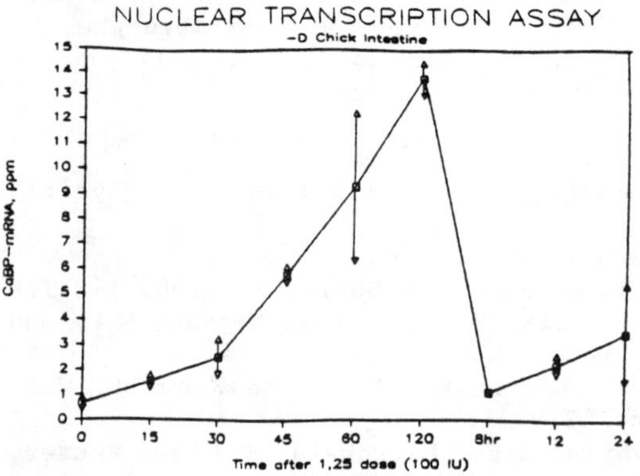

Figure 1.

RESULTS & DISCUSSION. Figure 1 shows the rate of transcription of CaBP-mRNA in chick intestinal nuclei following in vivo administration of 100 IU of 1,25-$(OH)_2D_3$. In the absence of hormone, there is no production of CaBP-mRNA. Transcription of the CaBP gene is significantly induced by 15-30 min after 1,25$(OH)_2D_3$ administration, reaching a peak by 2 hr. To our knowledge, this is the first demonstration of such a

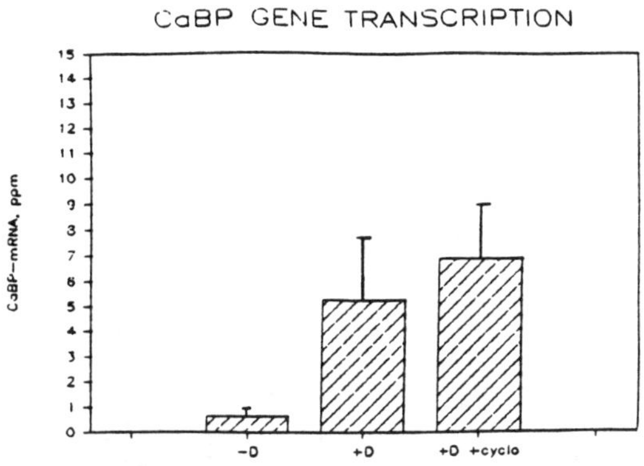

Figure 2.

rapid and direct effect of $1,25(OH)_2D_3$ on gene transcription. The data presented here confirm that $1,25(OH)_2D_3$ exerts its effects in a manner similar to other steroid hormones, i.e., by regulation of transcription of specific genes in target cells, presumably through a receptor-mediated mechanism (3,4). There is a significantly higher level of transcription of the CaBP gene in the +D chick intestine compared to the -D chick intestine (Fig. 2). Figure 2 also shows that cycloheximide treatment has no effect on the level of transcription of the CaBP gene in the +D chick intestine. Previous experiments have shown that cycloheximide inhibits CaBP-mRNA measured in dot blot preparations of total cellular RNA (2). The observation that cycloheximide does not have a direct effect on inhibiting transcription of CaBP-mRNA supports the hypothesis that a rapidly turned-over protein, which becomes depleted in the presence of cycloheximide, is necessary for maintaining stability of the CaBP-mRNA. There is evidence from other steroid-regulated systems for the existence of such a protein, based on the requirement for continual protein synthesis for production/accumulation of specific transcripts (5).

(Supported in part by USPHS grant AM-09012-021).

REFERENCES

(1) Theofan, G., Hall, A.K., King, M.W., and Norman, A.W. (1985) in: Vitamin D: Chemical, Biochemical and Clinical Update (Norman, A. W., Schaefer, K., Grigoleit, H.-G., and von Herrath, D., eds.) pp. 333-342, Walter de Gruyter, Berlin.
(2) Theofan, G., and Norman, A.W. (1985) in: Vitamin D: Chemical, Biochemical and Clinical Update (Norman, A.W., Schaefer, K., Grigoleit, H.-G., and von Herrath, D., eds.) pp. 379-380, Walter de Gruyter, Berlin.
(3) McKnight, G.S. and Palmiter, R.D. (1979) J. Biol. Chem. 254, 9050-9058.
(4) Taylor, R.N. and Smith, R.G. (1985) Biochemistry 24, 1275-1280.
(5) Vannice, J.L., Taylor, J.M., and Ringold, G.M. (1984) Proc. Natl. Acad. Sci. 81, 4241-4245.

ELISA DETECTION OF Z-DNA IN NEGATIVELY SUPERCOILED PLASMIDS

M.J. Thomas and J.S. Strobl
Department of Pharmacology and Toxicology, West Virginia University Medical Center, Morgantown, WV 26506

Z-DNA is a left handed helix which can form in regions of alternating purine-pyrimidine sequences under negatively supercoiled conditions. Although the *in vivo* formation of Z-DNA remains unproven, several investigators have hypothesized that Z-DNA may play a biological role (1). Antibodies against Z-DNA can be used to study the formation of Z-DNA *in vitro* (2,3). Previous studies have employed radiolabeled nucleotides or immunofluorescent techniques to monitor Z-DNA-antibody binding. This report describes a sensitive and DNA conformation-specific ELISA technique to detect Z-DNA-antibody binding that has been used to demonstrate Z-DNA antibody binding to the rat growth hormone promoter.

Two NZ white rabbits were immunized with brominated poly (dGdC)-poly(dGdC) which forms stable left-handed Z-DNA under physiologic ionic conditions (2). Crude sera was collected and non-specific antibodies to B-form DNA were removed by extensive absorption onto native calf thymus DNA-cellulose. To assay for Z-DNA, 5ug of each DNA sample, either synthetic polymer or plasmid, were electrophoresed at 100V in a .7% agarose gel in TAE buffer for 6 hours at 4°C. The gel was stained briefly in ethidium bromide (10 ug/100 ml H_2O) to visualize the DNA, and then equilibrated in electroblotting buffer (20 mM Sodium Acetate, pH 4). APT-paper was diazotized to activated DPT-paper according to the method of Alwine *et al* (4). The DNA was transblotted immediately onto DPT-paper, using a Bio-Rad Transblot apparatus immersed in ice water to keep the buffer at 4°C. Electroblotting was conducted for 1 hour at 15V (.22 Amps) and 4 hours at 40V (.68 Amps). All remaining steps were conducted at room temperature. The DPT-paper was immediately placed in 1% bovine serum albumin, 1% glycine in Tris-Buffer Saline, pH 7.5 (TBS), and gently shaken for 1.5 hours. Z-DNA specific antiserum was next diluted 1:600 in fresh TBS containing the DPT-paper and allowed to react for 1 hour with gentle agitation. After extensive washing to remove non-specifically bound antiserum, the DPT-paper was incubated for 1 hour in TBS plus a 1:500 dilution of peroxidase-conjugated anti-rabbit IgG. The DPT-paper was again washed extensively with TBS and then antibody binding sites were visualized by a peroxidase reaction performed in water:methanol (5:1) containing .05% 4-chloro-1-naphthol and .015% hydrogen peroxide.

Z-DNA antibodies reacted strongly with the immunogen, brominated poly(dGdC)-poly(dGdC), but very little with the B-form of this synthetic polymer, poly(dGdC)-poly(dGdC). Among the plasmids tested, the Z-DNA antibody was most reactive with pUC8 plasmids containing cloned inserts of alternating purine-pyrimidine sequence. pFP332 and pFP316 contain alternating G-C sequence inserts of 32 and 16 base pairs long, respectively. pFP124 contains the alternating purine-pyrimidine sequence G(CGCATGCG)$_3$C. As expected, the supercoiled forms of these plasmids were more reactive than the relaxed form because the insert DNA is stabilized in the Z-form by negative supercoiling (3). pUC8 without any alternating purine-pyrimidine sequence insert did not react with the Z-DNA antibody. The rat growth hormone promoter includes 11 base pairs of alternating purine-pyrimidine DNA sequence with one mismatch. Supercoiled pUC8 containing the 5'flanking region of the rat growth hormone gene reacted strongly with the Z-DNA antibody (See Fig. 1).

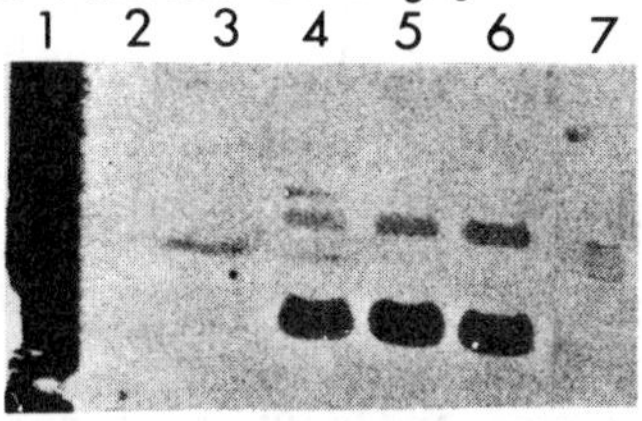

Figure 1. ELISA Detection of Z-DNA-Antibody Binding. Lane 1, Br-poly(dGdC)-poly(dGdC); Lane 2, poly(dGdC)-poly(dGdC); Lane 3, pUC8; Lane 4, pFP332; Lane 5, pFP316; Lane 6, pFP124; Lane 7, rat growth hormone promoter (in pUC8).

These results show that Z-DNA antibodies can react with negatively supercoiled plasmids containing alternating purine-pyrimidine sequences as short as 11 base pairs after covalent immobilization on DPT-paper. While these studies do not prove that alternating purine-pyrimidine sequences adopt a left-handed helix on DPT-paper, they do demonstrate that Z-DNA antibodies recognize an ultrastructural feature unique to the DNA helix when it is negatively supercoiled or brominated and contains a potential Z-DNA forming region. This technique offers a simple, non-radioactive method for detecting sequences of potential Z-DNA formation in supercoiled plasmids.

REFERENCES

(1) Rich, A., Nordheim, A., and Wang, A.H.-J. (1984) Annual Review of Biochemistry 53, 791-846.

(2) Lafer, E.M., Moller, A., Nordheim, A., Stollar, B.D., and Rich, A. (1981) Proceedings of the National Academy of Science 78, 3546-3550.

(3) Nordheim, A., Lafer, E.M., Peck, L.J., Wang, J.C., Stollar, B.D., and Rich, A. (1982) Cell 31, 309-318.

(4) Alwine, J.C., Kemp, D.J., Parker, B.A., Reiser, J., Stark, G.R. and Wahl, G.M. (1979) Methods in Enzymology 68, 220-242.

The authors wish to thank Dr. Eileen Lafer for providing Z-DNA bromination and immunization protocols; Dr. Fritz Pohl for providing pFP322, pFP316, and pFP124; and Dr. Bruce Caterson for suggesting the ELISA approach. Supported by a WVU Senate Research Grant and NIH Grant AM33631.

17 β-ESTRADIOL INDUCES PROLACTIN AND GROWTH-RELATED mRNAS AT DIFFERENT CONCENTRATIONS

C. Van Itallie and P.S. Dannies, Department of Pharmacology, Yale University School of Medicine, New Haven, CT 06510

Estradiol increases the growth rate of the rat pituitary tumor cell line, the GH_4C_1 cells, with a half-maximally effective concentration (EC50) that is at least 10-fold less than the EC50 value for the stimulation of prolactin production (1). Here we describe the construction of a cDNA library from this cell line and the identification of two estrogen-responsive clones within it. The estrogen dose-response relationship of the mRNAs corresponding to these two clones is compared with that for prolactin mRNA to determine if the separation of stimulatory effects on cell growth and prolactin is also seen at the level of mRNA.

cDNA LIBRARY: CONSTRUCTION AND SCREENING, GH_4C_1 cells were grown in medium with low estrogen horse serum plus insulin and 10^{-9} M estradiol for 8 d, collected and double stranded cDNA was made from poly A+ RNA (2,3). The cDNA was tailed and cloned into pBR322 and transfected into E. coli strain HB101 (4). About 700 ampS, tetR clones were differentially screened.

Screening was performed using ^{32}PcDNA prepared from mRNA from estrogen-treated and control GH cells; the labeled cDNA was used to screen replica plated colony grids (5). Out of 7 clones showing reproducible increases in hybridization signal after estrogen treatment, 2 were picked for further study. One, 1C28, hybridized with an 800 nucleotide mRNA; the second, 1D51, with an mRNA of 1800 nucleotides. Both clones hybridized with RNA from primary cultures from normal rat pituitary and from estrogen-induced tumors, and with the RNA from a fibroblast cell line (NRK cells). The hybridizing RNA from the rat pituitary cultures could be induced with estrogen treatment; that from the fibroblast cell line could not.

RESPONSE TO ESTROGEN. The dose response of the mRNA corresponding to 1C28 by estrogen can be seen in figure 1 and compared with the effects on cell growth and prolactin mRNA. Levels of mRNA were measured by the cytoplasmic hybridization technique (5); values correlated well with RNA dots. In this experiment, the effects of estrogen on both cell growth and 1C28 were biphasic; in other experiments, the maximal values occurred at same estrogen concentrations but 1C28 mRNA and cell number remained elevated at higher estrogen doses. In every case, induction of 1C28, 1D51 and cell growth were closely correlated. while prolactin mRNA peaked at at least 10-fold higher estrogen levels.

The time course for induction for 1C28 and prolactin mRNA showed that 1C28 is stimulated at least as early as is prolactin mRNA. In both cases the rate of increase is relatively slow; it takes 3-5 hrs to see mRNA induction.

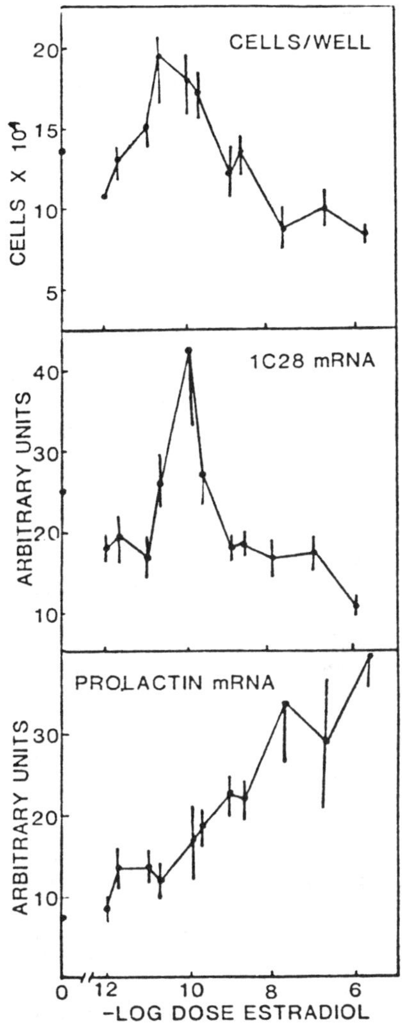

Fig. 1. Dose response of cell number, 1C28 mRNA and prolactin mRNA to increasing estradiol concentration. GH cells were plated at 2 x 104 cells/well and treated for 7 d. Cytoplasm from equal numbers of cells were spotted onto nitrocellulose, hybridized with the appropriate nick-translated probe and autoradiographed. Dots were quantitated by densitometric scanning. Each point is the mean of 3 determinations.

DISCUSSION. The most likely explanations for the observed separation in dose response are that there are differences either in the estrogen sensitivity in transcription of the genes which correspond to the induced mRNAs and/or that estrogen can differentially affect the stability of the transcripts, as has been seen in other systems (6).

The identities of these two estrogen-responsive proteins are not yet determined. Growth factors would be expected to induce a large number of proteins; estrogen is known to induce at least 9 proteins in MCF-7 cells (see 7). 1C28 and 1D51 are not specific to estrogen responsive tissues; however, their behavior may provide a useful probe for studying the mechanism underlying the separation in dose response in the stimulation of growth and prolactin production.

(1) Amara, J.F. and Dannies, P.S. (1983) Endocrinology 112, 1141-1143.
(2) Maniatis, T., Fritsch, E.F. and Sambrook, J. (1982) Molecular Cloning: A Laboratory Manual.
(3) Ticehurst, J.R., Racaniello, V.R. Baroudy, B.M., Baltimore D., Purcell, R.H. and Feinstone, S.M. (1983) Proc. Natl. Acad. Sci. USA 80, 5885-5889.
(4) Taub, F. and Thompson, E.B. (1982) Anal. Biochem. 126, 222-230.
(5) White, B. and Bancroft, F.C. (1982) J. Biol. Chem. 257, 8569-8572.
(6) Brock, M.L. and Shapiro, D.J. (1983) Cell 34, 207-214.
(7) Prud'homme, J.-F. et al. (1985) DNA 4, 11-21.

MOLECULAR CLONING OF THE HUMAN GLUCOCORTICOID RECEPTOR cDNA REVEALS THE CARBOXY-TERMINAL HALF IS RELATED TO THE V-ERBA ONCOGENE PRODUCT

Cary Weinberger*, Stanley M. Hollenberg*#, Michael G. Rosenfeld+ and Ronald M. Evans*

*The Salk Institute for Biological Studies, P.O. Box 85800, San Diego, CA 92037, #Department of Biology and +School of Medicine, University of California, San Diego, San Diego, CA 92093.

Steroid hormones modulate gene expression by binding to intracellular receptor proteins. The binding elicits a protein transformation resulting in transcriptional activation of limited sets of target genes (1). Using probes derived from clones expressing fusion proteins immunoreactive with human glucocorticoid receptor antibodies, we have isolated the full-length cDNA as a first step toward understanding the mechanism by which steroid receptors enhance gene transcription.

Expression Cloning of Human Glucocorticoid Receptor cDNAs

Initially, we constructed a cDNA library in λgt11 using poly(A)-containing cytoplasmic RNAs from IM-9 cells, a human B lymphoblastoid cell line expressing large amounts of glucocorticoid receptor. The library was screened with a rabbit polyclonal antiserum directed against the human receptor (2). Immunopositive clones were characterized by using the fusion proteins produced by each of the recombinants to specifically select antibodies. Antibodies extracted using three clones detected both 94 and 79 kd bands representing native and presumptive degradation products of the glucocorticoid receptor. The EcoRI inserts from these immunopositive clones cross-hybridized supporting the notion that an immunogenic region of the molecule had been identified.

Isolation and Characterization of Full-Length Receptor Clones

The largest immunopositive EcoRI insert was nick-translated and used to probe human fibroblast cDNA libraries (kindly provided by H. Okayama). Our studies indicate the receptor exists as two forms, GR alpha, 777 amino acids (MW=85.5 kd) and GR beta, 742 amino acids (MW=81.5 kd) differing by the substitution of the 50 carboxy-terminal amino acids in GR alpha by 15 amino acids in GR beta. The predicted amino acid sequence encoded by the cDNA reveals a basic, cysteine-rich domain in the central region of the molecule which may represent the DNA-binding region by analogy with TFIIIA, the Xenopus laevis 5S gene transcription factor.

Expression of the GR alpha polypeptide in vitro using SP6 transcription vectors indicates the immunoreactive polypeptide binds steroid and comigrates with protein isolated from intact cells. The beta receptor form, however, fails to bind steroid. DNA fragments derived from the entire cDNA detect sequences present on human chromosome 5 to which the human glucocorticoid receptor gene has been previously mapped. In addition, probes specific for the cysteine-rich region detect sequences found on chromosome 16. Multiple mRNAs are detected in many cell lines, some of which may result from alternative RNA processing.

Receptor Domain Structure and v-ErbA Homology

Several investigators have demonstrated that the receptor molecule can be divided into three domains: an immunogenic region toward which most antibodies are directed, a steroid-binding domain and a DNA-binding domain (3,4). Their studies have indicated the immunogenic domain may be localized on a half of the molecule distinct from the steroid- and DNA-binding domains. In addition, the steroid-binding domain can be found on a 22 kd fragment of the receptor. The immunopositive cDNA clones permit us to assign the immunogenic domain to the amino-terminal half of the receptor (Figure 1). DNA- and steroid-binding domains must then be found in the carboxyl half. Since the beta receptor form fails to bind steroid, the steroid-binding domain is assigned to the extreme carboxy terminus.

The receptor primary amino acid sequence was compared with other polypeptide sequences maintained in a database by R. Doolittle (Univ. of Calif., San Diego). Significant homology (approximately 22% over 385 amino acids) was revealed between the carboxy-terminal half of the receptor and the v-erbA oncogene product encoded by avian erythroblastosis virus. The v-erbA oncogene product is not required for erythroblast transformation, but seems to facilitate proliferation of transformed cells. Its functional relationship to the glucocorticoid receptor is unknown, although we postulate that the c-erbA proteins may act as transcriptional regulatory factors.

1. Gorski, J. and Gannon, F. Ann. Rev. Physiol. 38, 425 (1976).
2. Harmon, J. M. et al. Cancer Res. 44, 4540 (1984).
3. Carlstedt-Duke, J. et al. PNAS 79, 4260 (1982).
4. Sherman, M. R. et al. Fed. Proc. 37, 167 (1978).

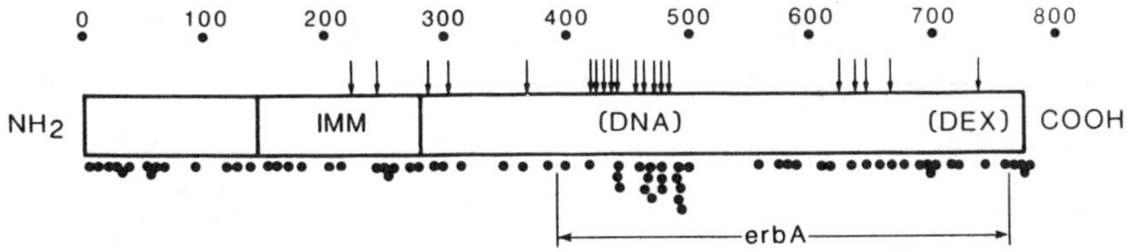

Figure 1. Schematic representation of the human glucocorticoid receptor primary amino acid structure and designation of oncogene homology. The cysteine residues found in the human glucocorticoid receptor are represented by arrows above the boxed coding region and basic amino acids (arginine and lysine) are denoted by filled circles. The immunogenic domain (IMM) determined from overlapping expression cDNA clones, the putative steroid binding region (DEX) and DNA binding domain (DNA) are indicated within the boxed receptor coding region. Numbers indicate amino acid residues. The relative position of the erbA homology is indicated below the receptor coding region.

POLYMORPHISM OF STEROID HORMONE RECEPTORS DETECTED BY HPLC

J.L. Wittliff, N.A. Shahabi, S.M. Hyder, D.M. Boyle, L. Myatt and L.A. van der Walt, J.G. Brown Cancer Center, University of Louisville School of Medicine, Louisville, KY 40292 USA

The origin and physiological significance of the multiple forms of receptors have been a major focus of our investigations[1]. Although certain of these components may represent distinct physiologic species, a few may arise due to proteolytic cleavage. Presumably, the latter possibility may occur during homogenization, prolonged incubation, and overnight centrifugation. To our knowledge, no one has provided conclusive evidence of the "native state" of estrogen (ER) and progestin receptors (PR) in breast and endometrial carcinomas.

To circumvent the problem of prolonged manipulation of receptor preparations, we developed the use of high performance liquid chromatography in size exclusion (HPSEC), ion-exchange (HPIEC), chromatofocusing (HPCF) and hydrophobic interaction (HPHIC) modes for the rapid separation of isoforms[2]. Receptor isoforms are defined as protein components in a target organ which exhibit a high ligand binding affinity and specificity for a single class of steroid hormones (e.g. estrogens) and may be identified based upon characteristics of size, shape, and surface ionic properties.

HPLC Methods: Currently, we employ an Altex (Beckman) HPLC system with extensive flow-through detection equipment for the following measurements: UV-visible absorbance (Altex or Hitachi), conductivity (Bio-Rad), pH (Pharmacia) and gamma radioactivity (Altex). Due to the thermal lability of receptor proteins the system was installed in a temperature-controlled chromatographic chamber (Puffer Hubbard). Optimizing a mode of analysis requires attention to the characteristics of the column employed, especially the pore size, hydrophobicity, and loading capacity. Details of the various separation modes are given in recent papers. (see ref. 2)

Table 1 - Comparison of Properties of Estrogen Receptors Separated by HPLC

Tissue	HPSEC (TSK-3000 SW)	HPIEC (AX-1000)	HPCF (AX-500)
MCF-7 Cells	68 A	55 and 180 mM phosphate	pH 6.3 and 4.3
Human Breast Carcinoma	>61 A and 29-32 A	52, 100, 190 mM phosphate	pH 6.3, 5.3 4.8-3.5 shoulder
Human Uterus	>61 A and 29-32 A	115 and 203 mM phosphate	pH 7.1, 6.6 6.15 and 5.3
Rabbit Endometrial Carcinoma	71 A	50 and 175 mM phosphate	pH 6.8, 6.4 and 5.6
Rat Lactating Mammary Gland	>61 A	90 and 205 mM phosphate	pH 6.8 and 6.5

Results: Table 1 provides a summary of results from our experience with ER from 5 different target organs. Note that a large molecular weight species (60-70A) was detected by HPSEC. Kinetics of its ligand binding and separation profile suggest this isoform may represent a precursor or aggregate of the receptor. A similar isoform of the PR was observed by HPSEC.

At least two charge isoforms of the ER were detected by HPIEC and HPCF. However, human uteri often exhibited 4 different isoforms by HPCF which shifted to highly acidic species with 10 mM sodium molybdate. When either [^{3}H]Tamoxifen or [^{3}H]Tamoxifen-4OH was substituted as a ligand for the ER of rat uterus, two isoforms were detected at 90 mM and 150 mM phosphate by HPIEC. PR exhibited one species primarily when separated by HPIEC or HPCF (Table 2) using either [^{3}H]R5020 or [^{3}H]Org-2058.

Table 2 - Summary of Properties of Progestin Receptors in Human Uterus

Ligand	HPSEC (TSK3000 SW)	HPIEC (AX-1000)	HPCF (AX500)
R5020	>80 A		
	35 A	100 mM phosphate	pH 5.7
ORG-2058	70 A		
	20 A	100 mM phosphate	pH 5.7

Summary: HPLC offers speed of analyses, sensitivity and high recov- eries. Technical advancements such as synthesis of ^{125}Iodine-labeled ligands of high specific radioactivity coupled with efficient flow-through detectors have facilitated our investigations of the properties of steroid hormone receptors. Factors we have found which may alter the profile of steroid receptor isoforms are stage of differentiation, endocrine status, age, tissue of origin, disease and administration of hormones or drugs.

Some of the cellular events which may give rise to receptor heterogeneity include proteolysis, phosphorylation, protein-protein interaction and protein-nucleic acid interaction. Regarding proteolysis, receptor isoforms may be generated by proteases released during homogenization. Another possibility is the processing of a high molecular weight precursor of the receptor which is an example of a physiologic event common in biology. Interchange between active and inactive receptor states may be modulated by phosphorylation or other posttranslational modification. Other means of deriving receptor isoforms could occur either due to aggregation during extraction or via association/dissociation of receptor subunits. While the latter represents examples of protein-protein interactions, it is possible that receptor-nucleic acid complexes may also be identified in tissue preparations. Our data suggest that the levels of receptor organization and interrelationship are more complicated than thought previously.

Acknowledgements: This research was supported in part by the Amer. Cancer Soc. and USPHS Grants CA-15697 and CA-32102 from the NCI.

References:

(1). Wittliff, J.L., Feldhoff, P.A., Fuchs, A. and Wiehle, R.D. (1981). Prog. Clin. Biol. Res., 74: 375-396.

(2) Wittliff, J.L., Shahabi, N.A., Hyder, S.M., van der Walt, L.A., Myatt, L., Boyle, D.M. and He, Y.-J. (1985) in Modern Methods in Protein Chemistry (L'Italien, J., ed.), Plenum Press (in press).

EXPRESSION OF U1 GENES IN SEA URCHIN EMBRYOS

Jin-Chen Yu, Michael Nash, Carlos Santiago and William Marzluff,
Dept. of Chemistry, Florida State University, Tallahassee, Fla.

There are at least two separate tandemly repeated units encoding U1 genes in the sea urchin L. variegatus (1). We have isolated separate and completely sequenced two different repeat units, pU1.1 (1) and pU1.2. Each 1400 base repeat unit encodes a single U1 gene. One of the repeats is present in four times the copy number of the other. The sequence of the two repeats are nearly identical (95%) for 500 bases 5' to the gene. The sequences 3' of the gene are highly divergent starting immediately after the CAAGAAGAA sequence required for formation of the 3' end of U1 RNA. The boundary of the conserved and divergent regions is a long polypyrimidine sequence. It is likely that gene conversion is maintaining the conservation of the 5' flanking region although it is possible that there is extensive selective pressure on this region.

We have taken two approaches to try to determine when these repeat units are expressed. The U1 RNAs in eggs and embryos have been sequenced using an oligonucleotide primer to prime reverse transcriptase with dideoxynucleotides. Using this approach we have detected a single nucleotide difference between the U1 RNA in eggs and in gastrula embryos from S. purpuratus demonstrating that a different gene set must be active in eggs and embryos (Fig. 1). The sequences of the U1 RNAs in L. variegatus eggs and embryos are identical, and match the sequence of the U1 RNA expected from pU1.1 and pU1.2. It is very possible that there are different gene sets in L. variegatus which encode the same RNA sequence.

Since the transcription unit of the U1 genes extends 3' to the genes (2), it is possible to determine whether a particular gene is expressed by analyzing the expression of a sequence 3' to the U1 gene. Subclones were constructed from unique regions 3' to the cloned U1 repeat units. Using these as probes and isolated nuclei active in U1 RNA synthesis (3) we have shown that the pU1.2 gene is actively transcribed in blastula nuclei but is much less actively expressed in nuclei from gastrula embryos. The pU1.1 gene is expressed much less actively. The data indicate that different U1 gene sets are expressed differentially duing sea urchin development.

References

Brown, D.T., Morris, G.M., Chodchoy, N., Sprecher, C.S. and Marzluff, W.F. (1985) Nuc. Acids. Res. 13 537-56.

Morris, G.M., Price D.H. and Marzluff, W.F. (1986) Proc. Nat. Acad. Sci., in press.

Morris, G.M. and Marzluff, W.F. (1985) Mol. Cell Biol. 5 1143-50.

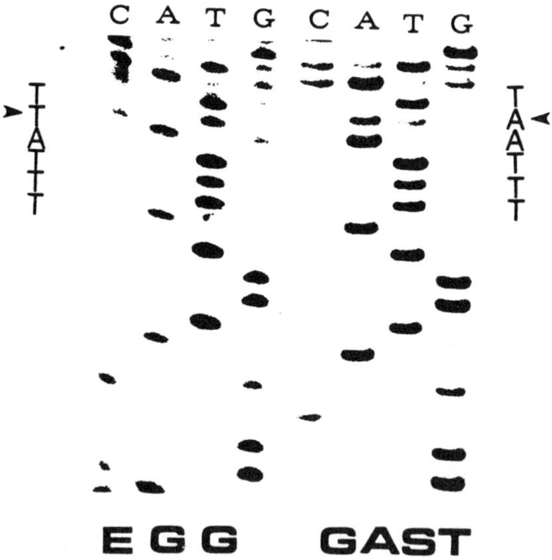

Fig. 1. Sequence of U1 RNA in S. purpuratus. Total RNA from egg or nuclear RNA from gastrula embryos was hybridized with an oligonucleotide complementary to the 3' end of U1 RNA. A cDNA was synthesized using reverse transcriptase and dideoxynucleotides. The single difference in sequence between the egg and gastrula U1 RNA is indicated.

CLONING OF BOVINE ESTROGEN RECEPTOR cDNA.

S. Zain, M. Salim, S. Rehman, and A.C. Notides Depts. of Radiation Biology and Biophysics, Biochemistry and Cancer Center, University of Rochester School of Medicine and Dentistry, Rochester, NY 14642 USA

Previous experiments described the mechanism of estradiol binding and the modulation of the active and nonactive states of estrogen receptor (ER) (1). The limiting factor in conducting crucial studies associated with the molecular properties of the receptor and the regulation of it's gene expression are due to the lack of the highly purified receptor protein. Recently, we purified the bovine ER to near homogeneity (2). In this report we present data on the preparation of an ER polyclonal antibody and bovine uterine mRNA/cDNA libraries in λgt11 expression vector. Using the anti-ER antibody we have isolated two cDNA clones expressing a chimera protein, of 110 Kd molecular weight and cDNA clones with an insert size of approximately 2.5 kb.

Anti-Estrogen Receptor Antibody Production and Its Characterization

The highly purified ER was subjected to SDS gel electrophoresis. Then the receptor band was cut out (200 μg) emulsified with Freund's complete adjuvant and injected into a young female rabbit at multiple sites over a one month period. After a month, 100 μg of receptor was injected in incomplete Freund's adjuvant over a one week period. The immunized rabbits generated anti-bovine ER antibodies with a good titre. The curve showed that at a 1:800 dilution of the sera removed 50 percent of the ER from the uterine cytosol. The species specificity of the sera is bovine > rabbit = rat > human. Sucrose gradient analysis showed that the antibody reacted with the 8S, 5S, and 4S forms of the ER but not the progesterone or androgen receptors. A Western blot of the bovine uterine cytosolic proteins showed a selective reactivity with the ER at 68 Kd and very weakly with a second unknown protein at 120 Kd (Fig. 1).

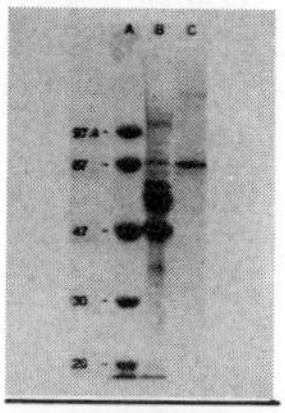

Fig. 1. A Western Blot of Bovine Uterine Proteins Using the Rabbit Anti ER Antibody: (A) Size markers (B) 35 percent $(NH_4)_2SO_4$ fraction of bovine uterus proteins stained with Coomassie Blue (C) Western blot of ER is the 68 Kd protein.

Preparation of the Calf Uterine cDNA Libraries and Isolation of Specific Clones

The total cellular RNA was isolated from calf uterine by a modified version of Chirgwin's procedure (3). The poly(A)$^+$ RNA was isolated by the method of Aviv and Leder (4). The double-stranded cDNA synthesis was conducted by a modification of Grubler and Hoffman's procedure using oligo-dT as the primer. The cDNA libraries were prepared in λgt11 vector and screened with the anti-bovine ER monospecific polyclonal antibody using the methods described by Young and Davis (5). Partial characterization of the cDNA insert and the specific protein product made in E. coli was conducted using restriction enzymology and Western blot analysis.

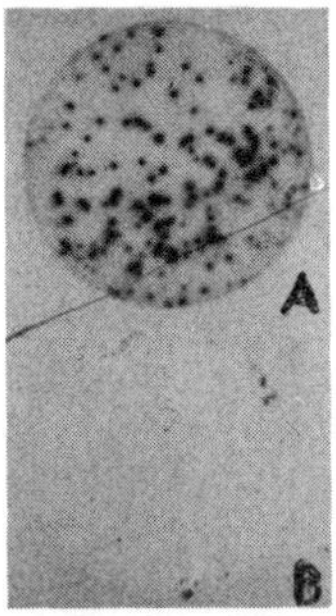

Fig. 2. Third Low Density Screening of Recombinant Phage U1ER35. A) The possible positive ER clone isolated from λgt11 expression library screened at high density using a polyclonal anti-ER antibody and (1^{125}) protein A, was confirmed after the third low density screening. (A) The I^{125} protein A from S. Aureis used as a secondary antibody shows no reactivity with the recombinant phages (B).

Cloning and Isolation of the ER Specific cDNA

We prepared two independent bovine uterine mRNA/cDNA libraries in λgt11 vector with 2 x 10^8 and 6 x 10^8 recombinant plaques/μg of cDNA plated. Screening of these libraries with the ER specific polyclonal antibody and ^{125}I-labeled protein A (S. aureus) as secondary antibody gave nine positive recombinant bacteriophage clones expressing ER specific sequences reactive with the anti ER antibody. The third low density screening of one of the recombinant phages U1ER35 is depicted in Fig. 2. Restriction endonuclease analyses of these clones revealed two of them have an insert of approximately 2.5 kb long (EcoR1 digestion pattern of U1ER35 is depicted in Fig. 3). Complete characterization of the insert and its protein product is underway.

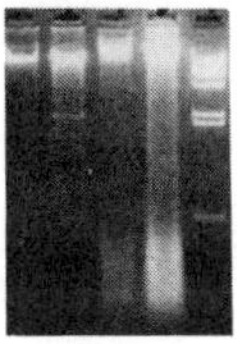

Fig. 3: EcoR1 Restriction Endonuclease Digestion to Size the cDNA Insert in Recombinant λgt11 U1ER35 phage. The recombinant phage DNA was isolated and digested with ECOR1 restriction enzyme. 1) Undigested DNA (2) U1ER35 DNA and ECOR1 (3,4) DNA from two clones whose expression products did not show reactivity to ER specific antibody (5) DNA size markers.

REFERENCES

1. Notides, A.C., Lerner, N., Hamilton, D.E. (1981) Proc. Natl. Acad. Sci. USA 78, 4926-4930.
2. Notides, A.C. Sasson S. and Callison, S. (1985) In: Molecular Mechanism of Steroid Hormone Action. Moudgil, V.K. ed., pp. 173-197.
3. Chirgwin, J.M., Przbyla, A., McDonald, R.J. and Ruffer, W.J. (1979) Biochemistry 18, 5294-5299.
4. Aviv, H. and Leder, P. (1972) Proc. Natl. Acad. Sci. USA 79, 1408-1412.
5. Young, R.A. and Davis, R.W. (1983) Science 22, 778-782.

Lymphokines, Interleukins, Interferons and Receptors

THYMOSINS: COMPONENTS OF BIDIRECTIONAL PATHWAYS BETWEEN THE BRAIN AND IMMUNE SYSTEM.

Nicholas R. Hall and Allan L. Goldstein
Department of Biochemistry, The George Washington University School of Medicine, Washington, D.C. 20037

The thymus gland performs a central role during the sequence of T-lymphocyte maturation. It is within this organ that T-cells become programmed to recognize self MHC determinants and to subsequently differentiate into effector cells of immunity. Contributing to certain aspects of this process are soluble products of thymic epithelial cells that are called thymosins. This family is comprised of relatively small and mostly acidic peptides that are able to modulate the course of host defense by direct action upon T-lymphocytes and by indirect effects via immunomodulatory neuroendocrine circuits (1).

THYMOSIN STIMULATES REPRODUCTIVE HORMONES. Our first observation that thymosin peptides are capable of stimulating reproductive hormones was made using an in vitro model system in which rat brain and pituitary tissue were superfused with thymosin preparations (2). This study revealed that thymosin fraction 5 (TF5) and thymosin β_4 (Tβ_4) were, in a dose dependent manner, capable of stimulating the release of luteinizing hormone (LH). However, this stimulation of LH did not occur at the level of the pituitary gland. It was subsequently found that the thymosin peptides were stimulating the release of luteinizing hormone releasing hormone (LHRH) at the level of the hypothalamus. A site of action within the brain was also suggested by the results of a study in which Tβ_4 was injected directly into the lateral cerebroventricle of chronically cannulated mice (3). In this study, the peptide caused a significant increase in LH but had no effect on the pituitary-adrenal axis as assessed by the measurement of corticosterone. Thymosin α_1 (Tα_1), which was used as a control peptide, did not stimulate LH release, indicating that the results were relatively specific.

Another reproductive hormone that we have recently found to be stimulated by TF5 is prolactin. However, in contrast to LH, prolactin can be released as a result of direct stimulation of the pituitary gland. Using a prolactin and growth hormone secreting pituitary cell line (GH3), TF5 was found to stimulate prolactin release in a time and dose dependent manner. Maximal release was observed after 30 minutes of incubation with doses of TF5 ranging from 10 to 1000 micrograms (4). In addition to prolactin, growth hormone was also released by these cells following incubation with TF5 (5). Tα_1 and Tβ_4 were not active using this assay system, suggesting that LHRH and prolactin are stimulated by different component peptides of TF5.

THYMOSIN STIMULATES ACTH AND β-ENDORPHIN RELEASE. The pituitary-adrenocortical axis can also be stimulated by TF5. Activation of this neuroendocrine axis was first demonstrated using prepubertal cynomolgus monkeys (Macacca fascicularis) (6). TF5 was found to stimulate the release of ACTH, β-endorphin and cortisol in a dose and time dependent manner. ACTH reached peak levels at approximately 60 minutes, while cortisol was maximally elevated at 90 minutes, suggesting that the steroid release was stimulated by the ACTH. TF5 is also capable of stimulating steroidogenesis in laboratory rodents. In a time and dose dependent manner, corticosterone release was significantly elevated in both mice and rats (7). Other studies have revealed that the site of action includes the anterior pituitary gland. This was not apparent using a superfusion model (8), however, it was when primary cultures of rat adenohypophyseal cells were treated with varying doses of TF5. Optimal stimulation was observed at 4 hours using 100 or more micrograms/ml of this thymosin preparation (9). Similar findings have been reported following studies in which AtT20 cells, an ACTH and β-endorphin secreting line were co-incubated with TF5 (10). In the latter series of studies, significant increases in β-endorphin were observed within 15 minutes after treating the cells with 200 micrograms/ml of TF5.

While these data identify the pituitary gland as a site of action where thymosin can stimulate the pituitary-adrenocortical axis, they do not preclude the possibility of a central nervous system site of action as well. Several types of evidence suggest that this may indeed be the case. First, TF5 is corticogenic when injected directly into the third cerebroventricle of chronically cannulated rats (11). Concentrations as low as 10 micrograms per animal were effective in stimulating a significant increase in adrenal weight. In a subsequent study, adult male mice were fitted with polyethelene guide tubes that were secured to the skull overlying the lateral cerebroventricle. The administration of as little as 1 microgram of $T\alpha_1$ was correlated with a significant elevation in serum corticosterone levels (3).

DISCUSSION. These results suggest that the thymus gland regulates not only the differentiation of lymphocytes, but also the release of pituitary hormones that modulate virtually all components of homeostasis. These include trophic hormones such as prolactin and growth hormone, reproductive hormones and glucocorticoids via the release of ACTH. Each of these hormonal systems, including β-endorphin, is known to have immunomodulatory effects and thus constitutes a potential circuit by which the immune system can regulate itself.

It is necessary to exercise caution in postulating a biological scenario by which these hormones regulate the course of host-defense, since a functional circuit between these hormones and the immune system has not been definitively established. However, some working hypotheses can be formulated that do incorporate at least certain of the observed findings.

With respect to activation of the pituitary-adrenal axis, it has been suggested that this may constitute a mechanism by which the immune system down-regulates itself, since under certain conditions glucocorticoids can be immunosuppressive (12). It is also noteworthy that during the course of an immune response, there occurs a significant rise in glucocorticoid levels in rodents (12). The present data suggest that this rise in steroid may be signalled by thymosin peptides or by lymphokines which have also been found to be corticogenic (13). At the time steroid levels peak, antibody production is also approaching the plateau phase. Thus, the various cellular interactions that ultimately give rise to antibody production have presumably ended or would no longer be needed. Elevated steroids would serve to inhibit the clonal expansion of additional lymphocytes and would thus serve to end the immune response.

Prolactin appears to exert a facilitative effect upon immune system measures, possibly during the early phase of an immune response (14). If, as the present data suggest, different thymosin peptides are responsible for the release of different pituitary hormones, a crucial component of this regulatory circuit would be the temporal relationship of these peptides' release. Under stressful conditions when normal circadian patterns of hormone release are disrupted, one would expect to observe an aberrant state of immunity. This is a phenomenon that is well documented in the scientific literature. Exactly how β-endorphin and LH fit into this scenario is not clear at the present time. Reproductive hormones exert differential effects upon the various cell types that comprise the immune system while contradictory influences following β-endorphin treatment have been reported.

Whether or not all of these hormones will prove to have a physiological role to play during the course of host-defense is too speculative to conclude based upon the available data. Nonetheless, the potential for pituitary hormone regulation of immunity with thymosin peptides providing feedback signals is strongly suggested by the discussed observations.

ACKNOWLEDGEMENTS. These studies were supported in part by grants and gifts from the National Cancer Institute (CA24974), Alpha 1 Biomedicals, Inc. and Hoffmann-LaRoche, Inc.

REFERENCES

1. Hall, N.R. and Goldstein, A.L. (1984). in Immune Modulation Agents and Their Mechanisms (Fenichel, R.L. and Chirigos, M.A., eds.) pp. 553-563. Marcel Dekker,New York.
2. Rebar, R.W., Miyake, A., Low, T.L.K. and Goldstein, A.L. (1981). Science. 214, 669-671.
3. Hall, N.R., McGillis, J.P., Spangelo, B.L., Palaszynski, E., Moody, T.and Goldstein, A.L. (1982). Dev. Immunology. 17, 653-660.
4. Spangelo, B.L., Hall, N.R. and Goldstein, A.L. (submitted to Endocrinology).
5. Spangelo, B.L. (1985). Doctoral Dissertation submitted to The George Washington University College of Arts and Sciences.
6. Healy, L., Hodgen, G.D., Schultz, H.M., Chrousos, G.P., Loriaux, D.L., Hall, N.R. and Goldstein, A.L. (1983). Science. 222, 1353-1355.
7. McGillis, J.P., Hall, N.R., Vahouny, G.V. and Goldstein, A.L. (1985). J. Immunology. 134, 3952-3955.
8. McGillis, J.P., Hall, N.R. and Goldstein, A.L. (1983). Soc. for Neuroscience Abstracts. 343.
9. McGillis, J.P. (1985). Doctoral dissertation submitted to The George Washington University College of Arts and Sciences.
10. Farah, J.M., Bishop, J.F., McGillis, J.P., Hall, N.R., Goldstein, A.L. and O'Donohue, T.L. (1985). Society for Neuroscience Abstracts. 886.
11. Hall, N.R., McGillis, J.P., Spangelo, B.L., Healy, D.L., Chrousos, G.P., Schulte, H.M. and Goldstein, A.L. (1985). in Neural Modulation of Immunity (Guillemin, R., Cohn, M., and Melnechuk, T., eds.) pp.179-193. Raven Press, New York.
12. Besedovsky, H.O. and Sorkin, E. (1977). Clin. Exp. Immunol. 27,1-12.
13. Besedovsky, H.O., del Ray, A. and Sorkin, E. (1981). J. Immunology. 126, 385-389.
14. Spangelo, B.L., Hall, N.R. and Goldstein, A.L. (1985). in Prolactin. Basic and Clinical Correlates (MacLeod, R.M., Thorner, M.O. and Scapagnini, U. eds.) pp.343-349. Liviana Press, Padova, Italy.

The Interleukin 2 Hormone Receptor System and Regulation of T Lymphocyte Function

T.R. Malek*, J. Miller**, R.N. Germain**,
J.D. Ashwell** and E.M. Shevach**

*Department of Microbiology and Immunology
University of Miami School of Medicine
Miami, Florida 33101

and

The Laboratory of Immunology
NIAID, NIH
Bethesda, Maryland 20205

INTRODUCTION. The expression of interleukin 2 (IL-2) and the IL-2 receptor in T lymphocytes is each dependent upon stimulation with antigen (1). The clonal expansion of the antigen-activated T cells requires the polypeptide growth factor IL-2 (1). IL-2 stimulates T lymphocyte proliferation by binding to the IL-2 receptor in a manner characteristic of hormones binding their receptors. IL-2 receptors have two classes of IL-2 binding sites that have been defined on the basis of their affinity for IL-2 (2). The lower affinity receptor (Kd of approximately 10^{-8}M) comprises 90-95% of the total receptor molecules in T cells, whereas the remaining receptor molecules exhibit a higher affinity (Kd of approximately 10^{-11}M). It is believed that only the high affinity IL-2 receptor is able to transmit a biological signal to T cells (2). In order to understand the mechanism by which IL-2 stimulates T cell growth and potentially regulates an immune response, we have determined the primary structure and the biosynthesis of the mouse IL-2 receptor and have investigated the role of IL-2 and specific antigen in the regulation of IL-2 receptor expression.

BIOCHEMICAL ANALYSIS OF THE MURINE IL-2 RECEPTOR. Biochemical studies of the murine IL-2 receptor from the IL-2 dependent CTL-L cell line indicated that the receptor is synthesized as a 32,000 dalton peptide that is rapidly glycosylated by the addition of N-linked glycans to short-lived intracytoplasmic precursors of 38,000 and 40,000 daltons. These precursors are then further processed to the mature cell surface receptor protein of 58,000 daltons (3,4). After removal of these N-linked sugars by digestion with endoglycosidase F, the mouse

IL-2 receptor exhibited considerable change heterogeneity. This result suggests that the mouse IL-2 receptor may undergo other posttranslational modifications such as the addition of O-linked sugars, phosphorylation, or sulfation. All these type of modifications have been shown for the human IL-2 receptor (5,6), although the biological role, if any, of these posttranslational modifications is unknown. Immunoprecipitation of the murine IL-2 receptor with anti-IL-2 receptor monoclonal antibodies has lead to identification of a molecule that exhibited a band on SDS-PAGE of 110,000 daltons. This molecule appeared to be related to the IL-2 receptor, and data suggest that it maybe a covalent, but non-disulfide bonded, homodimer of the IL-2 receptor. The functional relevance of the 110,000 dalton molecule is under investigation.

CLONING AND EXPRESSION OF THE MOUSE IL-2 RECEPTOR. A cDNA library from the murine IL-2 dependent CTL-L cell line was screened with a human IL-2 receptor probe, pIL-2R3 (7), and a 1.3 kilobase cDNA (mIL-2R8) that contained the entire 804 base pair coding region of the murine IL-2 receptor was isolated and sequenced (8). Comparison of the mouse and human (7,9) sequences revealed overall amino acid homology of 61% with distinct regions of sequence more high conserved. We found no other sequence homology for the mouse IL-2 receptor and other protein sequences except for a weak, but a statistically significant, homology with bovine factor X, a zymogen protease involved in the blood coagulation pathway. Computer-assisted comparison of the mouse and human receptor sequences against themselves and with each other revealed an internal repeat in each molecule that encompassed the amino acid positions 3-97 and 100-199. This internal repeat suggests the presence of two extracellular domains within the IL-2 receptor. The IL-2 receptor also contains a single transmembrane region and an 11 amino acid intracytoplasmic tail. Since this intracytoplasmic region is so short, it is unlikely that the IL-2 receptor will function as a protein kinase.

By inserting mIL-2R8 into the expression vector pcEXV-3, the IL-2 receptor was transiently expressed in COS 7 monkey kidney cells. These transfected cells were able to bind IL-2 and anti-IL-2 receptor monoclonal antibodies. More recently, a stable L cell transfectant was produced that expressed high levels of surface IL-2 receptors. Interestingly, all the receptors on these L cells had only low affinity IL-2 binding sites. This result suggests that the appearance of functional high affinity IL-2 receptors may be dependent upon a specific regulatory mechanism present in some, eg. T cells, but not all cell types.

REGULATION OF IL-2 RECEPTOR EXPRESSION BY ANTIGEN OR IL-2. Untransformed murine class II-restricted T cell clones are maintained by stimulation with antigen and IL-2, and these cells always expressed cell surface IL-2 receptors. We have used two of these cloned T cell lines (11.4 and A.E7) as a model to investigate the role of IL-2 or antigen stimulation on cell surface IL-2 receptor levels (10). The 11.4 T cell clone is specific for the random terpolymer antigen of L-glutamic acid, L-alanine, L-tyrosine, whereas A.E7 T cells are specific for the antigen pigeon cytochrome c. IL-2 stimulation resulted in a specific 3-4 fold increase in IL-2 receptor expression, whereas specific antigen stimulation increased IL-2 receptors 10 fold for both T cell clones. Studies by others have also demonstrated that IL-2 is able to upregulate IL-2 receptors on mitogen preactivated human perpherial T cells (11-13). We have also noted that after stimulation with antigen or IL-2, IL-2 receptor mRNA also increased. This result suggests that IL-2 receptor upregulation is due to synthesis of new molecules rather than causing a redistribution of IL-2 receptors already present in the cell.

By Scatchard analysis of IL-2 binding data, antigen and IL-2 were shown to each cause an increase in both high and low affinity IL-2 receptors. However, relative to the total increase in cell surface IL-2 receptors, IL-2 stimulation was less efficient in increasing the cell surface expression of IL-2 receptors that contained high affinity binding sites.

An unexpected result was obtained for the bioassay of IL-2 responsiveness of the A.E7 T cell clone when assayed after IL-2 receptors were increased by IL-2 or antigen stimulation. As expected, A.E7 cells that had been stimulated with antigen showed an increased sensitivity in their proliferative response to IL-2. In contrast, activation of A.E7 with IL-2 caused almost a 4-fold decrease in sensitivity of these cells to subsequent stimulation with IL-2, even though all had a modest increase in levels of high affinity IL-2 receptors. However, if one calculates the number of high affinity receptors that are occupied to achieve 50% of the maximal proliferative response, it was observed that A.E7 T cells preactivated with IL-2 needed a 3.5 fold increase and those preactivated with antigen required 2.1 fold increase in the absolute number of receptors occupied when compared to unstimulated A.E7 cells. Therefore, despite the functional dichotomy between sensitivities of IL-2 and antigen preactivated T cells, both exhibited a reduction, on a per receptor basis, in the ability to respond to IL-2. In other words, although activation of a T cell clone with IL-2 induced a modest increase in the number of high affinity IL-2 receptors, there was a concomitant decrease in the apparent ability of the receptors to effectively transduce a proliferative signal. The net result was a T cell less sensitive to stimulation with IL-2. Activation with antigen resulted in a dramatic increase in the number of high affinity receptors, so that even with an apparent decrease in responsiveness per IL-2 receptor, these T cells were more sensitive to IL-2 than unstimulated A.E7 cells.

Thus, it appears that IL-2 binding of the IL-2 receptor initiates both positive and negative feedback that will influence the magnitude of T cell clonal expansion. On the one hand, IL-2 receptor upregulation provides a mechanism for antigen-independent clonal expansion. On the other hand, the apparent decreased sensitivity of IL-2 activated cells to mount a subsequent IL-2 driven proliferative response, provides a means to limit clonal expansion since the cells need to bind an increased amount of IL-2 for a biological response.

REFERENCES

1. Smith, K.A., and F.W. Ruscetti. 1981. Adv. Immunology 31:137.
2. Robb, R.J., W.C. Greene, and C.M. Rusk. 1984. J. Exp. Med. 160: 1126.
3. Malek, T.R., R.J. Robb, E.M. Shevach. 1983. Proc. Natl. Acad. Sci. USA. 80:5694.
4. Ortega, -R., G., R.J Robb, E.M. Shevach, and T.R. Malek. 1984. J. Immunol. 133:1970.
5. Leonard, W.J., J.M. Depper, M. Kronke, R.J. Robb, T.A. Waldmann, and W.C. Greene. 1985. J. Biol. Chem. 260:1872.
6. Shackelford, D.A., and I.S. Trowbridge. 1984. J. Biol. Chem. 259:11,706.
7. Leonard, W., J. Depper, G. Crabtree, S. Rudikoff, J. Pumphery, R. Robb, M. Kronke, P. Svettik, N. Peffer, T. Waldmann, and W. Greene. 1984. Nature 311:626.
8. Miller, J., T.R. Malek, W.J. Leonard, W.C. Greene, E.M. Shevach, and R.N. Germain. 1985. J. Immunol. 134:4212.
9. Nikarde, T., A. Shimizu, H. Ishida, H. Sabe, K. Teshigawara, M. Maeda, T. Uchiyama, J. Yodoi, and T. Honjo. 1985. Nature 311:336.
10. Malek, T.R., and J.D. Ashwell. 1985. J. Exp. Med. 161:1575.
11. Reem, G.H., and H.H. Yeh. 1984. Science 225:429.
12. Welte, K., M. Andreeff, E. Platzer, K. Holloway, B.Y. Rubin, M.A.S. Moore, and R. Mertelsmann. 1984. J. Exp. Med. 160: 1390.
13. Smith, K.A., and D.A. Cantrell. 1985. Proc. Natl. Acad. Sci. USA 82:864.

MOLECULAR ANALYSIS OF THE GENE ENCODING THE HUMAN INTERLEUKIN-2 RECEPTOR

Warren J. Leonard
Cell Biology and Metabolism Branch, National Institute of Child Health and Human Development, NIH, Bethesda, MD 20892 U.S.A.

INTRODUCTION. When resting T lymphocytes are stimulated with antigen or mitogenic lectin, at least some of the cells are stimulated to synthesize and secrete the lymphokine, interleukin-2 (IL-2), previously known as T-cell growth factor (1,2). Another, possibly overlapping subpopulation of T cells are stimulated to express IL-2 receptors. These cells with receptors proliferate in the presence of IL-2, resulting in the expansion of T cell populations capable of mediating helper, suppressor and cytotoxic T cell functions. This is therefore an example of a hormone receptor system in which both the ligand and the receptor are absent in the resting state, but are expressed solely after stimulation of the cells. Although the specificity of the immune response is determined by the stimulating antigen, the IL-2/IL-2 receptor system appears to be responsible for the subsequent antigen independent cell proliferation. A schematic summary of this system is presented in Figure 1.

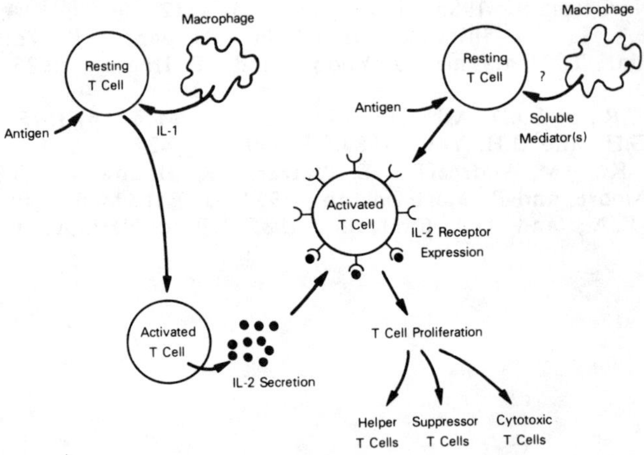

Fig. 1: A Model for T Cell Activation.

THE IL-2 RECEPTOR PROTEIN. IL-2 receptors are glycoproteins that may be sulfated and phosphorylated with apparent M_rs of 55,000 on normal activated T cells (3-5). The protein is synthesized as a proprotein of 272 amino acids and then processed to mature form of 251 amino acids (6-8). The protein has two N-linked carbohydrate addition sites, and is also known to contain O-linked carbohydrate. The protein contains a short (13 amino acid long) positively charged cytoplasmic domain. IL-2 receptors exist in both high and low affinity forms (K_ds of 10^{-12}M and 10^{-9}M, respectively) (9). Only the high affinity receptor has been associated with known biologic function, and only the high affinity receptor is internalized in response to the addition of IL-2 (10).

IL-2 receptors are present in large numbers on T cells infected with Human T Cell Lymphotrophic Virus I (HTLV-I); receptor number is five to twenty fold high than that found on normal activated peripheral blood T cells (11). It was these cell lines that facilitated the purification of IL-2 receptor protein and the cloning of cDNAs encoding the receptor (6-8).

GENOMIC ORGANIZATION OF THE IL-2 RECEPTOR. Using an IL-2 receptor cDNA, genomic phage clones spanning the IL-2 receptor gene (except part of the first intron) were isolated (12). All exons and exon-intron splice junctions were sequenced, and the map of the gene was determined. This information is depicted schematically in Figure 2.

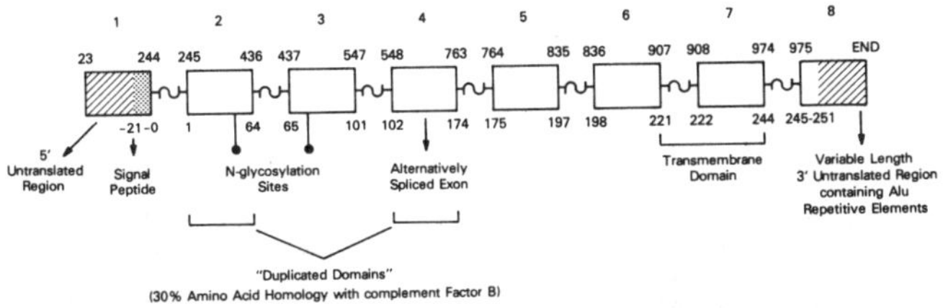

Fig. 2: Structure of the Human Interleukin-2 Receptor Gene. The 8 exons of the gene are indicated. Numbers above the boxes indicate the base numbers corresponding to the IL-2 receptor cDNA sequence published in ref. 6. Numbers below the boxes correspond to the numbers of the amino acids encoded by each exon.

As noted in the figure, the first exon consists of the 5' untranslated region and signal peptide. The second exon begins with amino acid 1 of the mature protein. Exons 2 and 4 share significant homology with each other suggesting an historical gene duplication event. These exons also share strong homology with the Ba fragment of complement factor B. The Ba fragment represents the binding domain rather than the serine protease region of factor B. Comparison of alignment scores of exon 4 to local regions of complement factor B versus 1000 random sequences showed the significance of homology to be 9.659 standard deviation units, similar to that of the low density lipoprotein receptor to coagulation factors IX and X. Exons 2 and 3 each contain one of the two N-linked carbohydrate addition sites; in addition, they and exons 5 and 6 contain clusters of serine and threonine residues, suggesting that O-linked carbohydrate may be added in these regions. Exons 5 and 6 encode the portion of the IL-2 receptor located just extracytoplasmic to the cell. Exon 7 encodes the transmembrane segment of the protein, and exons 7 and 8 each encode part of the cytoplasmic domain. Exon 8 contains at least three polyadenylation signal addition sites with repetitive alu sequences located between the second and third sites.

MULTIPLE mRNA SPECIES. Although encoded by a single gene, Northern blots using IL-2 receptor cDNAs reveal two major hybridizing regions of approximately 1550 and 3500 bases in T cells activated with phytohemagglutinin (PHA) and/or phorbol 12-myristate 13-acetate (PMA) (Figure 3). A series of S1 nuclease protection assays confirmed that these hybridizing signals consist of at least 6 potential mRNA species based on the use of three alternate polyadenylation addition sites combined with the ability to alternatively splice exon 4. All of these mRNAs exist in both normal activated peripheral blood T cells and in HTLV-I infected adult T cell leukemia cells. It is not clear at present whether the use of different polyadenylation sites results in mRNAs of greater stability or of greater translation efficiencies. Expression of the alternatively spliced IL-2 receptor mRNA species does not result in cell surface receptors capable of binding IL-2 or anti-IL-2 receptor antibodies; thus the physiologic role of this mRNA, if any, remains unknown.

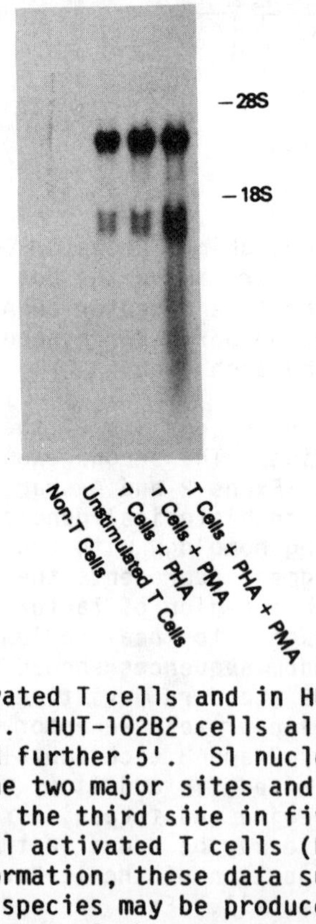

Figure 3: Northern blot of 10 ug of total cellular RNA from the indicated cell types, hybridized with ^{32}P-labeled IL-2 receptor cDNAs.

More recent data indicates that even more IL-2 receptor associate mRNA species are present (15). A synthetic oligonucleotide corresponding to the 5' end of the IL-2 receptor cDNA was end-labeled with ^{32}P, annealed to mRNA, and extended with reverse transcriptase. Such primer extension studies revealed two major transcription initiation sites in both normal activated T cells and in HUT-102B2 cells (an HTLV-I infected T cell line). HUT-102B2 cells also had a third, minor initiation site located further 5'. S1 nuclease protection assays have confirmed the two major sites and in addition have demonstrated the existence of the third site in five HTLV-I infected cell lines but not in normal activated T cells (Figure 4). Taken together with the earlier information, these data suggest that as many as 12 to 18 mature mRNA species may be produced from the IL-2 receptor gene. The significance of the extra apparent transcription initiation site in HTLV-I infected cells is under investigation.

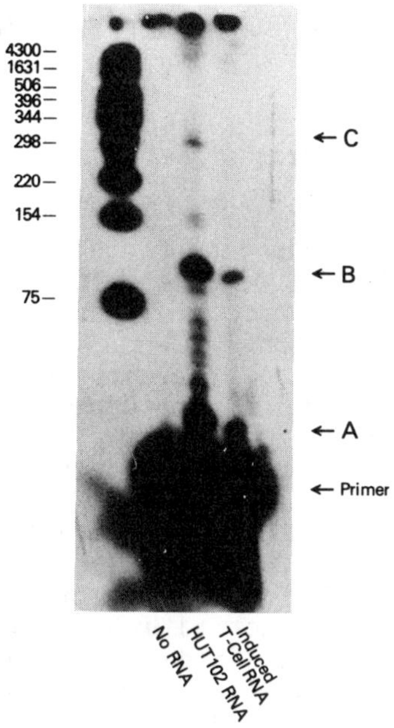

Figure 4: Primer extension experiment as described in the text with mRNA from HUT-102 cells or normal activated T cells. The two major transcription initiation sites are denoted A and B; C indicates the site detected in HTLV-I infected cells but not in normal activated T cells.

REFERENCES.

(1) Morgan, D.A., F.W. Ruscetti, R.C. Gallo (1976). Science 193, 1007-1008.

(2) Smith, K.A. (1980). Immunol. Rev. 51, 337-357.

(3) Leonard, W.J., J.M. Depper, T. Uchiyama, K.A. Smith, T.A. Waldmann, W.C. Greene (1982). Nature 300, 267-269.

(4) Leonard, W.J., J.M. Depper, R.J. Robb, T.A. Waldmann, W.C. Greene (1983). PNAS 80, 6957-6961.

(5) Leonard, W.J., J.M. Depper, R.J. Robb, M. Kronke, T.A. Waldmann, W.C. Greene (1985). J. Biol. Chem. 260, 1872-1880.

(6) Leonard, W.J., J.M. Depper, G.R. Crabtree, S. Rudikoff, J. Pumphrey, R.J. Robb, M. Kronke, P.B. Svetlik, N.J. Peffer, T.A. Waldmann, W.C. Greene (1984). Nature 311, 626-631.

(7) Nikaido, T., A. Shimizu, N. Ishida, H. Sabe, K. Teshigawara, M. Maeda, T. Uchiyama, J. Yodoi, T. Honjo (1984) Nature 311, 631-635.

(8) Cosman, D., D.P. Ceretti, A. Larsen, L. Park, C. March, S. Dower, S. Gillis, D. Urdal (1984) Nature 312, 768-770.

(9) Robb, R.J., W.C. Greene, C.M. Rusk (1984). J Exp. Med. 160, 1126-1146.

(10) Weissman, A., J. Harford, P. Svetlik, W. Leonard, J. Depper, T. Waldmann, W. Greene, R. Klausner (1985) PNAS, in press.

(11) Depper, J.M., W.J. Leonard, M. Kronke, T.A. Waldmann, W.C. Greene (1984) J. Immunol. 311, 1691-1695.

(12) Leonard, W.J., J.M. Depper, M. Kanehisa, M. Kronke, N.J. Peffer, P.B. Svetlik, M. Sullivan, W.C. Greene (1985) Science 230, 633-639.

INTERLEUKIN-2 RECEPTOR ON MALIGNANT CELLS: A TARGET FOR DIAGNOSIS AND THERAPY

T. A. Waldmann
National Cancer Institute, National Institutes of Health, Bethesda, MD 20892 U.S.A.

INTRODUCTION. The human body defends itself against foreign invaders such as bacteria and viruses by a defense system that involves antibodies and thymus-derived lymphocytes (T cells). The success of this response requires that human T cells change from a resting to an activated state. The sequence of events involved in the activation of human T cells begins with the interaction of appropriately processed and presented antigen with receptors on the surface of the T cells. Following the interaction of antigens with the T-cell antigen receptor, two principal events occur which are required for T-cell proliferation. First, following interaction with antigen and the macrophage-derived interleukin-1 (IL-1), T cells express the gene encoding interleukin-2 (IL-2) (1,2). In order to exert its biological effects, IL-2 must interact with high affinity-specific membrane receptors (3). Resting T cells do not express IL-2 receptors, but receptors are rapidly expressed on T cells following activation with antigen or mitogen. Thus, both the growth factor IL-2 and its receptor are absent in resting T cells, but following activation the genes for both proteins become expressed.

The specific membrane receptor for IL-2 on human lymphocytes has been identified using a monoclonal antibody (anti-Tac) we have developed that is directed towards this molecule (4,5). The anti-Tac monoclonal antibody was used to: (a) characterize the human receptor for IL-2 (5,6); (b) molecularly clone cDNAs for the human IL-2 receptor (7); (c) define the immunological events that require the interaction of IL-2 with its receptor (8); and as discussed below to: (d) characterize the expression of the Tac antigen (IL-2 receptor) in leukemias of mature T lymphocytes; and (e) treat patients with the Tac-expressing adult T-cell leukemia (ATL).

IL-2 RECEPTOR EXPRESSION IN ATL. We have analyzed the IL-2 receptor expression on three forms of T-cell leukemia: acute T-cell leukemia, the Sézary leukemia, and ATL (9). ATL is a leukemia of mature T cells that have a propensity to infiltrate the skin. Cases of ATL are clustered within families and geographically. Furthermore, ATL has been shown to be caused by the HTLV-I, a human type C retrovirus (10). The acute T-cell leukemic populations and nine of the 10 populations of Sézary leukemic T cells not associated with HTLV-I examined were Tac antigen negative (9). In contrast, all 15 populations of leukemic cells from patients with the ATL examined expressed the Tac antigen.

The IL-2 receptor expression on ATL cells differs from that on normal T cells. First, unlike normal T cells, ATL cells do not require prior activation to express the IL-2 receptors. Second, HTLV-I-infected leukemic T-cell lines characteristically express five- to tenfold more receptors per cell (270,000 to 640,000) than do maximally PHA-stimulated T lymphoblasts (30,000 to 60,000) (11). In addition, whereas normal human T lymphocytes maintained in long-term culture with IL-2 demonstrate a rapid decline in receptor number, ATL lines do not show a similar decline. Furthermore, a small proportion of HTLV-I-infected cell lines display aberrantly sized IL-2 receptors (12). Finally, in studies by Uchiyama and coworkers (13), IL-2 receptors on ATL cells, unlike normal activated T cells, were not modulated (down-regulated) by anti-Tac. It is conceivable that the constant presence of high numbers of IL-2 receptors on the ATL cells and/or the aberrancy of these receptors may play a major role in the pathogenesis of uncontrolled growth of these malignant T cells.

As noted above, the T-cell leukemias caused by HTLV-I, as well as all T-cell and B-cell lines infected with HTLV-I, universally express large numbers of IL-2 receptors. In addition to the GAG, POL, ENV, and LTR (long terminal repeats) sequences common to other groups of retroviruses, HTLV-I contains an additional genomic region between ENV and the LTR referred to as pX (14). Sodroski and colleagues (15) demonstrated that this pX or TaT region encodes a 42kd protein termed LOR (long open reading frame) that may act as a trans-acting regulator of transcription. They demonstrated that the LOR protein acts on receptors in the LTRs of HTLV-I, II, and III, stimulating transcription. The LOR protein could also play a central role in increasing the transcription of host genes such as the IL-2 receptor gene involved in T-cell activation and HTLV-I-mediated leukemogenesis.

TREATMENT OF ATL PATIENTS WITH THE ANTI-TAC MONOCLONAL ANTIBODY. We have initiated a clinical trial to evaluate the efficacy of intravenously administered anti-Tac monoclonal antibody in the treatment of patients with the ATL. The scientific basis for these studies is the observation that ATL cells express the Tac antigen whereas normal resting T cells and their precursors do not (9). Three patients with ATL have been treated wih intravenously administered anti-Tac. None of the patients suffered any untoward reactions, and none produced antibodies reactive with mouse immunoglobulin or the idiotype of the anti-Tac monoclonal. The two patients with a very rapidly developing form of ATL had a very transient response. However, therapy of the other patient was followed by a 6-month remission as assessed by routine hematological tests, immunofluorescence analysis of circulating T cells, and molecular genetic analysis of the arrangement of T-cell beta receptor genes. Approximately 6 months following the initial remission, the leukemia recurred. A new course of intravenous infusions of anti-Tac was followed by the virtual disappearance of the skin lesions and an over 90% reduction in the number of circulating leukemic cells. Three months subsequently leukemic cells again were demonstrable in the circulation. At this time the leukemia was no longer responsive to infusions of anti-Tac and the patient required chemotherapy.

These therapeutic studies have been extended in vitro by examining the efficacy of toxins coupled to anti-Tac in selectively inhibiting protein synthesis and viability of Tac-positive ATL cell lines.

The addition of anti-Tac antibody coupled to the A chain of the toxin ricin effectively inhibited protein synthesis by the HTLV-I-associated, Tac-positive ATL line HUT 102-B2. In contrast, conjugates of ricin A with a control monoclonal of the same isotype did not inhibit protein synthesis when used in the same concentration (16). In parallel studies performed in collaboration with David FitzGerald, Mark Willingham, and Ira Pastan (17), Pseudomonas exotoxin conjugates of anti-Tac inhibited the protein synthesis by HUT 102-B2 cells but not that by the Tac-negative acute T-cell line Molt-4, which does not express the Tac antigen. The Pseudomonas exotoxin conjugates of anti-Tac now are being used in the treatment of patients with ATL.

The action of toxin conjugates of monoclonal antibodies depends on their ability to be internalized by the cell and released into the cytoplasm. Anti-Tac bound to IL-2 receptors on leukemic cells is internalized slowly into endosomes (17). Furthermore, the toxin conjugate does not pass easily from the endosome to the cytosol as required for its action on elongation factor II. Thus, it was of value to develop an alternative cytotoxic reagent conjugable to anti-Tac that would be effective while bound to the surface of the leukemic cells. Bismuth-212 (^{212}Bi), an alpha-particle radionuclide conjugated to anti-Tac by use of a bifunctional chelate, was well suited for this role. Activity levels of 0.5 Ci or the equivalent of 12 rads/ml of alpha irradiation targeted by anti-Tac eliminated greater than 98% of the proliferative capacities of the HUT 102 cell with only modest effects on IL-2 receptor-negative lines. Thus, ^{212}Bi-anti-Tac is a potentially effective and specific immunocytotoxic reagent for the elimination of IL-2 receptor-positive cells.

In addition to its use in the therapy of patients with ATL, anti-Tac is being evaluated as a therapeutic agent to eliminate activated IL-2 receptor-expressing T cells in other clinical states, including organ allografts and certain autoimmune disorders. The reason for the use of an antibody to IL-2 receptors in recipients of renal and cardiac allografts is that anti-Tac inhibits the proliferation of T cells to alloantigens and prevents the generation of cytotoxic T lymphocytes in allogenic cell cocultures. Finally, the survival of cardiac allografts was prolonged in rodent recipients treated with an IL-2 receptor monoclonal antibody (18). In other studies anti-Tac is being evaluated for the therapy of patients who have diseases mediated by Tac-expressing T lymphocytes. For example, Zoumbos and coworkers (19) have demonstrated that a subset of patients with aplastic anemia has increased numbers of circulating Tac-positive cells. In this group of patients the Tac-positive but not Tac-negative T cells inhibited hematopoiesis in coculture with normal bone marrow cells. Furthermore, we have demonstrated that anti-Tac inhibits the generation of activated suppressor T lymphocytes. Thus, the development of the monoclonal anti-Tac directed toward the IL-2 receptor expressed on ATL cells, on host cells responding to foreign major histocompatibility antigens on organ allografts, and on the cells of certain patients with autoreactive T cells may permit the development of rational approaches for the treatment of these clinical conditions.

REFERENCES

(1) Morgan, D.A., Ruscetti, F.W. and Gallo, R.C. (1983) Science 193, 1007-1008.

(2) Smith, K.A. (1980) Immunol. Rev. 51, 337-357.

(3) Robb, R.J., Munck, A. and Smith, K.A. (1981) J. Exp. Med. 154, 1455-1474.

(4) Uchiyama, T., Broder, S. and Waldmann, T.A. (1981) J. Immunol. 126, 1393-1397.

(5) Leonard, W.J., Depper, J.M., Uchiyama, T., Smith, K.A., Waldmann, T.A. and Greene, W.C. (1982) Nature (Lond.) 300, 267-269.

(6) Leonard, W.J., Depper, J.M., Robb, R.J., Waldmann, T.A. and Greene, W.C. (1983) Proc. Natl. Acad. Sci. USA 80, 6957-6961.

(7) Leonard, W.J., Depper, J.M., Crabtree, G.R., Rudikoff, S., Pumphrey, J., Robb, R.J., Krönke, M., Svetlik, P.B., Peffer, N.J., Waldmann, T.A. and Greene, W.C. (1984) Nature (Lond.) 311, 626-631.

(8) Depper, J.M., Leonard, W.J., Waldmann, T.A. and Greene, W.C. (1983) J. Immunol. 131, 690-696.

(9) Waldmann, T.A., Greene, W.C., Sarin, P.S., Saxinger, C., Blayney, W., Blattner, W.A., Goldman, C.K., Bongiovanni, K., Sharrow, S., Depper, J.M., Leonard, W., Uchiyama, T. and Gallo, R.C. (1984) J. Clin. Invest. 73, 1711-1718.

(10) Poiesz, B.J., Ruscetti, F.W., Gazdar, A.F., Bunn, P.A., Minna, J.D. and Gallo, R.C. (1980) Proc. Natl. Acad. Sci. USA 77, 7415-7419.

(11) Depper, J.M., Leonard, W.J., Krönke, M., Waldmann, T.A. and Greene, W.C. (1984) J. Immunol. 133, 1691-1695.

(12) Leonard, W.J., Depper, J.M., Roth, J.S., Rudikoff, S., Waldmann, T.A. and Greene, W.C. (1983) Clin. Res. 31, 348A

(13) Uchiyama, T., Wano, Y., Tsudo, M., Umadome, H., Hori, T., Tamori, S., Yodoi, J. and Maeda, M. (1948) in Retroviruses in Human Lymphoma/Leukemia: The Fifteenth International Symposium of the Princess Takamatsu Cancer Research Fund. (Miwa, M., ed.), Japan Sci. Soc. Press, Tokyo, in press

(14) Seiki, M., Hattori, S., Hirayama, Y., Yoshida, M. (1983) Proc. Natl. Acad. Sci. USA 80, 3618

(15) Sodroski, J.G., Rosen, C.A. and Haseltine, W.A. (1984) Science 225, 381-385.

(16) Krönke, M., Depper, J.M., Leonard, W.J., Vitetta, E.S., Waldmann, T.A. and Greene, W.C. (1985) Blood 65, 1416-1421.

(17) FitzGerald, D.J.P., Waldmann, T.A., Willingham, M.C. and Pastan, I. (1984) J. Clin. Invest. 74, 966-971.

(18) Strom, T.B., Banet, L.V., Gauiton, G.N., Kelley, V.F., Thier, A.Y., Diamanstein, T., Tilney, N.L. and Kirkman, R.L. (1985) Clin. Res. 33, 561

(19) Zoumbos, N., Gascon, P., Trost, S., Djeu, J., Young, N. (1985) N. Engl. J. Med. 312, 257-265.

INTERFERON RECEPTOR AND INTERFERON-ACTIVATED GENES

M.Revel, J.Chebath, A.Kimchi, L.Shulman, O.Horovitz, B.Cohen, M. Goldberg* and M. Fellous*, Dept. of Virology, Weizmann Institute of Science, Rehovot, Israel and (*) Institut Pasteur, Paris, France

INTERFERONS AS CELL REGULATORY HORMONAL FACTORS AND GENE ACTIVATORS. Although Interferons (IFNs) were discovered by their antiviral effects this family of 20-25 Kd proteins clearly belongs to the group of polypeptide hormones and cellular factors providing signals to the cells to alter their gene expression program. In addition to preventing the replication of most viruses, IFNs regulate many cell functions, reducing or arresting cell growth and producing changes in structure, activity and differentiation of various cell types including the immune system (1,2). These biological effects are probably mediated by the induction of a group of 15-20 proteins whose genes are activated to a different extent by the three classes of IFNs (α,β and γ). The IFN-induced proteins include translation regulatory enzymes as the dsRNA-activated 2'-5' oligo A synthetase (OASE) and eIF2-protein kinase (1,3) surface antigens as HLA class I and II (1,4), and additional intracellular (5), membranal or secreted proteins, whose genes were recently cloned in several laboratories as listed in Table 1.

Classically, IFN production was seen mainly as a response to viral infection or exposure to double-stranded (ds) RNA, which activate the 15-20 IFN-α (leucocyte) and the major fibroblast IFN-β_1 genes on human chrom. 9 (1). However, mitogenic stimuli have also emerged as being physiological IFN inducers. Thus, the IFN-γ gene on human chrom. 12, is induced in T cells after activation of immune cells by mitogenic antigens, which also induce IFN-α in B and accessory cells (2,16). Moreover, some IFN-β is produced endogenously by cells undergoing transitions from growth to quiescence and differentiation (1,17). Such IFNs act as autocrine cell regulatory factors mediating some of the molecular changes occurring in these cells. Thus, anti IFN-β antibodies prevent the synthesis and accumulation of HLA class I and OASE during PMA-induced differentiation of human U937 histiocytes (17) and the Go arrest of cell proliferation and switch-off of the c-myc oncogene mRNA expression during CSF-induced differentiation of mouse M1 myelomonocytes (18). These effects of autocrine IFN resemble those of exogenously added IFN which induces the OASE and HLA genes (6,10) and inhibits several growth-related genes (c-myc, c-fos and ODC) in PDGF-stimulated fibroblasts and in some tumor cells as Daudi and Molt 4 (19,20). Inhibition of c-myc correlates with the ability of IFN to block cells in Go, and this control is lost in certain tumor cell lines or IFN-growth resistant variants of Daudi cells (20). PDGF itself induces IFN and OASE (21), which may provide a feed-back mechanism ensuring that proto-oncogenes are only transiently expressed. In synchronized cultures of embryonic mouse fibroblasts, IFN is endogenously produced during G1 and a sharp peak of OASE is observed at the end of the S phase (22). The endogenous IFN-β is not IFN-β_1, but may be the product of minor IFN-β genes not on chrom. 9 (1,23). An IFN-β_2 gene was cloned and expressed (24) and can be activated by IL-1 (25). Genes for autocrine IFN-β_1 remain to be identified but their existence has changed our concept of IFN activity and justifies its classification as a cellular

TABLE 1. Interferon-induced cloned cDNA and genes

Name of clone or gene	RNA size	Protein Mol.Wt.	Function	Induction	Ref.
(2'-5')oligo A synthetase (OASE)	3.6 kb	?	Ds RNA dependent Synthesis of ppp(A2'p)nA activator of RNase F.		6
E18	1.8 kb	46Kd		α,β > γ	
E16	1.6 kb	40Kd			
C56 pIF-2	2.0 kb	56Kd	Poly IC binding function unknown	α,β > γ	7,8
pIF-1	2.9 kb	42Kd 58Kd		α,β	8
1-8 gene family 9-27 related ?	0.8 kb	?		α,β,γ not in Daudi-R	9
6-16 10Q related ?	1.0 kb	13Kd excreted		α,β not in Daudi-R	9
MT-IIa	0.5 kb	7Kd	Metallothionein Metal detoxific.	IFN,Zn Dexamet.	9
Thymosin B4 6-26	0.8 kb	5.2Kd) 16Kd precursor	Induces terminal transferase in B lymphocytes		9
HLA-A,B,C	1.8 kb	44Kd	Heavy chain of Histocompatibility Class I antigens	γ > α,β	4,10
β_2-microglobulin	0.9 kb	14Kd	Small invariant HLA class I chain	γ > α,β	10
HLA-DR α	1.3 kb	34Kd	HLA class II Heavy and Light chains	γ >>α,β	4,11
HLA-DR β		29Kd			
pIF-γ-31	1.5 kb	12Kd precursor	excreted as 10Kd homology to Platelet factor 4	γ >>α	12
GBP	4.0 kb	67Kd	GTP, GDP binding	α,β,γ	13
15KD protein	0.7 kb	15Kd	cytoplasmic prot.	α,β	14
MTX (mouse)	3.2 kb	72Kd	specific inhibition of influenza virus	α,β	15

Unless indicated genes are from man. Daudi-R are resistant to antigrowth effect of IFN.

hormone.

THE HUMAN IFN TYPE I RECEPTOR. IFN-α and β (type I IFNs) act on cells through the same plasma membrane receptor, while the action of IFN-γ is mediated by a separate type II-IFN receptor (26). The type I IFN receptor has high affinity binding sites for IFN, (Kd 10^{-10} M) and contains a 110,000-Mr membrane protein which can be cross-linked to labeled IFNs (27). It is not clear if the IFN-receptor complex acts after internalization (26) or from the membrane, for example through an associated protein kinase (28). What is clear is that transcriptional activation of some of the IFN-induced genes of Table 1, follows within a few minutes of IFN binding to its cell receptor (8,9). Since the number of type I IFN receptors per cell is usually very low (2-5,000), isolation and characterization of this protein is difficult. Fortunately somatic cell genetic offers a way to study the human typeI IFN receptor, thanks to its marked species specificity. Mouse cells do not respond to HuIFN, but mouse-human hybrids containing human chrom. 21 as the only human DNA respond well to HuIFN-α or β (29). Polyclonal and monoclonal (McAB) antibodies against such 21^+ hybrid cells produced in mice inhibit HuIFN-α,β antiviral effect on human cells (27,30), block binding of these IFNs but not IFN-γ to the cells and immunoprecipitate the type I IFN-receptor complex (27). Anti IFN-receptor McAB A20, inhibit the induction of OASE by 16 U/ml IFN-β_1 in FS11 fibroblasts and abolish the OASE rise in differentiating U937 cells (18), confirming that both endogenous and exogenous IFN-β act on the same 21-encoded receptor molecule.

DNA-MEDIATED TRANSFER OF THE HUMAN TYPE I RECEPTOR GENE. To clone the gene for the HuIFN-receptor, we transformed mouse LM TK^- cells by either sheared human DNA co-transfected with a Herpes TK gene, or by a cosmid library of human DNA fragments (average size 45 kb) linked to the Herpes TK gene (31). We then made use of the IFN-dependent increase in cell surface MHC antigens to sort HuIFN responders in a fluorescence activated cell sorter (Orthodiagnostic cytofluorograph 50H). Since H2 antigens are a 100 times more abundant than the IFN receptors, this provides a strong amplification of the signal expected for the transferred HuIFN receptor. A pool of TK^+ cells transformed by the cosmid DNA library (CT-0 cells) was treated by HuIFN for 20 hrs, fixed, stained with McAB 12-41 (Ha-K^k specific) and the 1-2% most fluorescent cells were sorted. After two such cycles, we subcloned the sorted cells (CT2) by dilution and isolated clones (CT2-5,11,36) which responded to Hu-rIFN-αc or β_1 by a significant increase in H2, OASE and VSV virus inhibition (32). These cells bound specifically HuIFN, the number of sites being 20% that of human cells (32). McAB anti-HuIFN type I receptor inhibited the HuIFN-β_1 induced the increase in H2 in CT2 clones but did not impair the response to mouse IFN, indicating that the human and murine receptor systems coexist in the membrane of these transformants. Total DNA from clone CT2-36 was transfected again in LM TK^- recipients and about 50% of the secondary TK^+ transformants responded to HuIFN by OASE induction and VSV inhibition (32). Thus, the gene encoding the type I HuIFN receptor was transferred together with its neighboring Herpes TK gene to the secondary transformant clones. Human DNA sequences present in the HuIFN sensitive transformants are under investigation. Our experiments show, therefore, that the type I HuIFN-dependent antiviral response, increase in MHC antigens, induction of OASE and high-affinity binding sites can be transferred together at about $2x10^{-5}$ frequency into mouse cells via 40-50 kb fragments of human DNA, several hundred times smaller than chrom. 21 which should contain the type I IFN receptor gene.

REFERENCES: 1) Revel, M. (1984) in Antiviral Drugs and Interferon:The molecular basis of their activity (Becker,Y.ed.) Martinus Nijhoff Publ. Boston, pp 357-433; 2) DeMaeyer-Guignard, J. & DeMaeyer, E. (1985) in Interferon 6 (Gresser,I. ed.) Acad.Press, London pp 69-91; 3) Lengyel, P. (1982) Ann.Rev.Biochem. 51:251-252; 4) Rosa, F. & Fellous, M. (1984) Immunology Today 5:261-262; 5) Weil, J. et al. (1983) Nature 301:437-439; 6) Benech, P., Mory, Y., Revel, M. & Chebath, J. (1985) EMBO J. 4:2249-2256; 7) Chebath, J. et al. (1983) Nucleic Acids Res. 13:1267-1281; 8) Larner, A.C. et al. (1984) Proc.Natl.Acad.Sci. USA 81:6733-6737; 9) Friedman, R. L. et al. (1984) Cell 38:745-755; 10) Wallach, D., Fellous, M. & Revel, M. (1982) Nature 299:834-836; 11) Rosa, F. et al. (1983) EMBO J. 2:1585-1589; 12) Luster, A.D., Unkeless, J.C. & Ravetch, J.V. (1985) Nature 313:672-676; 13) Cheng, Y.-S.E., Colonno, R.J. & Yin, F.H. (1983) J.Biol.Chem. 258:7746-7750; 14) Knight, E., Fahey, D. & Blomstrom, D.C. (1985) J. Interferon Res. 5:305-313, and private commun; 15) Staeheli, P., Dreiding, P., Haller, O. & Lindeman, J. (1985) J.Biol.Chem. 260:1821-1825; 16) Stanton, G.J., Langford, M.P. & Weigert, D.A. (1982) Texas Rep.Biol.Med. 41:84-88; 17) Yarden, A. et al. (1984) EMBO J. 3:969-973; 18) Kimchi, A. et al. unpublished; 19) Einat, M., Resnitzky, D. & Kimchi, A. (1985) Nature 313:597-600; 20) Kimchi, A., Einat, M. & Resnitzky, D. (1985) in The Interferon System, Serono Symposia, Raven Press, New York, vol 24, pp 429-438; 21) Zullo, J.N., Cochran, B.H., Huang, A.S. & Stiles, C.D. (1985)Cell in press; 22) Mallucci, L., Chebath, J., Revel, M., Wells, V. & Benech, P. (1985) in The Interferon System, Serono Symposia, Raven Press, New York, vol 24 pp 165-170; 23) Sagar, A.D., Sehgal, P.B., Slate, D.L. & Ruddle, F.H. (1982) J.Exp.Med. 156:744-755; 24) Zilberstein, A., Ruggieri, R. & Revel, M. (1985) in The Interferon System, Serono Symposia, Raven Press, New York, vol 24 pp 73-83; 25) Content, J. et al. (1985) Eur.J.Biochem. in press; 26) Baglioni, C. (1985) in Advances in Gene Technology: Molecular Biology of the Immune System, Proceedings of 17th Miami Winter Symposium, ICSU Short Reports, Cambridge Univ. Press, vol 2 pp 53-56; 27) Raziuddin, A. et al. (1984) Proc.Natl.Acad.Sci. USA 81:5504-5506; 28) Eid, P. & Mogensen, K.E. (1985) in The Interferon System, Serono Symposia, Raven Press, New York, vol 24 pp 221-225; 29) Slate, D.L. et al., (1978) J.Virol. 25: 319-325; 30) Revel, M., Bash, D. & Ruddle, F.H. (1976) Nature 260:139-141; 31) Lindenmaier, W., Hauser, H., DeWilke, I.G. & Schutz, G. (1982) Nucleic Acids Res., 10:1243-1256; 32) Chebath, J. et al.(1985) in The Interferon System, Serono Symposia, Raven Press, New York, vol 24 pp 201-211.

BLOCKING OF FUNCTION OF MOUSE INTERFERON GAMMA BY SYNTHETIC PEPTIDES AND CORRESPONDING EPITOPE-SPECIFIC ANTISERA

J M Carter*, B Torres**, J Russell**, and H M Johnson**

*Department of Biochemistry and Molecular Biology, and **Department of Comparative and Experimental Pathology, University of Florida, Gainesville, Florida 32610

Mouse interferon gamma (MuIFN) contains 133 amino acids in its sequence. In order to examine the molecule for important domains, we prepared two synthetic peptides: one corresponding to the N-terminal 40 amino acids, and the other one corresponding to the C-terminal 40 amino acids. These peptides were used to prepare antisera in rabbits. The peptides and the antisera were then examined for ability to inhibit binding and activity of recombinant mouse interferon gamma (rMuIFN). Our results suggest that the N-terminal region of MuIFN is most important for activity, whereas both termini may be involved in binding.

METHODS. Production of Antisera. N-terminal peptide was coupled to keyhole limpet hemocyanin via glutaraldehyde (1) or bis-diazotized benzidine (2). C-terminal peptide was conjugated via m-maleimidobenzoic acid N-hodroxysuccinimide ester (3). Conjugated peptides were emulsified in Freund's complete adjuvant and injected intramuscularly and subcutaneously in New Zealand white rabbits. Blood was taken from the ear veins and allowed to clot. Sera were aliquoted and stored at -70 C°.

Blocking of Anti-viral activity. Sera were screened for neutralizing antibodies by viral plaque assay. Results are shown in table I, below. Only those sera which neutralized MuIFN were further characterized.

Table I: Neutralization of rMuIFNγ anti-viral activity by rabbit antisera against synthetic peptides. (5)

units of rMuIFN	titer anti-C ter	titer anti-N ter
8	1:10,000	1:10,000
20	1:3,000	1:30

Blocking of macrophage priming. Those sera which tested positive in the anti-viral assay were then examined for ability to neutralize rMuIFN in macrophage priming for tumor cell killing, as measured by release of chromium isotope from the target cells. Results of these experiments are displayed in figure I, on the facing page. In this figure anti-peptide antisera are compared to antisera against whole rMuIFN. Normal rabbit serum is included as a control.

Blocking by Synthetic Peptides. In similar experiments, the peptides themselves were used to inhibit rMuIFN macrophage priming. These results are shown in figure 2, on the facing page.

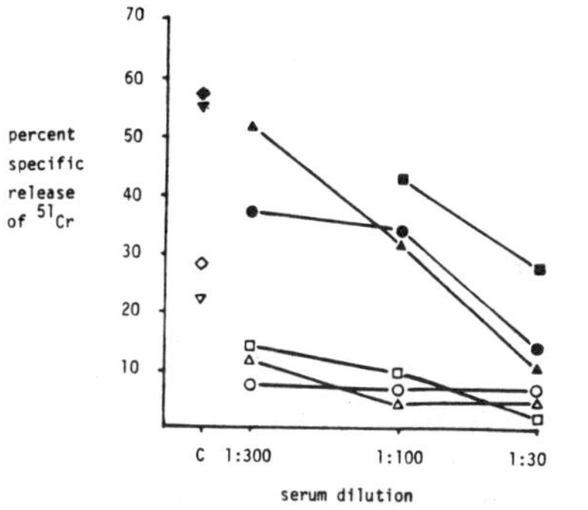

Figure 1: Blocking of macrophage priming by antisera. (4)

△ 1 unit rIFN + anti-rIFN ▲ 10 units rIFN + anti-rIFN
○ 1 unit rIFN + anti-C ter ● 10 units rIFN + anti-C ter
□ 1 unit rIFN + anti-N ter ■ 10 units rIFN + anti-N ter
◇ 1 unit rIFN ◆ 10 units rIFN
▽ 1 unit rIFN + NRS ▼ 10 units rIFN + NRS

RESULTS. The titer of the N-terminal specific antisera was lower in table I, however the ability of these antisera to neutralize macrophage priming appeared to be comparable to that of the C-terminal specific antisera in figure I. This suggests that the N-terminal region of MuIFN may be more important for activity. Figure 2, below supports this idea, since the N-terminal peptide preparation was more effective at competing with rMuIFN than the C-terminal peptide.

Figure 2: Blocking of macrophage priming by synthetic peptides. (4)

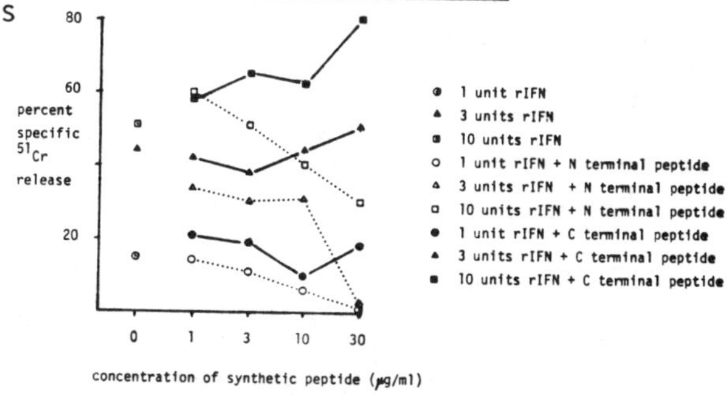

Current investigations are utilizing overlapping sub-fragments of the N-terminal peptide along with polyclonal and monoclonal antibodies. Also, we are attempting to develop a binding assay for use with the peptides and antibodies.

REFERENCES

(1) Morris Reichlin, Methods in Enzymology 70:159 (1980).
(2) Handbook of Experimental Immunology Vol I, Ed 2, p 20.14, ed D M Weir, Blackwell Sci Publ, Oxford (1973).
(3) Fu-Tong Liu, M Zinnecker, T Hamaoka, D Katz, Biochemistry 18:690 (1979).
(4) Marlyn P Langford, D A Weigent, G J Stanton, S Baron, Methods in Enzymology 78:339 (1981).
(5) J L Pace, S W Russell, J Immunol 126:1863 (1981).

CLONING, SEQUENCE AND EXPRESSION OF BOVINE INTERLEUKIN-2

D. P. Cerretti[1], K. McKereghan[1], A. Larsen[1], M. A. Cantrell[1], D. Anderson[1], S. Gillis, D. Cosman[1], and P. E. Baker[2]
Immunex Corporation, Departments of Molecular Biology[1] and Animal Health[2], 51 University Street, Seattle, Washington 98101

Interleukin-2 (IL-2) is a lymphokine which induces proliferation of responsive T-cells (1) and certain B-cells (2) via receptor-specific binding *in vitro*. More recently, human and murine IL-2 have been cloned from cDNA libraries and functional lymphokine expressed in recombinant vector systems (3,4). Using a human IL-2 probe, we have isolated the bovine homologue from a cDNA library. The cDNA library was made with RNA isolated from mitogen stimulated lymph node cells.

Cloning and Sequence of Bovine IL-2 cDNA. Screening of a bovine cDNA library with a ^{32}P-labeled DNA fragment encoding human IL-2 resulted in several positive clones. One of these, pBIL2-4, was selected for further analysis. The DNA sequence is shown in Fig. 1. pBIL2-4 contains a cDNA insert of 775 bp with an open-reading frame of 155 amino acids, starting with an initiator Met codon at nucleotide 18 and ending with a termination codon at nucleotide 485. This protein would have a predicted molecular weight of 19,555 daltons. Comparison of the amino acid sequence with that of human IL-2 (5) indicates that the amino-terminal residue of mature bovine IL-2 is Ala-21. The mature protein would be composed of 135 amino acids and have a predicted molecular weight of 15,452 daltons.

Figure 1

```
                                                  5'--CCTCAACTCCTGCCACA    17

Met Tyr Lys Ile Gln Leu Leu Ser Cys Ile Ala Leu Thr Leu Ala Leu Val Ala Asn Gly    20
ATG TAC AAG ATA CAA CTC TTG TCT TGC ATT GCA CTA ACT CTT GCA CTC GTT GCA AAC GGT    77
 *
Ala Pro Thr Ser Ser Ser Thr Gly Asn Thr Met Lys Glu Val Lys Ser Leu Leu Leu Asp    40
GCA CCT ACT TCA AGC TCT ACG GGG AAC ACA ATG AAA GAA GTG AAG TCA TTG CTG CTG GAT   137

Leu Gln Leu Leu Leu Glu Lys Val Lys Asn Pro Glu Asn Leu Lys Leu Ser Arg Met His    60
TTA CAG TTG CTT TTG GAG AAA GTT AAA AAT CCT GAG AAC CTC AAG CTC TCC AGG ATG CAT   197
                                      ▲
Thr Phe Asp Phe Tyr Val Pro Lys Val Asn Ala Thr Glu Leu Lys His Leu Lys Cys Leu    80
ACA TTT GAC TTT TAC GTG CCC AAG GTT AAC GCT ACA GAA TTG AAA CAT CTT AAG TGT TTA   257

Leu Glu Glu Leu Lys Leu Leu Glu Glu Val Leu Asn Leu Ala Pro Ser Lys Asn Leu Asn   100
CTA GAA GAA CTC AAA CTT CTA GAG GAA GTG CTA AAT TTA GCT CCA AGC AAA AAC CTG AAC   317

Pro Arg Glu Ile Lys Asp Ser Met Asp Asn Ile Lys Arg Ile Val Leu Glu Leu Gln Gly   120
CCC AGA GAG ATC AAG GAT TCA ATG GAC AAT ATC AAG AGA ATC GTT TTG GAA CTA CAG GGA   377

Ser Glu Thr Arg Phe Thr Cys Glu Tyr Asp Asp Ala Thr Val Asn Ala Val Glu Phe Leu   140
TCT GAA ACA AGA TTC ACA TGT GAA TAT GAT GAT GCA ACA GTA AAC GCT GTA GAA TTT CTG   437

Asn Lys Trp Ile Thr Phe Cys Gln Ser Ile Tyr Ser Thr Met Thr End                   155
AAC AAA TGG ATT ACC TTT TGT CAA AGC ATC TAC TCA ACA ATG ACT TGA TCACTAAGTGCCTCT   500
```

Expression of Recombinant Bovine IL-2. To determine whether the cDNA insert in pBIL2-4 encoded a protein with IL-2 activity, a plasmid was designed to direct synthesis of mature bovine IL-2 in *E. coli* under transcriptional control of the lambda P_L promoter. Upon heat induction of the promoter, 2.8×10^6 U/ml of IL-2 activity was detected when assayed on a bovine IL-2 responsive

T-cell line, BT2 (6). This corresponds to 24 µg of recombinant IL-2 per ml of E. coli culture, based on the specific activity (1.2 x 10^5 U/µg) of purified recombinant bovine IL-2 produced in yeast (Urdal et al., submitted). Only background activity (< 0.1 U/ml) was detected in a control plasmid lacking IL-2 sequences.

The amino acid sequence of bovine IL-2 aligned with the amino acid sequences of human (3) and murine (4) IL-2 is shown in Fig. 2. The bovine analog is more homologous to the human (approximately 65%) than to the murine (approximately 50%) sequence and this homology is disbursed throughout. However, one region, the amino terminus of mature IL-2 (Fig. 2, star), has seven identical amino acids in all three proteins. In addition, the positions of all three Cys residues (Fig. 2, arrows) are conserved, including the two Cys residues (Fig. 2, heavy arrows) thought to be involved in the formation of an active conformation (4). Bovine IL-2, like the human analog, lacks the unusual stretch of 12 Gln residues that is present in the murine polypeptide, but is unique in that it has one potential N-linked glycosylation site (Fig. 2, triangle). This is due to an insertion of an Asn residue at position 70 which is absent in the human and murine analogs.

Figure 2

```
                                        *
human     MYRMQLLSCI ALSLALVTNS APTSSSTKKT QLQ....... .......LEH
bovine    MYKIQLLSCI ALTLALVANG APTSSSTGNT MKE....... .......VKS
murine    MYSMQLASCV TLTLVLLVNS APTSSSTSSS TAEAQQQQQQ QQQQQQHLEQ

                                                    ▲          ⬇
          LLLDLQMILN GINNYKNPKL TRMLTFKFYM PKK.ATELKH LQCLEEELKP
          LLLDLQLLLE KVKNPENLKL SRMHTFDFYV PKVNATELKH LKCLLEELKL
          LLMDLQELLS RMENYRNLKL PRMLTFKFYL PKQ.ATELKD LQCLEDELGP

                                                      ⬇
          LEEVLNLAQS KNFHL.RPRD LISNINVIVL ELKGSETTFM CEYADETATI
          LEEVLNLAPS KNLNPREIKD SMDNIKRIVL ELQGSETRFT CEYDDATVNA
          LRHVLDLTQS KSFQLEDAEN FISNIRVTVV KLKGSDNTFE CQFDDESATV

                     ↓
          VEFLNRWITF CQSIISTLT
          VEFLNKWITF CQSIYSTMT
          VDFLRRWIAF CQSIISTSPQ
```


References

1. Gillis, S. and Smith, K.A. (1977) Nature (London) 268, 154-156.
2. Mittler, R. et al. (1985) J. Immunol. 134, 2393-2399.
3. Taniguchi, T. et al. (1983) Nature (London) 302, 305-310.
4. Kushima, N et al. (1985) Nature (London) 313, 402-404.
5. Clark, S.C. et al. (1984) Proc. Natl. Acad. Sci. USA 81, 2543-2547.
6. Senta-Picha, K. and Baker, P.E. (1985) Immunology, in press.

EFFECT OF INTERFERON -γ ON GROWTH OF A431 CELLS AND EXPRESSION OF EGF RECEPTORS

*E.H. Chang, *T. Masnyk, *R. Black, and +J.B. Harford
*Dept. Pathology, USUHS and +Cell Biology and Metabolism Branch, NICHD, Bethesda, Md 20814

Treatment with interferon (IFN) has been reported to have a broad spectrum of effects on mammalian cells in culture. In certain transformed cell lines wherein a given viral or cellular oncogene is overexpressed, IFN treatment has been reported to selectively reduce the expression of the oncogene. This observation has been made in cell lines that overexpress either src (1), myc (2), or ras (3) and in two of these instances, the reduction in oncogene expression was accompanied by morphological reversion of the transformed phenotype of the cells under study (1,3). Other genes are expressed to higher levels upon IFN treatment. The enzyme 2'-5' A synthetase has been shown to be elevated in a variety of cultured cells in response to treatment with IFN. It is abundantly clear that IFN is a biological response modifier whose effects are dependent on the nature of the cell to which it is applied. The inability to generalize regarding the effects of IFN is further complicated by the fact that there are different types of IFN (α, β, γ) and the purity of IFN preparations is not uniform.

We have observed that IFN-γ has a marked effect on the ability of A431, a human epidermoid carcinoma cell line, to grow in culture. At concentrations of 200U/ml, IFN-γ induced an elongated cell morphology and growth inhibition was apparent within 3 days. By 4 days, massive cell death was seen and no survivors were detected at 6 days of IFN-γ treatment. Analogous treatment with preparations of IFN-α or IFN-β did not result in this massive killing of A431 cells. Little, if any, alteration in cell morphology was apparent even at concentrations of IFN-α or IFN-β of 400U/ml. Cell growth was only slightly inhibited after 10 days of treatment with IFN-α or IFN-β. The specific killing of A431 cells has been seen with several preparations of IFN-γ including highly purified recombinant IFN-γ.

A431 cells express levels of the EGF receptor that have been reported to be as much as 30-fold elevated over those seen in untransformed cells (4). The EGF receptor is the cellular homologue of the v-erb-B oncogene (5,6). Using northern analyses with v-erb-B as a probe, we have examined the effect of IFN-γ treatment on the expression of the transcript of the EGF receptor. The 10kb mRNA encoding this receptor was found to be 3- to 7-fold elevated after 3 days of IFN-γ treatment. Once again, this effect was dependent on IFN type in that analogous treatment with IFN-α or IFN-β had only insignificant effects on EGF receptor mRNA levels. Other mRNA species were examined for comparison. Expression of the ras gene was also elevated 4- to 5-fold by treatment with IFN-γ but not by IFN-β treatment. In contrast, levels of the transcripts of the genes encoding actin or the transferrin receptor were unaltered or slightly decreased by IFN-γ treatment. The 1.6kb and 1.8kb mRNA species corresponding to 2'-5'A sythetase were elevated 8-fold by IFN-γ treatment but this effect was not IFN type dependent in that IFN-α and IFN-β treatment resulted in elevations of 2'-5' A synthetase transcript levels of 2-fold and 4-fold respectively. Metabolic labeling of A431 cells with [^{35}S]methionine and immunoprecipitation of the EGF receptor indicated that the receptor protein as well as its mRNA was elevated by IFN-γ treatment.

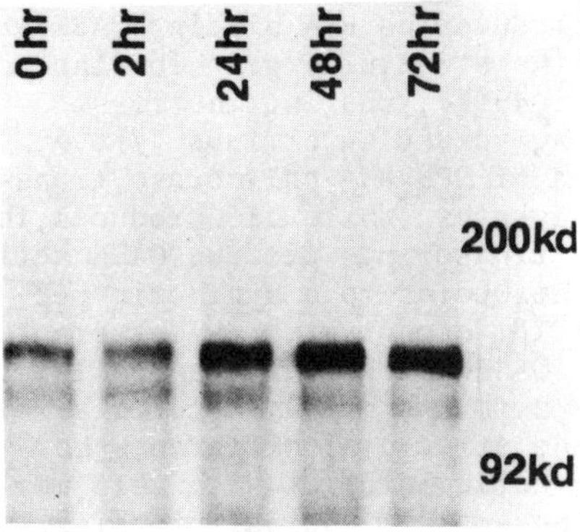

FIGURE 1 - Increase in EGF receptor biosynthesis in reponse to interferon-γ treatment. A431 cells were treated for the indicated times with 200U/ml of IFN-γ before being incubated for 16 hours with 50 μCi/ml of [^{35}S]methionine in methionine-free growth medium. Cells were lysed in a detergent containing buffer and the EGF receptor immunoprecipitated from 2 x 10^7cpm of trichloroacetic acid-precipitable protein. The immunoprecipitates were subjected to SDS-PAGE. The relevant portion of the autoradiograph of the gel is shown.

REFERENCES

1. Lin, S.L., et al. (1983) Molec. Cell Biol. 3, 1656-1664.
2. Jonak, G.J. and Knight, E., Jr. (1984) Proc. Natl. Acad.Sci. USA, **81**,1747-1750.
3. Samid, D., et al. (1984) Biochem. Biophys. Res. Commun. **119**,21-28.
4. Merlino, G.T., et al. (1984) Science **224**, 417-419.
5. Downward, J., et al. (1984) Nature **307**, 521-527.
6. Fabricant, R.N., et al. (1977) Proc. Natl. Acad. Sci. USA **74**, 565-569.

THE IFN-INDUCED (2'-5') OLIGO A SYNTHETASE GENE PRODUCES DIFFERENT FORMS OF THE ENZYME

J.Chebath, P.Benech, L.Mallucci* and M.Revel. Dept. of Virology, The Weizmann Institute of Science, Rehovot, Israel, (*) Guy's Hospital, London Bridge, England.

One of the proteins most markedly and specifically induced in cells by all interferons (IFNs) is the enzyme (2'-5') oligo A synthetase (OASE) which polymerizes ATP into short ppp(A2'p)nA oligomers (1-3). The enzyme binds and requires ds RNA for its activity, the requirement being fulfilled by poly(rI)(rC) and by certain cellular RNAs (4). The (2'-5') oligo A nucleotides act in turn by binding and activating a latent ribonuclease RNase F or L and this pathway has been implicated in IFN's antiviral and anti cell-growth effects (3 for review). We have isolated cDNA clones for the OASE mRNA from human SV80 fibroblasts (5) and found multiple species of IFN-induced OASE mRNAs of 1.6, 1.8, and 3.6 kb with smaller amounts of 2.7 and 4 kb RNAs. These transcripts seem to originate from a single gene of 13 kb comprising 8 exons (6,7). The two mRNAs of 1.6 kb (E16) and 1.8 kb (E18) are produced by differential splicing within the 7th exon, and produce two active forms of the enzyme differing in their C-termini (6,7). The E16 product is a 38 kb protein with a hydrophobic C-terminus. Antibodies to a E16 C-terminal synthetic peptide immunoprecipitate this IFN-induced 38 Kd protein. A complete E16 cDNA was fused to the lac z gene of λgt11 and E. coli lysogen extracts produced ds RNA binding OASE activity, demonstrating that IFN induces the structural gene for the enzyme. The E18 cDNA predicts a protein of 46 Kd, sharing the first 346 aa of E16 but with a different 54 aa long acidic C-terminus (7). A 46 Kd protein is formed upon translation of SP6 RNA polymerase transcripts of the E18 cDNA in reticulocyte lysates, while E16 produces the smaller 38 Kd protein. Both E18 and E16 transcripts produce OASE activity when injected into frog oocytes. Antibodies to a synthetic peptide from the region common to E16 and E18 demonstrated by Western blots the induction of the two forms of OASE by IFN in human cells. OASE activity is found in different compartments of human cells as cytoplasm, ribosomes and nucleus (3,8). The structural difference between the two enzymes suggests that E16 could interact with cell membranes while E18 could bind to basic ribosomal or nuclear proteins.

Analysis of various types of human cells showed that the IFN-induced OASE RNAs are differentially expressed in a cell-specific manner (5,6). Fibroblasts (SV80, FS11) contain all the OASE RNA species, but in B-lymphoblastoid cells as Namalva or Daudi, only the 1.8 kb E18 RNA accumulates. In contrast, in amniotic WISH cells, in HeLa cells and in the histiocytic lymphoma U937 cells, the E16 RNA is the predominant form induced by IFN with some 3.6 kb RNA but almost no E18 RNA. The 3.6 kb RNA has the same 3' end as the E18 RNA but appears to be a uncompletely spliced precursor, suggesting a deficient processing in these cells. Protein analysis by Western immunoblots confirms that WISH cells produce the 38 Kd E16 protein, while Daudi cells make the larger E18 protein. The difference between the WISH and Daudi OASE is further shown by a pronounced difference in ds RNA requirement for optimal OASE activity: WISH cell extracts require 100 times more poly (rI)(rC) than

Daudi cell extracts. The E. coli produced E16 enzyme has the same ds RNA optimum as the WISH cell extracts, suggesting that this may be a property of the E16 protein. Gel filtration of human cell extracts separates native OASE from SV80 and HeLa cells in two peaks of 80-100 Kd and 30-40 Kd respectively (8,9). The small form requires high ds RNA concentrations for activation, while the large form works with low ds RNA (9). The relation between these two forms and the multiple gene products observed is, however, not entirely clear. The large form could be a dimer, or represent a larger enzyme whose cDNA was not yet identified. Thus, a 100 Kd polypeptide was reported in purified OASE preparations from HeLa cells (10). In Daudi and WISH cells, the antibodies that we made against the peptides derived from the E16-E18 sequence, detect also another IFN-induced polypeptide of 67 Kd. It is possible that the large enzyme is the product of one of the OASE RNAs of 2.7, 3.6 or 4 kb observed by hybridization with the cloned cDNAs. The function of these different forms of OASE in the antiviral and antigrowth effects of IFN will be important to determine.

Large and small forms of OASE are also seen in mouse cells, the small enzyme (30Kd) being mainly nuclear and coded by a 1.7 kb RNA, while the large enzyme cytoplasmic would be cytoplasmic and encoded by a 4 kb RNA (11). By cross-hybridization with human cDNA, we could identify these two OASE RNA forms in mouse cells and show that they are differentially expressed (13). In this case, however, differential expression could be demonstrated in the same cells under two distinct conditions. Addition of virally-induced mouse IFN-α,β to L cells or embryonic fibroblasts induced predominantly the 1.7 kb OASE RNA. In contrast, in synchronized cultures of the embryonic fibroblasts, the large 4 kb RNA accumulated during the S phase to decrease again sharply when cells moved into G2. The OASE activity in extracts of these cells, rose sharply toward the end of the S phase to levels similar to those induced by exogenous IFN, and decreased again in G2. This indicates that the 2 forms of mouse IFN-induced OASE mRNA are active mRNAs and play different roles in the cells.

REFERENCES: 1) Kerr, I.M. & Brown, R.E. (1978) Proc.Natl.Acad.Sci. USA 75:256-260; 2) Zilberstein, A., Kimchi, A., Schmidt, A. & Revel, M. (1978) Proc.Natl.Acad.Sci. USA 75:4734-4738; 3) Revel, M. (1984) in Antiviral Drugs and Interferons: The molecular basis of their activity (Becker, Y. ed.) Martinus Nijhoff Publ., Boston, pp 357-433; 4) Revel, M. et al. (1980) Ann.N.Y.Acad.Sci. 350:459-472; 5) Merlin, G. et al. (1983) Proc.Natl.Acad.Sci. USA 80:4904-4908; 6) Benech, P., Merlin, G., Revel, M. & Chebath, J. (1985) Nucleic Acids Res., 13:1267-1281; 7) Benech, P., Mory, Y., Revel, M. & Chebath, J. (1985) EMBO J. 4: 2249-2256; 8) Nilsen, T.M., Wood, D.L. & Baglioni, C. (1982). J. Biol. Chem. 257:1602-1605; 9) Ilson, D.H., Torrence, P.F. & Vilcek, J. (1985) J. Interferon Res., in press; 10) Yang, K. et al. (1981) J. Biol.Chem. 256:9324-9328; 11) St. Laurent et al. (1983) Cell 33:95-102; 12) Mallucci, L. et al. (1985) in The Interferon System, Serono Symposia, Raven Press, New York, vol 24 pp 165-170.

INCREASED PHOSPHORYLATION OF VIMENTIN IN ACTIVATED MACROPHAGES

E.S. Didier, M.M. Soong, S. Fan and W.A.F. Tompkins
Department of Pathobiology, University of Illinois, Urbana, IL 61801

During the process of activation into a tumoricidal state, macrophages (MP) undergo changes that include increased spreading, ruffling, and adherence (1,2,3). Mecham et al. (4) also observed an extension of the cytoskeleton in activated MP which correlated with tumoricidal capacity. Subsequently, Fan et al. (5) described two proteins (pp58 and pp60) extracted from the cytoskeleton-rich fraction with ATP (thus enriching for actin) which were more highly phosphorylated in activated MP than resident MP. In addition, the increased phorphorylation of pp58 and pp60 correlated with increased tumoricidal capacity. Many cell processes are regulated by phophorylation-dephosphorylation reactions and we hypothesized that the activation of MP is in part, at least, regulated by the phosphorylation of these two proteins.

Attempts thus were made to identify one of these phosphoproteins (pp58). Our initial studies focussed on the possibility that pp58 may be the intermediate filament of MP, vimentin. Vimentin is a phosphoprotein and would be expected to exist in the cytoskeleton-rich fraction (6). Although the 55 KD vimentin protofilament remained in the ATP-insoluble fraction of the cytoskelton-rich extract while pp58 was extracted into the ATP-soluble fraction, it was possible that pp58 was the soluble precursor of vimentin reported by Blikstad and Lazarides (7). In addition, the reported molecular weights of vimentin range from 52 to 58 KD. (6,8) which may reflect the existence of different forms of vimentin.

Immunoprecipitation of the cytoskeleton-rich fraction of activated MP from vaccinia virus-infected $C3H_{HeN}$ with BALB/c anti-3T3 fibroblast vimentin serum revealed major proteins of 58 KD and 55KD, as well as several minor bands of approximately 40, 30, 14, and 13 KD. Vimentin is associated with a specific Ca^{+2}-dependent protease (9) and it was possible that these minor bands represented breakdown products of vimentin. To examine this, the cytoskeleton-rich extract of the activated MP was electrophoresed, blotted onto nitrocellulose (10) and incubated with either monoclonal antibodies specific for vimentin or the polyclonal anti-vimentin serum. The blots were then incubated with ^{125}I-labeled Protein A and exposed on film. The autoradiograms revealed binding to bands of the same molecular weights as precipitated by the polyclonal antiserum suggesting that the minor bands immunoprecipitated were vimentin breakdown products.

Partial proteolytic peptide maps of ^{32}P-labeled pp58 and vimentin from vaccinia virus-infected $C3H_{HeN}$ mice were compared to determine more conclusively whether $pp58^{mac}$ was vimentin. The cytoskeleton-rich extracts (not ATP-extracted) were electrophoresed and the protein bands were excised and subjected to <u>Staphylococcus aureus</u> V-8 protease digestion as described by Cleveland (11). The results expressed in Figure I indicated that pp58 and vimentin (55 KD) shared similar partial peptide digest maps. Pp58 expressed identical peptides as vimentin plus two additional bands which accounted for the slightly higher molecular weight. That pp58 is slightly larger than the observed vimentin subunit might be explained by the possibility that pp58 is the precursor to vimentin or may be a modified form of the protofilament. Pulse-chase experiments may help us to resolve this.

Our results suggest that one of the two phosphoproteins expressed in the cytoskeleton-rich fraction of activated MP is vimentin. The role of vimentin phoshorylation is presently unknown. This model, however, presents an interesting system for studying the role of the cytoskeleton and the role of phosphorylation in regulating MP-mediated tumor-cell lysis.

Figure 1

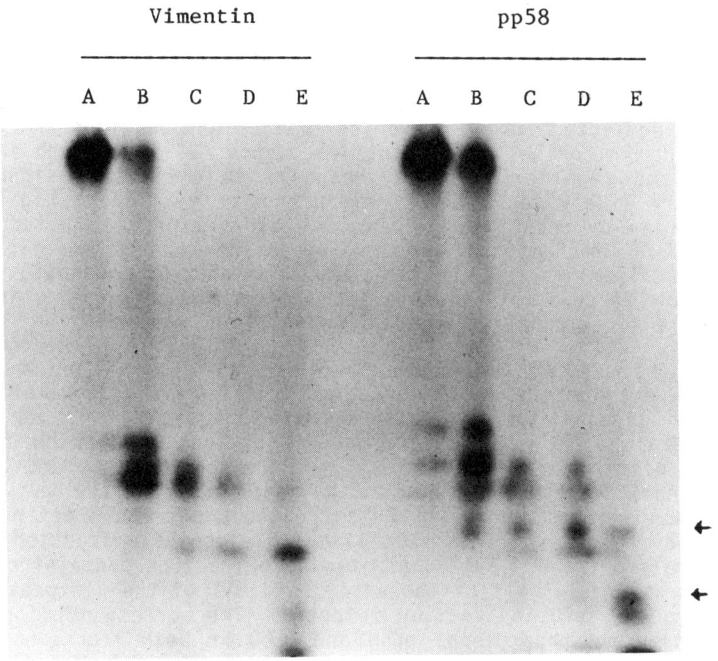

Adherent peritoneal MP were obtained from vaccinia virus-infected $C3H_{HeN}$ mice, and labelled for 2 hr with [^{32}P]-orthophosphoric acid. The cytoskeleton-rich fraction (Triton X-100 treated) was analyzed by SDS-PAGE. The vimentin (55KD) and 58KD bands were excised and subjected to partial peptide digestion with V-8 protease. A) no enzyme, B) 20 ng, C) 100 ng, D) 200 ng, E) 1 ug.

References:

1. North, R.J. (1978) J. Immunol. 121:806-808.
2. Karnovsky, M.L. and J.K. Lazdins (1978) J. Immunol. 121:809-813.
3. Cohn, Z.A. (1978) J. Immunol. 121:813-816.
4. Mecham, J.O., M.M. Soong, C.A. Cain, S. Koehm, J. Goff, and W.A.F. Tompkins (1985) J. Immunol. 134:3516-3523.
5. Fan, S., M.M. Soong, H. Duy, E.S. Didier, and W.A.F. Tompkins (1985) (submitted for publication).
6. Lazarides, E. (1982) Ann. Rev. Biochem. 51:219-250.
7. Blikstad, I. and E. Lazarides (1983) J. Cell Biol. 96:1803-1808.
8. Franke, W.W., E. Schmid, S. Winter, M. Osborn, and K. Weber (1979). Exp. Cell Res. 123:25-46.
9. Yoshida, H., T. Murachi, and I. Tsukahara (1984) Fed. Eur. Biochem. Soc. 170:259-262.
10. Thomas, P.S. (1980) Proc. Nat'l. Acad. Sci. 77:5201-
11. Cleveland, D.W., S.G. Fisher, M.W. Kirshner, and V.K. Laemmli (1977) J. Biol. Chem. 252:1102-1106.
12. Supported by U.S. P.H.S. N.C.I Training Grant No. CA24930.

PHOSPHORYLATION OF CYTOSKELETON ASSOCIATED PROTEINS IN RESPONSE TO MACROPHAGE ACTIVATION SIGNALS

S. Fan, M. M. Soong, E. S. Didier, and W. A. F. Tompkins
Department of Pathobiology, University of Illinois, Urbana, IL 61801

Macrophages (MP) play crucial roles in controlling neoplastic diseases and are essential in regulating immune responses (1,2). MP functions are modulated by soluble T cell lymphokines, including interferon (3). Although the intracellular mechanisms regulating the MP response to activating signals are not known, they are likely to involve protein phosphorylation, a highly conserved general mechanism by which a cell controls its response to external stimuli. In the case of MP, Mecham et al. (4) showed an increased association of calmodulin with microfilaments (MF) in the process of activation and postulated that phosphorylation of cytoskeleton associated proteins participates in the tumoricidal response to external stimuli.

To address this question we employed murine peritoneal MP and the C57BL/6 MP line B6102 to examine the phosphorylation profiles of cytoskeleton extracts. MP adhered to plastic for 16-24 hr and labeled with [^{32}P] for 60 min and were then extracted by a two-step procedure designed to enrich for actin MF and their associated proteins (5,6). TX-100 extraction yielded an insoluble cytoskeleton-nuclear fraction in which the major proteins are the 58 Kd intermediate filament vimentin, the 43 Kd microfilament protein actin and several smaller nuclear histones. Treatment of the TX-insoluble fraction with an ATP buffer to depolymerize MF yielded an insoluble fraction containing most of the vimentin, approximately half of the actin, and all of the histones. The major protein in the ATP soluble fraction is actin. The corresponding autoradiogram showed two major phosphoproteins pp58 and pp60 in both fractions. Both pp58 and pp60 are most intense in the ATP-soluble actin-rich fraction. Similar results were observed with elicited peritoneal MP from $C3H_{HeN}$ and C57BL/6 mice and the B6102 MP cell line. Neither pp58 or pp60 were observed in a number of other cell types, including thymocytes and fibroblasts.

Having identified 2 major phosphoproteins in the actin-rich fraction of murine peritoneal MP, we were interested in determining if a correlation existed between phosphorylation of these proteins and cytotoxicity. Peritoneal exudate cells were collected from untreated (resident MP), proteose peptone-injected (elicited MP), or vaccinia virus-infected (activated MP) $C3H_{HeN}$ mice. After labeling with [^{32}P] for 30 and 60 min, the ATP-soluble fraction was processed by SDS-PAGE and analysed by autoradiography. Figure 1A shows that the major protein in the ATP-soluble fraction is actin and that comparable amounts are found in all preparations. The autoradiogram of the same gel (Fig 1b) shows the the major phosphoproteins in all preparations to be pp58 and pp60. These 2 phosphoproteins in elicited MP (Lanes 3 [30'] and 4 [60']) and activated MP (Lanes 5 [30'] and 6 [60']) are more highly phosphorylated, than those from elicited MP (Lanes 3 [30'] and 4 [60']), which in turn are more phosphorylated than their counterparts in resident macrophages.

Relative [^{32}P] incorporation in pp60 and pp58 were normalized against actin concentration to yield a phosphorylation-Index. The P-Indices generated from Figure 1 confirmed that pp58 and pp60 were phosphorylated to the highest level per unit of actin in activated MP (Table 1). Furthermore, the level of MP cytotoxicity correlated positively with the increased phosphorylation of pp58 and pp60 (Table 1).

Table 1. [^{32}P]-phosphate-uptake into pp60 and pp58 in C3H/HeN macrophages.

Macrophage Population[a]	Labeling Time	P-Index[b] pp60	P-Index[b] pp58	% Specific Lysis[c]
Resident macrophage	30'	0.09	0.03	8.4 +/- 1.2
	60'	0.16	0.16	
Elicited macrophage	30'	0.26	0.16	5.6 +/- 0.8
	60'	0.65	0.49	
Activated macrophage	30'	0.44	0.30	38.6 +/- 1.9
	60'	1.19	0.85	

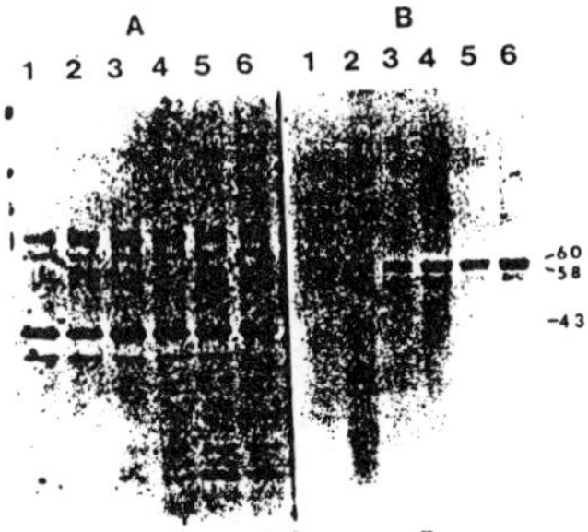

Figure 1

a. Macrophages were obtained as described (4).
b. The P-Index for a phosphoprotein in a sample is its integrated absorbance peak (from the autoradiogram) divided by the integrated absorbance peak for actin (from the stained gel). The relative actin concentration in each sample of a stained electrohoretogram was determined by the actin band's absorbance at 560 nm; the relative [^{32}P] activity in pp60 and pp58 in each sample was detemined from the autoradiogram by the corresponding band's absorbance at 680 nm.
c. Macrophage cytotoxicity was measured in quadruplicate against ^{51}Cr labeled SV3T3 targets at an effector to target ratio of 20:1 (4).

These results lend support to the argument that pp58 and pp60 play a role in expression of cytotoxicity by MP. Further, the data suggest that pp58 and pp60, at least in their phosphorylated states, are associated with the cytoskeleton. We do not know if pp60 and pp58 are restricted to the cytoskeleton or exist in other cell fractions, as well. Furthermore, we do not know if pp58 and pp60 are phosphorylated while in association with the cytoskeleton or translocate to the cytoskeleton from some other compartment following phosphorylation. While pp58 does not appear to coextract with the major fraction of the 58 Kd vimentin protein, Didier et al. (unpublished) has presented evidence based on peptide analysis that pp58 is, indeed, vimentin and may represent a more easily solubilized phosphorylated form of the intermediate filament protein. Further, Soong et al. (unpublished) has evidence that pp60 has kinase activity and antigenic similarities to avian pp60^{src}, suggesting it may be a type of proto-oncogene product. With the development of antibody probes for pp58 and pp60, their cellular distribution, phosphorylation patterns, and role in expression of specific MP functions can be further elucidated.

References:

1. Mackaness (1962). J. Exp. Med. 127:915.
2. Unanue and Cerrotini (1970). J. Exp. Med. 131:711.
3. Schultz and Kleinschmidt (1983). Nature 305:235.
4. Mecham, Soong, Cain, Koehm, Goff, and Tompkins (1985). J. Immunol. 134:3516.
5. Phillips, Jennings, and Edwards (1980). J. Cell. Biol. 86:77.
6. Schloss and Goldman (1980). J. Cell Biol. 87:633.
7. Supported by U. S. PHS NCI Training Grant No CA24930.

B LYMPHOCYTE ENRICHED POPULATIONS PRODUCE IMMUNOREACTIVE ENDORPHIN THAT BINDS TO DELTA OPIATE RECEPTORS AND MAY PLAY A ROLE IN ENDOTOXIC SHOCK.

D. Harbour-McMenamin, E.M. Smith, and J.E. Blalock
Department of Microbiology, University of Texas Medical Branch, Galveston, Texas 77550.

We have previously reported that bacterial lipopolysaccharide (LPS) treated leukocytes synthesize de novo molecules that are similar if not identical to γ-endorphin and corticotropin (ACTH 1-24) (1). We postulated that the leukocyte-derived endorphin may be an extrapituitary source of the endogenous opioid component associated with the pathophysiologic responses, hypotension and hyperthermia, observed in endotoxic shock. Holaday and coworkers have shown that this opioid component specifically binds to delta opiate receptors which then induces the pathophysiologic responses (2). They have shown that these responses can be mimicked in vivo by treatment with DADLE, a delta receptor agonist and abrogated by ICI M154,129, a delta antagonist. In this report, we characterize the immune cell making the immunoreactive (ir)-endorphin molecules and show that this material binds to delta opiate receptors.

(I) Immunofluorescence of Fractionated Leukocytes. Leukocytes from LPS sensitive C3HeB/FeJ mice were prepared by Ficoll/Hypaque density centrifugation. Macrophages were removed by adhesion to plastic. The T cell populations were prepared by passing through nylon wool according to standard protocol (3). Subsequent staining of this population with monoclonal anti-Thy 1.2 antibody showed approximately 77% T cells by immunofluorescence. The adherent B lymphocytes were dissociated from the nylon wool and stained with monoclonal antibody to the heavy chain of the IgM (μ) antibody. Fluorescence with the anti-mu antibody yielded 82% B cells. The fractionated cells were cultured at a concentration of $1X\ 10^7$ cells/ml for 48 hours in the presence or absence of trichloroacetic acid extracted LPS. Table 1 shows the results of indirect immunofluorescent staining of the fractionated cells using antibody to γ-endorphin. The results demonstrate that significant immunofluorescence with the antibody to γ-endorphin occurs only in the LPS treated B lymphocyte enriched population.

Table 1
Comparison of the fluorescence of C3HeB/FeJ fractionated leukocytes after staining with monospecific or monoclonal antisera.

C3HeB/FeJ Cells	Treatment	Antisera: Normal Rabbit Serum	Anti-gamma Endorphin	Anti-Thy1.2	Anti-mu
T-cells	LPS	4 ± 2*	3 ± 2	N.D.	N.D.
	Mock	6 ± 3	4 ± 2	77 ± 7	N.D.
B-cells	LPS	15 ± 8	47 ± 4	N.D.	N.D.
	Mock	4 ± 2	10 ± 4	N.D.	82 ± 10

*% positive fluorescing cells ± SD

(II) Opiate Receptor Binding Assay. NG108 cells were plated in 96 well polystyrene microtiter plates at a concentration of $1X\ 10^5$ cells per well. The sample ligands were added in 100 λ volumes in triplicate and incubated for 30 minutes at 4°C. The cells were washed with PBS containing 1% FBS followed by incubation with

Table 2
Binding of ir-Endorphin to the delta opiate receptor

Sample		Specifically Bound (^{3}H)-DADLE	% Inhibition of Specific (^{3}H)-DADLE Binding
		CPM±SD	
T	Mock	1067 ± 90	4.7
	LPS Treated	1054 ± 137	9.1
B	Mock	1025 ± 68	18.9
	LPS Treated	782 ± 121	99.3
β-endorphin	10^{6}	833 ± 64	83.5
	10^{-8}	940 ± 135	52.5
	10^{-10}	1035 ± 157	15.5
DADLE	(δ agonist)	920 ± 49	54.2
DAGO	(μ agonist)	1139 ± 73	0
Media		995 ± 184	28.9

Table 2. Opiate Receptor Binding to Delta Opiate Receptor Bearing NG108 Cells. Sample ligands are as follows: T or B lymphocyte culture supernates at a 1:2 dilution, culture media alone, 50 μg/ml of DAGO (D-Ala^2, N-Me-Phe^4, Met(0)^5-ol)-Enkephalin, 50 μg/ml of DADLE (D-Ala^2-D-Leu^5)-Enkephalin, 10^{-5}M Naloxone, B-endorphin. The labeled ligand was H^3 DADLE, AMERSHAM, specific activity 76.8 mCi/mg.

the labeled ligand for 15 minutes at 4°C. The cells were washed 3 times and each well was counted in liquid scintillation fluid. Table 2 shows results of radioreceptor assays indicating significant binding of the NG108 delta receptor with the delta agonist DADLE but not the mu agonist DAGO. As shown, there is significant inhibition of the labeled delta agonist with the supernate of the B cell enriched population treated with LPS and no significant inhibition with the T cell-derived material.

In conclusion, our results show that the major cell type making the ir-endorphin that specifically binds to delta opiate receptors is probably a B-lymphocyte. This strongly suggests that B cells, which may or may not respond mitogenically to the LPS, produce a component of the endogenous opioid response seen in endotoxic shock. Lolait et al. have shown that a subpopulation of macrophages also synthesize endorphins, and we have preliminary evidence to confirm this observation in peritoneal macrophages treated with LPS (unpublished observations). The data provided herein lend further evidence that the interactions between the immune and neuroendocrine system are bidirectional (4). The fact that the leukocyte-derived endorphin binds to delta receptors concurs with the work of Holaday et al. and also indicates that the immune system can directly communicate with the neuroendocrine system and possibly modulate its functions.

REFERENCES

(1) Harbour-McMenamin, D., Smith, E.M., Blalock, J.E. (1985) Infect. Immun. 48(3), 813-817.
(2) Holaday, J.W. (1984) in Neuroendocrine Perspectives, Volume 3 (Muller, E.E., MacLeod, R.M., eds.) pp. 161-199, Elsevier Science Publishers.
(3) Henry, C., et al. (1980) in Selected Methods in Cellular Immunology (Mishell, B.B. and Shigi, S.M., eds.) pp. 182-185. W.H. Freeman and Co., San Francisco.
(4) Blalock, J.E. et al. (1985) J. Neuroimmunol. 10, 31-40.

PHOSPHORYLATION OF COMPONENTS OF THE MURINE T CELL ANTIGEN RECEPTOR COMPLEX

J.B. Harford*, L.E. Samelson*, M.D. Patel*, S. Jaken+, and R.D. Klausner

*Cell Biology and Metabolism Branch, NICHD and +Center for Drugs and Biologics, FDA, Bethesda, Maryland 20892

Introduction

The antigen receptors of several murine and human MHC-restricted T cell clones have been isolated and characterized with clone-specific monoclonal antibodies (1-4). In all cases, this receptor appears to be a disulfide-linked heterodimeric glycoprotein containing an α and β chain, each of approximately 43 kd. Evidence suggests that the human T cell antigen receptor is noncovalently associated with additional proteins termed the T3 complex (5,6). Reports indicating that analogous proteins may be associated with the murine T cell antigen receptor have recently appeared (7-9). Using several radiolabeling techniques, we have identified and partially characterized four polypeptides that are specifically co-precipitated with a monoclonal antibody that binds the antigen receptor of the murine T cell hybridoma 2B4. Here, we describe recent findings regarding the phosphorylation of certain components of the murine T cell antigen receptor complex.

Immunoprecipitation of a Receptor-Associated Complex

When 2B4 cells are radiolabeled using 3-(trifluoromethyl)-3-(m-[^{125}I]-iodopenyl) diazirine (^{125}I-TID), the α chain of the antigen receptor is labeled and precipitated with A2B4-2, a monoclonal antibody recognizing the clonotypic receptor structure (9). In addition, A2B4-2 specifically precipitates from labeled 2B4 cells, four other polypeptides. These consist of two glycoproteins migrating on SDS-PAGE after reduction at 21 kd and 25 kd, and two nonglycosylated proteins of 26 kd and 16 kd. The latter polypeptide (termed zeta) appears to exist in the complex as a disulfide-linked homodimer of 32 kd and has no reported analogue in the human antigen receptor complex.

Phosphorylation of the Complex in 2B4 Cells

None of the six receptor complex chains are labeled during up to 4 hr of incubation with ^{32}P in the absence of stimulation. However, antigen or concanavalin A activation of the 2B4 cells results in rapid phosphorylation of the 21 kd polypeptide associated with the murine T cell antigen receptor (9). The phosphorylation of this polypeptide that is induced by antigen requires antigen-presenting cells bearing the relevant MHC-encoded Ia molecules. Treatment of ^{32}P-loaded cells with phorbol esters also results in rapid phosphorylation of the 21 kd polypeptide of the complex. In addition, the 26 kd chain of the complex is phosphorylated in response to treatment with phorbol esters. The phosphate moities acquired on the 21 kd and 26 kd chains in response to phorbol esters have apparent half-lives of 40 min and 2 min respectively. The phosphorylation induced by antigen is inhibited by dibutyryl cAMP whereas that induced by phorbol esters is not. Analysis of the ^{32}P-labeled complex on two dimensional gels and by peptide mapping suggests that antigen stimulation results in phosphorylation of the 21 kd chain at a site not phosphorylated in response to phorbol esters. The only detected [^{32}P]amino acid in the 21 kd polypeptide is phosphoserine irrespective of the mode of stimulation.

Phosphorylation of the Complex In Vitro

When the A2B4-2 immunoprecipitates of unlabeled 2B4 cells are exposed to [γ-^{32}P]ATP and a highly purified preparation of protein kinase C from rabbit brain cytosol, polypeptides of 26 kd and 21 kd are phosphorylated. No such phosphorylation is seen in control immunoprecipitates of 2B4 cells or when the exogenous protein kinase C is omitted. The in vitro phosphorylation is dependent upon calcium and added phosphatidyl serine and can be shown to be stimulated by addition of phorbol dibutyrate. Two dimensional gel patterns of the [^{32}P]polypeptides phosphorylated in vitro resemble those of [^{32}P]polypeptides from 2B4 cells treated with phorbol esters.

References

1. Allison, J.P. et al. (1982) J. Immunol. 129, 2293-2300.
2. Meuer, S.C. et al. (1983) J. Exp. Med. 157, 705-719.
3. Haskins, K. et al. (1983) J. Exp. Med. 157, 1149-1169.
4. Samelson, L.E. et al. (1983) Proc. Natl. Acad. Sci. USA 80, 6972-6976.
5. Borst, J. et al. (1983) Eur. J. Immunol. 13, 576-580.
6. Kanellopoulos, J.M. et al. (1983) EMBO J. 2, 1807-1814.
7. Allison, J.P., and Lanier, L.L. (1985) Nature 314, 107-109.
8. Samelson, L.E., and Schwartz, R.H. (1984) Immunol. Rev. 81, 131-144.
9. Samelson, L.E. et al. (1985) Proc. Natl. Acad. Sci. USA 82, 1969-1973.

PURIFICATION TO HOMOGENEITY OF HUMAN INTERLEUKIN-3 FROM NORMAL PHA-STIMULATED LEUKOCYTES.

G. Krystal, C.J. Eaves, C. Macdonald, and A.C. Eaves
Terry Fox Laboratory, B.C. Cancer Research Centre, 601 West 10th Avenue, Vancouver, B.C. V5Z 1L3

Murine interleukin-3 (IL-3) is a potent lymphokine produced by stimulated T cells and active on a variety of primitive and mature hemopoietic cells of murine origin (1-3). Search for the human analog has to date been elusive due to significant differences between species in the amino acid sequence of this factor and difficulties in obtaining sufficient human material for purification.

In preliminary studies we found that serum-free media conditioned by PHA-stimulated leukocytes (PHA-LCM) from normal human donors could stimulate the proliferation of B6SUtA cells, a murine IL-3-dependent cell line derived from mouse marrow (4). Subsequent dose-response studies with PHA-LCM and murine IL-3 showed that the effects of these two preparations on B6SUtA cells were additive. Using the B6SUtA cell response as an assay, we have now purified the human leukocyte derived stimulator to homogeneity using a 4 step procedure, involving phenyl sepharose, Concanavalin A sepharose, Sephadex G100 superfine and DEAE high pressure liquid chromatography (Table 1). SDS-PAGE of the purified material revealed a single silver-stained band with a molecular weight of 23.5 kd under both reducing (5% 2-ME) and non-reducing conditions. Elution of gel slices and B6SUtA bioactivity tests demonstrated that the activity was localized in the slices corresponding to 23.5 kd. Chromatography on C18-HPLC of a trypsin digest of pure material revealed the presence of 4 peptides. Three of these yielded unique amino acid sequences, none of which showed homology with any previously sequenced hemopoietins or with any of the sequences in either the Dayhoff protein data bank or the Genbank data base (version #36) (Biogen, personal communication).

This factor, which we have called human interleukin-3 is thus clearly different from murine IL-3 and from the following human factors: EPA (5), GM-CSF (6), M-CSF (7), IL-2 (8) or Ep (9). Further studies of the full range of biological activities of human IL-3 are in progress.

REFERENCES

(1) Ihle, J.N., et al (1983) J. Immunol. 131, 282.
(2) Garland, J.M., and Crompton S. (1983) Exp. Hematol. 11, 757.
(3) Palacios, R. (1982) J. Immunol. 129, 2586.
(4) Greenberger, J.S., et al. (1983) Proc. Natl. Acad. Sci. U.S.A. 80, 2931.
(5) Gasson, J.C., et al. (1985) Nature 315, 768.
(6) Miyatake, S., et al. (1985) EMBO J. 4, 2561.
(7) Kawasaki, E.S., et al. (1985) Science 230, 291.
(8) Taniguchi, T., et al. (1983) Nature 302, 305.
(9) Jacobs, K., et al. (1985) Nature 313, 806.
(10) Bradford, M.M. (1976) Anal. Biochem. 72, 248.
(11) Krystal, G., et al. (1985) Anal. Biochem. 148, 451.

TABLE I

PURIFICATION OF HUMAN IL-3

Step	Volume (ml)	Total Protein* (mg)	Total Units (U)**	Specific Activity (U/mg)	Overall Yield (%)
PHA-LCM	5,000	2,000	500,000	250	100
Amicon Concentrated PHA-LCM	300	1,950	900,000	460	180
Phenyl Sepharose Material	700	420	280,000	670	56
Concentrated Con A Sugar Eluate	1.0	5	3,000	600	0.6
Sephadex G100 Superfine Material	8.0	0.24	2,000	8,330	0.4
DEAE-HPLC Eluate	4.0	0.024	600	25,000	0.12

* Protein determined using the Coomassie dye binding technique (10) for concentrations above 2 μg/ml and a soluble silver method (11) for concentrations below 2 μg/ml, both assays being standardized with BSA.

** 1 U/ml is defined as the human IL-3 concentration stimulating half-maximal ^{3}H-thymidine incorporation into B6SUtA cells.

INTERFERON RESPONSIVE AND NON-RESPONSIVE MHC VARIANTS OF A MURINE THYMOMA.

Patrick MACHY*, Bernt ARNOLD**, Salvador ALINO***, Barbara DALTON* and Lee D. LESERMAN****.
*Smith Kline and French Laboratories, 1500 Spring Garden Street, Philadelphia, PA 19101, U.S.A. **Deutsches Krebsforschungszentrum, Im Neuenheimer, Feld 280, D-6900, Heidelberg, F.R.G. ***Facultad de Medicina, Departamento de Histologia, Universidad del Pais Vasco, Leonja, Vizcaya, Espagna. ****Department of Genetics, Stanford University School of Medicine, Stanford, CA 94305, U.S.A.

INTRODUCTION. Numerous studies indicate that cytotoxic T cells recognize tumor cells by virtue of antigens expressed with class I molecules of the major histocompatibility complex (MHC) (1). Although other mechanisms exist for the elimination of tumor cells not expressing MHC determinants (2), the expression of class I molecules by tumor cells aids in generating an optimal immune response against them. Therefore, non-expression of class I molecules might confer a selective advantage on a tumor population (3). While evaluating the therapeutic potential of methotrexate (MTX)-containing liposomes directed via surface-bound monoclonal antibodies specific for murine MHC molecules, we found variants of RDM4 thymoma cells which expressed very low levels of the target H-2K molecule and escaped killing by the targeted drug (4). Because it is known that interferons (IFN) enhance the induction of MHC molecules (5), we evaluated the ability of IFN γ, α/β to render this population susceptible to killing by anti-H-2K-targeted liposomes. Two types of variants were selected: IFN responsive cells that were killed and IFN non-responsive cells that remained resistant to the targeted drug. These results suggest that while IFN may improve the efficacy of targeted chemotherapy, it does not prevent development of non-responsive mutants lacking the target molecule.

RESULTS. IFN augment expression of H-2K molecule. Immunoselected H-2K low expressor variant cells (type 1) from RDM4 (4), when incubated with mouse recombinant IFN γ for 48h, augmented the expression of the H-2K molecule (Fig.1a). This effect is time- and IFN dose-dependent and is specifically inhibited by an anti-IFN γ monoclonal antibody (kindly provided by Santo Landolfo). The same result was obtained with highly purified mouse IFN α/β (Fig.1b).

Immunoselection in the presence of IFN. When the H-2K low expressor variants were incubated with IFN, they became susceptible to killing by MTX-containing liposomes or immunotoxins targeted to the H-2K determinant. A second variant cell (type 2) was selected by this procedure, which was not killed by the targeted drugs. In these cells IFN γ (Fig.1a) or IFNα/β (Fig.1b) failed to augment expression of the H-2K molecule. These two cell types expressed the same amount of IFN receptors and they responded to IFN by expressing H-2D molecules encoded by a gene present on the same chromosome (6). Therefore, the inability of IFN to enhance H-2K expression was not due to a lack of normal response to IFN, nor to a loss of chromosome encoding H-2K (6). The evalua-

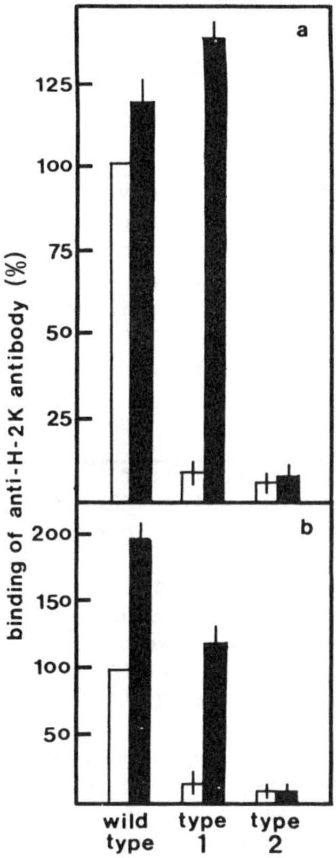

tion of class I MHC gene transcripts, in IFN non-responsive cells indicates that the control is at the transcriptional level (6).

Figure 1. Effect of IFN on the recovery of the H-2K molecule. Cells incubated with 100 units/ml of IFN γ (a) or 2000 units/ml of IFN α/β (b) were tested for the presence of the H-2K molecule by incubation with a radiolabeled anti-H-2K monoclonal antibody. The % refer to the binding of the antibody as compared to RDM4 wild type not incubated with IFN. (□)-IFN, (■)+IFN.

DISCUSSION. Phenotypic diversity with respect to cell surface molecules in tumor populations is of selective advantage for tumors in exploitation of local microenvironmental conditions or in their ability to escape from host defences. In an immunocompetent host, class I molecules represent priviledged targets for immune surveillance. MHC molecules are sensitive to induction by IFN (5). This has stimulated interest in the use of IFN to augment host immune responses against tumors. However, in the present study, negative selection by targeted drugs, in the presence or absence of IFN, despite eliminating the majority of tumor cells, did not prevent eventual out-growth of tumor cells lacking the target molecule. Recent data suggest that low levels of MHC expression correlate with high levels of oncogenes and tumorigenicity (7). The tumorigenic potential of these variant thymoma cells is currently under investigation.

ACKNOWLEDGMENTS. We thank Dr. A. Truneh for fruitful discussions.

REFERENCES.

1- Doherty, P.C., Knowles, B.B. and Wettstein, P.J. (1984). Adv. Cancer Res. 42, 1-66.
2- Zinkernagel, R.M. and Oldstone, M.B.A. (1976). Proc. Natl. Acad. Sci. U.S.A. 73, 3666-3670.
3- Anderson, A.R. and Beverley, P.C.L. (1983). Immunol. Today. 4, 211-213.
4- Machy, P. and Leserman, L .D. (1984). EMBO. J. 3, 1971-1977.
5- Lindahl, P., Levy, P. and Gresser I. (1973). Proc. Natl. Acad. Sci. U.S.A. 70, 2785-2788.
6- Machy, P., Arnold, B., Alino, S. and Leserman L.D. (1985). J. Immunol. Submitted.
7- Doyle, A., Martin, W.J., Funa, K., Gazdar, A., Carney, D., Martin, S.E., Linnoila, I., Cuttita, F., Mulshine, J., Bunn, P. and Minna, J. (1985). J. Exp. Med. 161, 1135-1151.

PROPERTIES OF SPECIFIC INTERLEUKIN 1 (IL 1) RECEPTOR ON HUMAN EPSTEIN BARR VIRUS TRANSFORMED B LYMPHOCYTES

K. Matsushima, T. Akahoshi, and J. J. Oppenheim
Laboratory of Molecular Immunoregulation, BRMP, DCT, NCI, Frederick, MD 21701-1013

We have previously reported the production of (IL 1) activity (thymocyte comitogenic, fibroblast proliferation, and acute phase protein induction activities) by various types of human B lymphocytes (1,2,3). It has also been reported that IL 1 augments B cell proliferation and maturation (4), we have studied the expression of IL 1 receptor on human EBV-B lymphocyte cell lines to examine the hypothesis that IL 1 may be an autostimulatory signal in B lymphocyte transformation.

(II) Specific Binding of Human ^{125}I-labeled IL 1- β to EBV-B Cell line. Purified human IL 1-β from a human myelomonocytic cell line (THP-1) cells was labeled with ^{125}I by the Bolton-Hunter method ($2X10^8$ cpm/μg) (5). There was no apparent loss of biological activity after labelling. Analytical SDS-PAGE showed only a 17 KD band by autoradiography. One of four treated EBV-B cell lines (consisting of two high IL 1 producers and two low IL 1 producers), a pre-B cell line (VDS-0) specifically bound the highest amount of ^{125}I-IL 1-β. Therefore, VDS-0 cells were used to study the IL 1 receptor in more detail. Investigations of the kinetics of ^{125}I-IL 1-β binding to 1×10^7 cells/0.2 ml at 4°C, indicated that maximum binding was reached within 20 min. Scatchard plot analysis of the binding data yielded a Kd of $2.4\text{-}5.9 \times 10^{-10}$ M, the IL 1 concentration required to reach half-saturation of binding sites, with approximately 110-220 binding sites/cell. To further confirm the specificity of the binding of ^{125}I-IL 1-β to VDS-0 cells the competitive effects of unlabeled recombinant α-interferon, lymphotoxin, tumor necrosis factor and phorbol myristic acid was examined. None of these inhibited the binding of ^{125}I-IL 1β to VDS-0 cells. However, F $(ab)_2$' fragments of rabbit anti-human IL 1 and partially purified acidic human IL 1 (IL 1-α) did inhibit the binding of ^{125}I-IL 1-β to VDS-0 cells. These data suggest that the binding of ^{125}I-IL 1-β is specific and that IL 1-α and IL 1-β bind to the same receptor on B cells.

(II) Biochemical properties of human IL 1 receptor on EBV-B lymphocytes. First, to determine the MW of receptor on VDS-0 cells for IL 1, ^{125}I-IL 1-β was chemically cross-linked to VDS-0 cells using disuccinimidyl suberate. SDS-PAGE analysis of VDS-0 cells that were incubated with ^{125}I-IL 1-β yielded only a 76 KD band by autoradiography. In the presence of excess unlabeled IL 1-β, this 76 KD band disappeared. Assuming one IL 1-β molecule (17 KD) binds to one IL 1 receptor molecule, the MW of the IL 1 receptor was estimated to be 59 KD. Second, we determined the MW of solublized IL 1 receptors by HPLC gel filtration. IL 1 receptors were extracted from isolated membranes of VDS-0 cells by 8 mM CHAPS at 4°C and chromatographed on an HPLC TSK 3000 column. Binding to ^{125}I-IL 1-β could be detected only in 60 KD fractions, supporting the estimated molecular weight of IL 1 receptor obtained by chemical crosslinking. We also determined the pI of solubized IL 1 receptor to be 7.3 by HPLC chromatofocusing.

Conclusion: We have described a specific IL 1 receptor on human EBV-B lymphocytes with a MW of 60 KD and pI of 7.3. Since many human EBV-B lymphocytes constitutively produce IL 1, express specific receptors for IL 1, and are stimulated to proliferate more by IL 1, IL 1 may be an autostimulatory factor which may contribute to the immortalization of B lymphocytes by EBV.

Acknowledgement: We gratefully acknowledge Dr. R. Newton (DuPont) for providing anti-human IL 1 antibody; Dr. G. Tosato for providing EBV-B lines; Drs. C. Faltynek, K. Elliot for reviewing this manuscript; and the editorial services of Ms. L. Shaw.

REFERENCES

(1) Matsushima, K., Kuang, Y-D., Tosato, G., Hopkins, S.J., and Oppenheim, J.J. (1985) Cell Immunol. 94, 406-417.

(2) Matsushima, K., Tosato, G., Benjamin, D., and Oppenheim, J.J. (1985) Cell Immunol. 94, 418-426.

(3) Matsushima, K., Procopio, A., Abe, H., Ortaldo, J.R., and Oppenheim, J.J. (1985) J. Immunol. 135, 1132-1136.

(4) Howard, M., Mizel, S.B., Lachman, L., Ansel, J., Johnson, B. and Paul, W.E. (1983) J. Exp. Med. 157, 1529-1563.

(5) Matsushima, K., Durum, S.K., Kimball, E.S., and Oppenheim, J.J. (1985) Cell Immunol. 92, 290-301.

INTERACTION OF HUMAN INTERFERON-α WITH CELLULAR RECEPTORS

L.M. Pfeffer and D.B. Donner*
The Rockefeller University and Memorial-Sloan Kettering Cancer Center*, New York, New York 10021, U.S.A.

Interferons (IFNs) are a family of cellular proteins, whose binding to specific cell surface receptors appears to be required to induce antiviral and antiproliferative activity. Detailed characterization of the interactions between IFNs and their receptors has been aided by the production of sufficiently large quantities of pure IFNs by recombinant DNA technology. The Daudi line of human lymphoblastoid cells is highly sensitive to the biological activity of leukocyte IFN (IFN-α) and, in general, appears to bind more IFN-α than other human cells.[1] In the present study we have characterized the binding of IFN-α to Daudi cells, the dissociation of the IFN-receptor complex, and the association of the IFN-receptor complex with the Triton X-100 insoluble matrix.

<u>IFN-α Binding</u>. ^{125}I was coupled to IFN-α by using limiting amounts of chloramine T. Iodinated IFN-α, separated from free ^{125}I by gel filtration on a Sephadex G-25 column, was found to retain essentially full (>90%) biological activity. Aliquots of 1 x 10^6 cells/ml of tissue culture medium were incubated for 100 min with 100 u/ml of [^{125}I]IFN-α. The specific binding of [^{125}I]IFN-α to Daudi cells was measured at 4°, 15° and 37°. The cell-associated radioactivity was determined after centrifugation of cells through a mixture of phthalate oil at 10,000 x g for 1 min. The specificity of binding was assayed by adding a 40-fold excess of unlabeled IFN-α to one set of tubes in the binding assay. It was observed that apparent binding to cells increased as a function of temperature. Approximately 20-fold more IFN was bound at 37° than at 4°, and 40% more IFN was bound at 37° than at 15°.

Dilute acid extraction (0.2 M acetic acid and 0.5 M NaCl for 6 min at 4°) has been used to quantitate the amount of ligand internalized during binding assays.[2] This assay is based on the ability of acidic conditions to effect release of cell surface-bound but not of internalized ligand. The acid extraction procedure showed that the apparent increase in binding at 37°, relative to the binding at 15°, was due to internalization of surface bound IFN-α. 48% of the cell-associated radioactivity after a 60-min incubation at 37° was internalized IFN-α, while <2% was internalized after a 60 min incubation at 15°. The rate of internalization of IFN at 37° was linear up to 90 min of incubation. When the amount of internalized IFN-α was subtracted from the total cell-associated radioactivity at 37°, the binding of IFN-α to the cell surface at 37° closely resembled that of binding at 15°. Scatchard analysis of the IFN-α binding data at 15° yielded a linear plot with a binding constant of 2 x 10^{-11} M and 2,300 IFN-α binding sites per cell.

<u>Dissociation and Triton X-100 insolubility of the IFN-receptor complex</u>. Cells were incubated with 100 u/ml of [^{125}I]IFN-α for 100 min at 15°. Afterwards a 40-fold excess of unlabeled IFN-α was added

to promote dissociation of [^{125}I]IFN from the IFN-receptor complexes. The amount of [^{125}I]IFN-α remaining specifically bound was then measured as a function of dissociation time at 15°. The reaction was stopped by centrifugation of the cells through phthalate oils. The dissociation of [^{125}I]IFN from Daudi cells was resolved into a fast and a slow component. ~20% of the bound IFN dissociates within 5 min, while ~35% of the IFN remains bound after 120 min.

A ligand-induced conversion of fast to slowly dissociating ligand-receptor complexes has been reported for nerve growth factor (NGF) bound to rat PC12 cells.[3] In that system, the alteration in the binding properties of the receptor is accompanied by association of NGF-receptor complex with the Triton-insoluble matrix and is enhanced by treatment with agents, such as wheat germ agglutinin (WGA) and concanavalin A, that crosslink cell surface components. To determine the effects of WGA on the dissociation of the IFN-receptor complex and the association of the IFN-receptor complex with Triton-insoluble matrix, cells were incubated for 100 min at 15° with 100 u/ml of [^{125}I]IFN-α. The cells were then pelleted at 4°, resuspended in the same volume of tissue culture medium, and incubated with 50 μg/ml of WGA for 30 min at 15°. In the absence of WGA, only 20% of IFN bound to Daudi cells was associated with the Triton X-100 insoluble pellet. In contrast, when cells were first incubated with [^{125}I]IFN and subsequently treated with WGA, 70% of the cell-bound IFN-α became Triton insoluble. The increase in Triton insolubility correlated with decreased dissociation of the IFN-receptor complex, with 60% of the IFN remaining bound in the WGA-treated cells after 2 hrs of dissociation while in controls 20% remained bound.

Conclusions. Daudi cells have 2,300 high affinity cell surface receptors for IFN-α (K_d=2 x 10^{-11} M) at 15°. Surface-bound IFN-α is rapidly internalized at 37° but not at 15°. The dissociation of IFN-receptor complexes can be resolved into a fast and a slow component. The slow component reflects association of the IFN-receptor complex with the Triton-insoluble matrix. Addition of WGA, which crosslinks cell surface components, decreases the dissociation of the IFN-receptor complex and increases the fraction of the complex that is Triton insoluble. Thus, IFN-α binding to specific cell surface receptors on Daudi cells alters the affinity of the receptors and leads to the association of the IFN-receptor complex with the Triton-insoluble matrix.

Acknowledgements. This work was supported by program project grant CA13213, and research grants AM22121 and AM30788 from the NIH. DB Donner is a recipient of a Career Development award from the NIADDK. We thank Dr. N. Stebbing (AMGEN, Inc.) for generously providing purified human IFN-α and Dr. I Tamm for his encouragement and support in these studies.

References

1. Branca AA & Baglioni C. Nature 294:768 (1981).
2. Haigler HT, McKanna JS & Cohen S. J. Cell Biol 81:382 (1979).
3. Landreth GE & Shooter E. Proc. Natl. Acad. Sci. USA 77:4751 (1980).

STRUCTURAL FEATURES OF THE HUMAN INTERLEUKIN-2 RECEPTOR

D. A. Shackelford and I. S. Trowbridge
The Salk Institute, La Jolla, California 92037

The human interleukin-2 (IL-2) receptor is a 50-55,000-dalton glycoprotein expressed on activated T lymphocytes (1). It is also found in lesser amounts on activated B lymphocytes. The amino acid sequence of the receptor has been deduced from the nucleotide sequence of cDNA clones (2-4). The sequence of the receptor predicts a 219-amino acid extracellular domain followed by a 19-amino acid hydrophobic transmembrane segment, and a 13-amino acid carboxy terminal intracellular domain.

The IL-2 receptor on HUT102B2 cells has been shown to be rapidly phosphorylated *in vivo* in response to the tumor-promoting phorbol ester TPA (5). It has been shown that TPA activates protein kinase C by replacing diacylglycerol normally produced by the turnover of inositol phospholipids in response to various extracellular signals (6). To demonstrate directly that the IL-2 receptor is a substrate for protein kinase C, the IL-2 receptor immunoprecipitated from HUT102B2 with the anti-Tac antibody was incubated with purified protein kinase C *in vitro* (Fig. 1). The IL-2 receptor was phosphorylated on serine and to a lesser extent on threonine as observed *in vivo* (7). To unequivocally establish the site of phosphorylation, the peptide YQRRQRKSRRTI corresponding to the C-terminus was synthesized and phosphorylated *in vitro* by protein kinase C. The tryptic peptide map of the phosphorylated synthetic peptide was identical to that of the IL-2 receptor phosphorylated *in vitro* by protein kinase C or *in vivo* by TPA stimulation of cells. Thus the major site of phosphorylation was identified as serine-247 and threonine-250 was a minor site.

A minor protein of M_r = 35,000 (previously called p27) was coprecipitated with the IL-2 receptor from ^{125}I-labeled HUT102B2 cells as were other minor species (5). The protein could be metabolically labeled with $^{32}PO_4$ and was sensitive to digestion with neuraminidase but resistant to endoglycosidase F. One possibility was that this protein was a proteolytic fragment of the IL-2 receptor containing the C-terminus of the molecule. To investigate this point, the IL-2 receptor immunoprecipitated with anti-Tac was subjected to partial proteolysis by trypsin. The receptor could be quantitatively cleaved into two fragments which migrated under reducing conditions as M_r = 35-38,000 and M_r = 26-28,000 (Fig. 2). The two fragments were disulphide bonded since under nonreducing conditions the trypsin-treated receptor comigrated with the uncleaved receptor. The 35-38,000-dalton fragment (C) appears to be the C-terminal portion of the receptor including the cytoplasmic domain since it retains the phosphate label. The 26-28,000-dalton fragment contains two N-linked oligosaccharides as demonstrated by digestion with endoglycosidase F and therefore represents the N-terminal portion of the molecule. Both fragments have carbohydrate moieties since both are sensitive to neuraminidase. These results provide direct biochemical evidence that the extracellular portion of the IL-2 receptor may be folded into two discrete domains roughly corresponding to the two homologous regions defined by amino acid residues 1-102 and 103-174 (4). The number and location of the binding sites for IL-2 on the receptor are presently unknown.

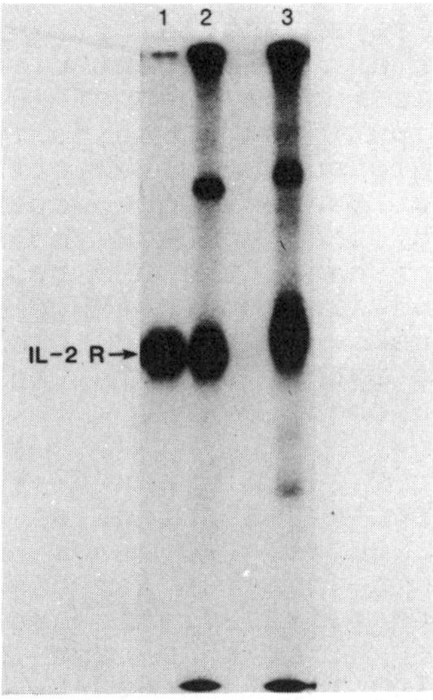

Fig 1. Phosphorylation of the IL-2 receptor by protein kinase C *in vitro*. The IL-2 receptor was immunoprecipitated with anti-Tac antibody from (1) ^{125}I-labeled HUT102B2 cells, (2) HUT102B2 cells or (3) CEM cells induced with 50 ng/ml TPA for 2 days. The samples for lanes (2) and (3) were phosphorylated *in vitro* by protein kinase C as described (8). The samples were analyzed by SDS-PAGE in the absence of reducing agents.

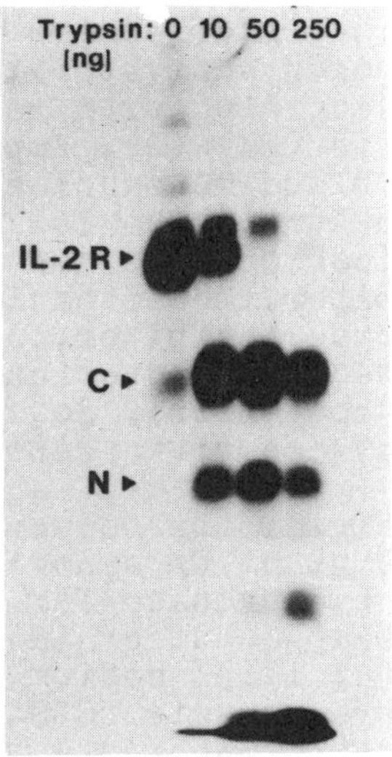

Fig. 2. Limited proteolysis of IL-2 receptor. The IL-2 receptor was immunoprecipitated with anti-Tac from ^{125}I-labeled HUT102B2 cells. The immunoprecipitates were incubated with trypsin as indicated in the figure for 1hr at 37°C. The samples were analyzed by SDS-PAGE in the presence of 2-mercaptoethanol.

References

1. Leonard, W. J., et al. (1982) Nature **300:**267-269.
2. Leonard, W. J., et al. (1984) Nature **311:**626-631.
3. Nikaido, T., et al. (1984) Nature **311:**631-635.
4. Cosman, D., et al. (1984) Nature **312:**768-771.
5. Shackelford, D. A., and Trowbridge, I. S. (1984) J. Biol. Chem. **259:**11706-11712.
6. Nishizuka, Y. (1984) Nature **308:**693-697.
7. Shackelford, D. A., and Trowbridge, I. S., manuscript submitted.
8. Cochet, C., Gill, G. N., Cooper, J. A., and Hunter, T. (1984) J. Biol. Chem. **259:**2553-2558.

INTERLEUKIN-1 INDUCTION OF SYNOVIAL FLUID AND SYNOVIAL CELL PLASMINOGEN ACTIVATORS

W. Yang, Department of Biology, Rutgers University, Camden, New Jersey, USA

The interleukin-1 (IL-1) stimulates synovial cell plasminogen activator (PA) production and this event might be associated with cartilage destruction in rheumatoid arthritis (RA) (1). Employing highly purified human peripheral blood mononuclear IL-1 I have found that IL-1 stimulates human synovial cell PA production in a dose dependent fashion that can be prevented by the cyclo-oxygenase inhibitor,indomethacin. On the other hand, the phosphodiesterase inhibitor,theophylline, and dibutyryl c-AMP enhance the IL-1 induction of synovial cell PA about 2-fold (data not shown). So, the IL-1 induction of synovial cell PA may occur via generation of endogenous c-AMP.

Fig. 1 the molecular weight forms of RA synovial fluid PA. 9 uL of RA synovial fluid is treated with 1 uL of 1 mg/ml hyaluronase for 30 minutes, mixed with 10 uL of Laemmli sample buffer (2) without reducing reagent for one well of 17.5% sodium dodecyl sulfate-polyacrylamide gel electrophoresis (SDS-PAGE), run the gel at 18 mA for 16-18 hours, washed in 2.5% Triton X-100 for 1 hour, rinsed in distilled water 3 times, cut into 2.2 mm slices, and assayed for PA activity. Fig. 2 estimation of molecular weight of synovial cell PA. PA was obtained from synovial cells in culture that were stimulated by mononuclear cell factor (IL-1) and run as in Fig. 1 .

Fig. 1

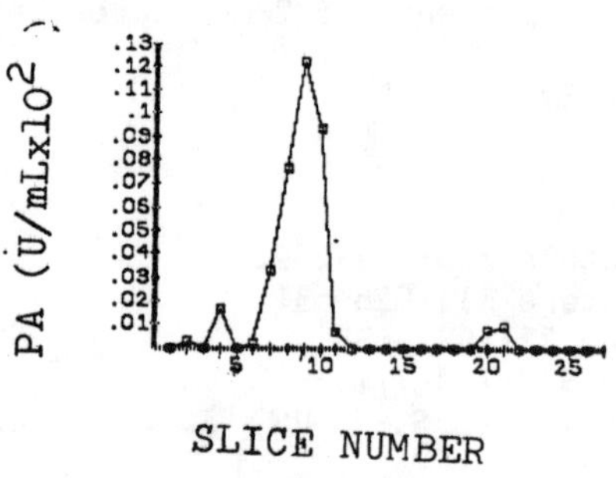

Fig. 2

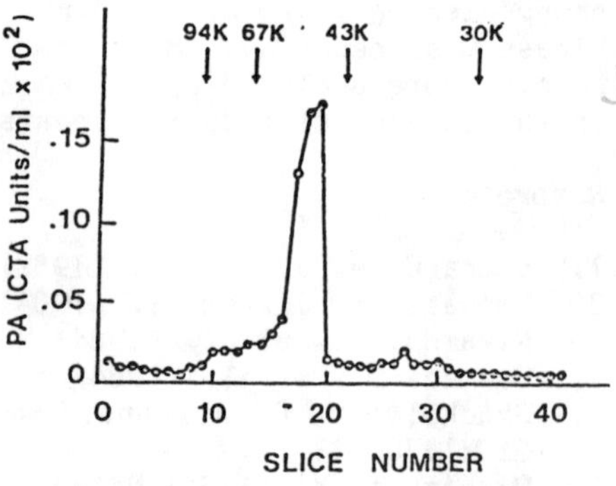

PA is a serine protease which acts very specifically to convert the zymogen,plasminogen into the active protease, plasmin. At least two immunologically distinct forms have been described tissue-type PA and urokinase. Tissue-type PA usually has a molecular weight of 72,000 dalton. Urokinase contains two enzymatically active fractions with molecular weights of 55,000 and 33,000 daltons.

SDS-PAGE study indicates three molecular weight forms of PA are present in RA synovial fluid: the high molecular forms, 88,000 and 72,000 daltons and a low molecular form of 55,000 dalton. Since the 55,000 molecular form and the 72,000 molecular form resemble tissue-type PA and urokinase in size, their presence in RA synovial fluid could reflect synovial pannus activity associated with articular cartilage destruction. The physiological and / or origin of the 88,000 dalton form are unknown.

REFERENCES

(1) Mochan,E. and Uhl,J. JAOA 84:211,1984
(2) Laemmli,U. K. Nature 227:680,1970

EXPRESSION OF TRANSFECTED HUMAN GAMMA INTERFERON GENOMIC DNA IN MOUSE FIBROBLASTS

H. A. Young, L. Varesio and P. Hwu
Lab. of Mol. Immunoregulation, BRMP, DCT, NCI/FCRF, Frederick, MD.

Gamma interferon is an important immunoregulatory lymphokine which is normally produced only in T cells and large granular lymphocytes (for a review, see 1). We have investigated the biological activity of human gamma interferon genomic DNA by linking an 8.6 kb BamH1 human genomic DNA fragment containing the entire gamma interferon coding region with the shuttle vector, pSV-2 neo (2) and transfecting this DNA into a mouse T cell line and NIH 3T3 cells. This results in the production of gamma interferon by the transfected mouse T cells (but not mouse fibroblasts) and gamma interferon levels can be increased by both phorbol esters and interleukin 2 in the T cells (3). We now report that expression of the human gamma interferon in transfected mouse fibroblasts can be induced by cycloheximide and that brief(0.5 hr) additional treatment of the cells with actinomycin D enhances interferon production over ten fold. We have also assessed the biological activity of the gamma interferon genomic DNA after sequences 5' to the TATA box have been removed.

mRNA Production. We have shown that transfected mouse fibroblasts contain 1-5 copies of the human gamma interferon DNA per cell but did not synthesize any gamma interferon and did not contain gamma interferon mRNA in the cytoplasm (3). In an attempt to stimulate gamma interferon mRNA synthesis, the transfected fibroblasts were treated with the protein synthesis inhibitor, cycloheximide since this drug has been shown to induce expression of the transfected human beta interferon gene upon introduction into heterologous cells (4,5). As shown in Figure 1, induction of gamma interferon cytoplasmic RNA was observed after 1 hr of cycloheximide treatment, with maximum levels observed between 3-4 hours after treatment. No hybridization was observed with untreated or non-transfected cells.

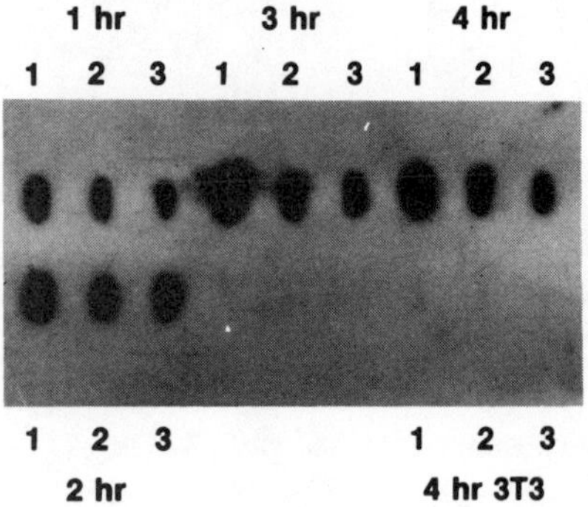

Figure 1. Slot Blot Analysis of Cycloheximide Treated Transfected Mouse Fibroblasts RNA.

1. 10μg; 2. 5μg; 3. 2 μg. Hybridization of RNA with ^{32}P-labeled human gamma interferon cDNA

Effect of inducers on gamma interferon mRNA. Since gamma interferon mRNA could now be detected after cycloheximide treatment, the effect of the presence of either phorbol myristate acetate (20 ng/ml) or poly inosinic acid•cytosinic acid (poly I:C) (10 μg/ml) on the induction process was analyzed. The inducers were present during and after the cycloheximide treatment but, as shown in Figure 2, no increases in levels of mRNA were observed in the presence of either inducer and no increase in gamma interferon was detected in the culture medium (data not shown).

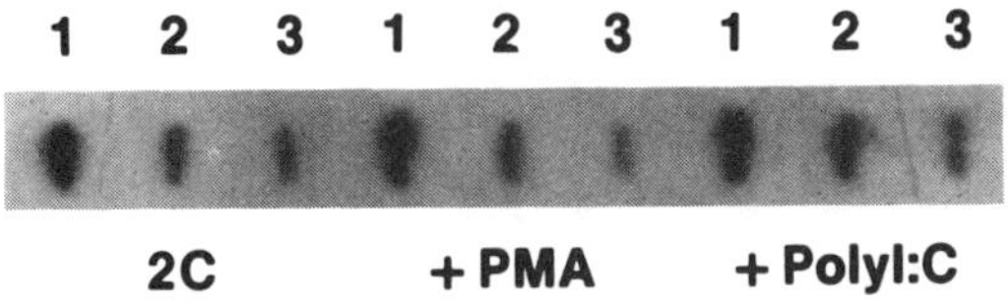

Figure 2. Slot Blot Analysis of PMA and Poly I:C Treated Transfected Mouse Fibroblast RNA.

1 10μg; 2 5μg; 3 2.5μg

Gamma interferon production. When 10 μg/ml of cycloheximide was used,no gamma interferon was observed in the culture medium 18-20 hours after removal of the drug (Table 1). However, lowering the cycloheximide to 1 μg/ml during the 4 hour treatment resulted in low but detectable levels of gamma interferon in the culture medium. Furthermore, when actinomycin D (0.5 μg/ml) was added during the final 30 minutes of cycloheximide treatment in an attempt to "super-induce" the gamma interferon levels, significant enhancement of gamma interferon was observed (Table 1).

Table 1. Levels of Human Gamma Interferon in Culture Medium

Cells	Inhibitors Cyclo	Inhibitors Act D	Time (hrs)	Supernatant CPM	Units/ml
Fibroblast	-	-	4	519 ± 77	0
Clone 2C	1 μg/ml	-	4	2371 ± 355	4.4
	10 μg/ml	-	4	510 ± 75	0
	-	+	4	480 ± 72	0
	1 μg/ml	+	4	20990 ± 3148	>50

Gamma interferon values are based on a radioimmunoassay obtained from Centocor, Inc. This assay is linear to 50 units/ml and does not cross react with any mouse interferon.

In conclusion, we have been able to induce expression of transfected human gamma interferon genomic DNA in NIH 3T3 cells through the use of the protein synthesis inhibitor, cycloheximide. Furthermore, we have been able to enhance production over ten fold by brief treatment with actinomycin D. The mechanisms underlying this induction process are under investigation and will provide important information as to how cells regulate specific gene expression.

REFERENCES

(1) Trinchieri, G. and Perussia, B. (1985) Immunology Today 6, 131.
(2) Southern, P.J. and Berg, P. (1982) J. Mol. Appl. Genet. 1, 327.
(3) Young, H.A. Dray, J.F. and Farrar, W.L. (1986) In press.
(4) Maroteaux, L., Chen, L., Mitrani-Rosenbaum, S., Howley, P.M. and Revel, M. (1983) J. Virol. 47, 89.
(5) Ringold, G.M., Dieckmann, B., Vannice, J.L., Trahey, M., and McCormick, F. (1984) Proc. Natl. Acad. Sci. U.S.A. 81, 3964.

AUTHOR INDEX